Psychiatric Certification Review Guide for the Generalist and Clinical Specialist in Adult, Child, and Adolescent Psychiatric and Mental Health Nursing

Editor

Clare Houseman, Ph.D., R.N.,C.S.
Associate Professor
College of Nursing
Old Dominion University
Private Practice
Avery-Finney Associates
Norfolk, Virginia

SECOND EDITION

Health Leadership Associates
Potomac, Maryland

Health Leadership Associates

Manuscript Editor: Virginia Layng Millonig
Managing Editor: Mary A. Millonig
Production Manager: Martha M. Pounsberry
Editorial Assistants: Cheryl C. Patterson
                   Bridget M. Jones
Cover and Design: Merrifield Graphics
Composition: Port City Press, Inc.
Printing/Binding: Port City Press, Inc.

Printed in the United States of America

Health Leadership Associates, Inc. ● P.O. Box 59153 ● Potomac, Maryland 20859

Library of Congress Cataloging-in-Publication Data

Psychiatric certification review guide for the generalist and clinical
    specialist in adult, child, and adolescent psychiatric and mental
    health nursing
         p.   cm.
   ISBN 1-878028-19-7 (pbk.)
   1. Psychiatric nursing.   2. Psychiatric nursing—Examinations,
questions, etc.
RC440.P72985   1998
610.73'68'076—dc21
DNLM/DLC
for Library of Congress   98-12134
                                        CIP

10 9 8 7 6 5 4 3 2 1

To my son Gregg Magier whose presence brings joy to my life, to my parents Anthony and Phyllis Woodell for their continued unquestioning support of my efforts, and to Blake Rochelle a special partner in my life.

Contributors

TEST TAKING STRATEGIES AND TECHNIQUES

Clare Houseman, Ph.D., R.N.,C.S.
Associate Professor
College of Nursing
Old Dominion University
Private Practice
Avery-Finney Associates
Norfolk, Virginia

Nancy A. Dickenson Hazard, M.S.N., F.A.A.N.
Executive Officer
Sigma Theta Tau International
Indianapolis, Indiana

THE ESSENTIALS OF CARE

Clare Houseman, Ph.D., R.N.,C.S.
Associate Professor
College of Nursing
Old Dominion University
Private Practice
Avery-Finney Associates
Norfolk, Virginia

MAJOR THEORETICAL FRAMEWORKS FOR PSYCHIATRIC NURSING

Clare Houseman, Ph.D., R.N.,C.S.
Associate Professor
College of Nursing
Old Dominion University
Private Practice
Avery-Finney Associates
Norfolk, Virginia

Joan Donovan, Ph.D., R.N.,C.S.
Private Practice
Richmond, Virginia

MENTAL DISORDERS DUE TO SUBSTANCE ABUSE

Therese K. Killeen, M.S.N., R.N.,C.S.
Clinical Nurse Specialist
Institute of Psychiatry
Medical University of South Carolina
Charleston, South Carolina

ANXIETY AND STRESS RELATED DISORDERS

Karma Castleberry, Ph.D., R.N.,C.S.
Professor
School of Nursing
Radford University
Consultant
St. Albans Psychiatric Hospital
Radford, Virginia

SCHIZOPHRENIA AND OTHER PSYCHOTIC DISORDERS

Mary Ann Camann, M.N., R.N.,C.S.
Assistant Professor
Department of Nursing
Kennesaw State University
Kennesaw, Georgia

Mary Fultz Spencer, M.N., R.N.,C.S.
Psychotherapist
Glenwood Psychiatric Associates,
Raleigh, North Carolina

MOOD DISORDERS

Mary D. Moller, M.S.N., R.N.,C.S., A.R.N.P.
Administrator
Suncrest Wellness Center
Adjunct Instructor
Washington State University
Spokane, Washington

BEHAVIORAL SYNDROMES AND DISORDERS OF ADULT PERSONALITY

Richardean Benjamin-Coleman, Ph.D., M.P.H., R.N.,C.S
Assistant Professor

School of Nursing
Old Dominion University
Norfolk, Virginia

COGNITIVE MENTAL DISORDERS

Jane Bryant Neese, Ph.D., R.N.,C.S.
Assistant Professor
Family and Community Nursing
College of Nursing and Health Professions
University of North Carolina at Charlotte
Charlotte, North Carolina

Anita Thompson-Heisterman, M.S.N., R.N.,C.S.
Instructor in Nursing
School of Nursing
University of Virginia
Charlottesville, Virginia

Ivo L. Abraham, Ph.D., R.N.,C.S., F.A.A.N.
Principal
Epsilon Group LLC
Charlottesville, Virginia

BEHAVIORAL AND EMOTIONAL DISORDERS OF CHILDHOOD AND ADOLESCENCE

Michele L. Zimmerman, M.A., R.N.,C.S.
Associate Professor
School of Nursing
Old Dominion University
Psychotherapist
Avery-Finney Associates
Norfolk, Virginia

THE LARGER MENTAL HEALTH ENVIRONMENT

Janice V. R. Belcher, Ph.D., R.N.,C.S.
Assistant Professor
Miami Valley College of Nursing and Health
Wright State University
Dayton, Ohio

Reviewers

Preface

This is the second edition of a book developed especially for nurses preparing to take Certification Examinations offered by the American Nurses Credentialing Center (ANCC). Major revisions were needed in a number of areas to accommodate changes in the field of psychiatric nursing and to incorporate newer references that may have become available since the previous text was published. The book is inclusive in that it contains both basic and advanced content so that nurses seeking certification as generalists as well as nurses seeking certification as clinical specialists in adult, and child and adolescent psychiatric and mental health nursing will find the guide useful for review.

Basic content has been highlighted in shaded blocks throughout the text (indicating content applicable for both the generalist and clinical specialist) whereas content areas not shaded are directed toward the clinical specialist. *The two exceptions are the Test Taking Strategies chapter which is essential information for all nurses who are taking certification examinations and the Childhood and Adolescence chapter which is directed exclusively toward the Clinical Specialist.*

The purpose of the book is twofold. It will assist individuals engaged in self study preparation for Certification Examinations, and may be used as a reference guide in the practice setting.

Many nurses preparing for certification examinations find that reviewing an extensive body of scientific knowledge requires a very difficult search of many sources that must be synthesized to provide a review base for the examination. The purpose of this publication is to provide a succinct, yet comprehensive review of the core material.

The book has been organized to provide the reviewer with test taking strategies and techniques. This is followed by chapters on The Essentials of Psychiatric Nursing Care, Major Theoretical Frameworks for Psychiatric Nursing, Mental Disorders Due to Substance Abuse, Anxiety and Stress Related Disorders, Schizophrenia and Other Psychotic Disorders, Mood Disorders, Behavioral Syndromes and Disorders of Adult Personality, Cognitive Mental Disorders, Behavioral and Emotional Disorders of Childhood and Adolescence and The Larger Mental Health Environment.

Following each chapter are test questions, which are intended to serve as an introduction to the testing arena. In addition a bibliography is included for those who need a more in depth discussion of the subject matter in each chapter. These references can serve as additional instructional material for the reader.

Psychiatric Nursing

The editor and contributing authors are certified nurses who are respected experts in the field of psychiatric nursing. They have designed this book to assist potential examinees to prepare for success in the certification examination process. It may also be used as a reference source in the clinical area.

It is assumed that the reader of this review guide has completed a course of study in psychiatric nursing. The Psychiatric Nursing Certification Review Guide for the Generalist and Clinical Specialist in Adult, Child, and Adolescent Psychiatric and Mental Health Nursing is not intended to be a basic learning tool.

Certification is a process that is gaining recognition both within and outside the profession. For the professional it is a means of gaining special recognition as a certified psychiatric nurse which not only demonstrates a level of competency, but may also enhance professional opportunities and advancement. For the consumer, it means that a certified nurse has met certain predetermined standards set by the profession.

CONTENTS

4   **Mental Disorders Due To Substance Abuse**   *Therese K. Killeen*

5   **Anxiety and Stress Related Disorders**   *Karma Castleberry*

6   **Schizophrenia and Other Psychotic Disorders**   *Mary Fultz Spencer*
                                                                 Mary Ann Camaan

7   **Mood Disorders**   *Mary D. Moller*

8   **Behavioral Syndromes and Disorders of Adult Personality**

Richardean Benjamin-Coleman

9   Cognitive Mental Disorders

Jane Bryant Neese
Anita Thompson-Heisterman
Ivo L. Abraham

10   Behavioral and Emotional Disorders of Childhood and Adolescence

Michele L. Zimmerman

11   The Larger Mental Health Environment

Janice V. R. Belcher

Test Taking Strategies and Techniques

Clare Houseman
Nancy A. Dickenson Hazard

We all respond to testing situations in different ways. What separates the successful test taker from the unsuccessful one is knowing how to prepare for and take a test. Preparing yourself to be a successful test taker is as important as studying for the test. Each person needs to assess and develop their own test taking strategies and skills. The primary goal of this chapter is to assist potential examinees in knowing how to study for and take a test.

STRATEGY #1 Know Yourself

When faced with an examination, do you feel threatened, experience butterflies or sweaty palms, have trouble keeping your mind focused on studying or on the test questions? These common symptoms of test anxiety plague many of us, but can be used advantageously if understood and handled correctly (Divine & Kylen, 1979). Over the years of test taking, each of us has developed certain testing behaviors, some of which are beneficial, while others present obstacles to successful test taking. You can take control of the test taking situation by identifying the undesirable behaviors, maintaining the desirable ones and developing skills to improve test performance.

Technique #1:   From the following descriptions of test taking personalities, find yourself (Table 1). Write down those characteristics which describe you even if they are from different personality types. Carefully review the problem list associated with your test taking personality characteristics. Write down the problems which are most troublesome. Then make a list of how you can remedy these problems from the improvement strategies list. Be sure to use these strategies as you prepare for and take examinations.

STRATEGY #2 Develop Your Thinking Skills

Understanding Thought Processes: In order to improve your thinking skills and subsequent test performance, it is best to understand the types of thinking as well as the techniques to enhance the thought process.

Everyone has a personal learning style, but we all must proceed through the same process to think.

Thinking occurs on two levels—the lower level of memory and comprehension and the higher level of application and analysis (ABP, 1989). Memory is the ability to recall facts. Without adequate retrieval of facts, progression through the higher levels of thinking cannot occur easily. Comprehension is the ability to understand memorized facts. To be effective, comprehension skills must allow the person to translate recalled information from one context to another. Application, or the process of using information to know why it occurs, is a higher form of learning. Effective application relies on the use of understood memorized facts to verify intended action. Analysis is the ability to use abstract or logical forms of thought to show relationships and to distinguish the cause and effect between the variables in a situation.

Table 1

Test Taker Profile

Type	Characteristics	Pitfalls	Improvement Strategies
The Rusher	• Rushes to complete the test before the studied facts are forgotten	• Unable to read question and situation completely	• Practice progressive relaxation techniques
	• Arrives at test site early and waits anxiously	• At high risk for misreading, misinterpreting and mistakes	• Develop a study plan with sufficient time to review important content
	• Mumbles studied facts	• Difficult items heighten anxiety	• Avoid cramming and last minute studying
	• Tense body posture	• Likely to make quick, not well-thought-out guesses	• Take practice tests focusing on slowing down and reading and answering each option carefully
	• Accelerated pulse, respiration and neuromuscular excitement		• Read instructions and questions slowly
	• Answers questions rapidly and is generally one of the first to complete		
	• Experiences exhaustion once test is over		
The Turtle	• Moves slowly, methodically, deliberately through each question	• Last to finish; often does not complete the exam	• Take practice tests focusing on time spent per item
	• Repeated rereading, underlining and checking	• Has to quickly complete questions in last part of exam, increasing errors	• Place watch in front of examination paper to keep track of time
	• Takes 60 to 90 seconds per question versus an average of 45 to 60 seconds	• Has difficulty completing timed examinations	• Mark answer sheet for where one should be halfway through exam based on total number of questions and total amount of time for exam
			• Study concepts not details
			• Attempt to answer each question as you progress through the exam

Psychiatric Nursing

Type	Characteristics	Pitfalls	Improvement Strategies
The Personalizer	• Mature person who has personal knowledge and insight from life experiences	• Risk in relying on what has been learned through observation and experience since one may develop false understandings and stereotypes	• Focus on principles and standards that support nursing practice
		• Personal beliefs and experiences are frequently not the norm or standard tested	• Avoid making connections between patients in exam clinical situations and personal clinical experience
		• Has difficulty identifying expected standards measured by standardized examination	• Focus on generalities not experiences
The Squisher	• View exams as threat, rather than an expected event in education	• Procrastinates studying for exams	• Establish a plan of progressive, disciplined study
	• Preoccupied with grades and personal accomplishment	• Unable to study effectively since waits until last minute	• Use defined time frames for studying content and taking practice exams
	• Attempts to avoid responsibility and accountability associated with testing in order to reduce anxiety	• Increased anxiety over test since procrastinating study impairs ability to learn and perform	• Use relaxation techniques • Return to difficult items • Read carefully
The Philosopher	• Academically successful person who is well disciplined and structured in study habits	• Over analysis causes loss of sight of actual intent of question	• Focus on questions as they are written
	• Displays great intensity and concentration during exam	• Reads information into questions answering with own added information rather than answering the actual intent of question	• Work on self confidence and not on question. Initial response is usually correct
	• Searches questions for hidden or unintended meaning		• Avoid multiple rereadings of questions
	• Experiences anxiety over not knowing everything		• Avoid adding own information and unintended meanings
			• Practice, practice, practice with sample tests
The Second Guesser	• Answers questions twice, first as an examinee, second as an examiner	• Altering an initial response frequently results in an incorrect answer	• Reread only the few items of which one is unsure. Avoid changing initial responses

Type	Characteristics	Pitfalls	Improvement Strategies
The Lawyer	• Believes second look will allow one to find and correct errors	• Frequently changes answers because the pattern of response appears incorrect (i.e., too many "true" or too many correct responses)	• Take exam carefully and progressively first time, allowing little or no time for rereading • Study facts • Avoid reading into questions
	• Frequently changes initial responses (i.e., grades own test)		
	• Attempts to place words or ideas into the question (leads the witness)	• Veers from the obvious answer and provides response from own point of view	• Focus on distinguishing what patient is saying in question and not on what is read into question
	• Occurs most frequently with psychosocial or communication questions which ask for the most appropriate response	• Reads a question, jumps to a conclusion then finds a response that leads to predetermined conclusion	• Avoid formulating responses aimed at obtaining certain information
			• Choose responses that allow patient to express feelings, which are intended to clarify, and identify feeling tone of patient or which avoid negating or confronting patient feelings

From: "Making the grades as a test-taker," by N. Dickenson-Hazard, (1989) *Pediatric Nursing, 15,* p. 303. Adapted from: *Nurse's guide to successful test-taking* by M. B. Sides and N. B. Cailles, 1989. Philadelphia: J. B. Lippincott, Co., pp 59–70, 199–203. Copyright 1989 by A. J. Jannetti, Inc. Reprinted by permission.

As related to testing situations, the thought process from memory to analysis occurs quite quickly. Some examination items are designed to test memory and comprehension while others test application and analysis. An example of a memory question is as follows:

Clients' initial response to learning that they have a terminal illness is generally:

a) Depression
b) Bargaining
c) *Denial*
d) Anger

To answer this question correctly, the individual has to retrieve a memorized fact. Understanding the fact, knowing why it is important or analyzing what should be done in this situation is not needed. An example of a question which tests comprehension is as follows:

Shortly after having been informed that she is in the terminal stages of breast cancer, Mrs. Jones begins to talk about her plans to travel with her husband when he retires in two years. The nurse should know that:

a) The diagnosis could be wrong and Mrs. Jones may not be dying
b) *Mrs. Jones is probably responding to the news by using the defense mechanism of denial*
c) Mrs. Jones is clearly delusional
d) Mrs. Jones is not responding in the way most clients would

In order to answer this question correctly, an individual must retrieve the fact that Denial is often the first response to learning about a terminal illness and that Mrs. Jones' behavior is indicative of denial.

In a higher level of thinking examination question, individuals must be able to recall a fact, understand that fact in the context of the question, apply this understanding to explaining why one answer is correct after analyzing the answer choices as they relate to the situation (Sides & Cailles, 1989). An example of an application analysis question is as follows:

Mr. Smith has just learned that he has an inoperable brain tumor. His comment when the nurse speaks to him later is "This can't possibly be true. Mistakes are made in hospitals all the time. They might have mixed up my test results." The nurse's most appropriate response would be:

a) Refer Mr. Smith for a psychiatric consultation
b) *Neither agree nor disagree with Mr. Smith's comment*
c) Confront Mr. Smith with his denial
d) Agree with Mr. Smith that mistakes can happen and tell him you will see about getting repeat tests

To answer this question correctly, the individual must recall the fact that denial is often the initial response to learning about a terminal illness; understand that Mr. Smith's response in this case is evidence of the normal use of denial; apply this knowledge to each option, understanding why it may or may not be correct; and analyze each option for what action is most appropriate for this situation. Application/analysis questions require the examinee to use logical rationale, which demonstrates the ability to analyze a relationship, based on a well defined principle or fact. Problem solving ability becomes important as the examinee must think through each question option, deciding its relevance and importance to the situation of the question.

Building your thinking skills: Effective memorization is the cornerstone to learning and building thinking skills (Olney, 1989). We have all experienced ''memory power outages'' at some time, due in part to trying to memorize too much, too fast, too ineffectively. Developing skills to improve memorization is important to increasing the effectiveness of your thinking and subsequent test performance.

Technique #1: Quantity is NOT quality, so concentrate on learning important content. For example, it is important to know the various pharmacologic agents appropriate for the management of chronic obstructive pulmanary disease (COPD), not the specific dosages for each medication.

Technique #2: Memory from repetition, or saying something over and over again to remember it usually fades. Developing memory skills which trigger retrieval of needed facts is more useful. Such skills are as follows:

Acronyms: These are mental crutches which facilitate recall. Some are already established such as PERRL (pupils equal, round, reactive to light), or PAT (paroxysmal atrial tachycardia). Developing your own acronyms can be particularly useful since they are your own word association arrangements in a singular word. Nonsense words or funny, unusual ones are often more useful since they attract your attention.

Acrostics: This mental tool arranges words into catchy phrases. The first letter of each word stands for something which is recalled as the phrase is said. Your own acrostics are most valuable in triggering recall of learned information since they are your individual situation associations. An example of an acrostic is as follows:

Kissing **P**atty **P**roduces **A**ffection stands for the four types of nonverbal messages: **K**inesics, **P**aralanguage, **P**roxemics and **A**ppearance

ABCs: This technique facilitates information retrieval by using the alphabet as a crutch. Each letter stands for a symptom, which when put together creates a picture of the clinical presentation of the disease. For example, the characteristics of the disease and symptoms of osteoarthritis using the ABC technique is as follows:

a) Aching or pain
b) Being stiff on awakening
c) Crepitus
d) Deterioration of articular cartilage
e) Enlargements of distal interphalangeal joints
f) Formation of new bone at joint surface
g) Granulation inflammatory tissue
h) Heberden's nodes

One letter: Recall is enhanced by emphasizing a single letter. The major symptoms of Schizophrenia are often remembered as follows:
Affect (flat)
Autism
Auditory hallucinations

Imaging: This technique can be used in two ways. The first is to develop a nickname for a clinical problem which when said produces a mental picture. For example, "a wan, wheezy pursed lip" might be used to visualize a patient with pulmonary emphysema who is thin, emaciated, experiencing dyspnea, with a hyperinflated chest, who has an elongated expiratory breathing phase. A second form of imaging is to visualize a specific patient while you are trying to understand or solve a clinical problem when studying or answering a question. For example, imagine an elderly man who is experiencing an acute asthma attack. You are trying to analyze the situation and place him in a position which maximizes respiratory effort. In your mind you visualize him in various positions of side lying, angular and forward, imaging what will happen to the man in each position. A second form of imaging is to visualize a specific situation while you are trying to answer a question. For example if you are trying to remember how to describe active listening or physical attending skills see yourself in a comfortable environment, facing the other person, with open posture and eye contact.

Rhymes, music & links: The absurd is easier to remember than the most common. Rhymes, music or links can add absurdity and humor to learning and remembering (Olney, 1989). These retrieval tools are developed by the individual for specific content. For example, making up a rhyme about diabetes may be helpful in remembering the predominant female incidence, origin of disease, primary symptoms and management as illustrated by:

> There once was a woman
> > whose beta cells failed
> She grew quite thirsty
> > and her glucose levels sailed
> Her lack of insulin caused her to
> > increase her intake
> And her increased urinary output
> > was certainly not fake
> So she learned to watch her diet
> > and administer injections
> That kept her healthy, happy
> > and free of complications.

Words which rhyme can also be used to jog the memory about important characteristics of phenomena. For example, the stages of group therapy can be remembered and characterized by the following according to Tuckman (1965):

> Forming
> Storming
> Norming
> Performing

Setting content to music is sometimes useful to remembering. Melodies which are repetitious jog the memory by the ups and downs of the notes and the rhythm of the music.

Links connect key words from the content by using them in a story. An example given by Olney (1989) for remembering the parts of an eye is IRIS watched a PUPIL through the LENS of a RED TIN telescope while eating CORN-EA on the cob.

Additional memory aids may also include the use of color or drawing for improving recall. Use different colored pens or paper to accentuate the material being learned. For example, highlight or make notes in blue for content about respiratory problems and in red for cardiovascular content. Drawing assists with visualizing content as well. This is particularly helpful for remembering the pathophysiology of the specific health problem.

The important thing to remember about remembering is to use good recall techniques.

Technique #3:   Improving higher level thinking skills involves exercising the application and analysis of memorized fact. Small group review is particularly useful for enhancing these high level skills. It allows verbalization of thought processes and receipt of input about content and thought process from others (Sides & Cailles, 1989). Individuals not only hear how they think, but how others think as well. This interaction allows individuals to identify flaws in their thought process as well as to strengthen their positive points.

Taking practice tests is also helpful in developing application/analysis thinking skills. These tests permit the individual to analyze thinking patterns as well as the cause and effect relationships between the question and its options. The problem solving skills needed to answer application/analysis questions are tested, giving the individual more experience through practice (Dickenson-Hazard, 1990).

STRATEGY #3 Know The Content

Your ability to study is directly influenced by organization and concentration (Dickenson-Hazard, 1990). If effort is spent on both of these aspects of exam preparation, examination success can be increased.

Preparation for studying: Getting organized. Study habits are developed early in our educational experiences. Some of our habits enhance learning while others do not. To increase study effectiveness, organization of study materials and time is essential. Organization decreases frustration, allows for easy resumption of study and increases concentrated study time.

Technique #1:   Create your own study space. Select a study area that is yours alone, free from distractions, comfortable and well lighted. The ventilation and room temperature should be comfortable since a cold room makes it difficult to concentrate and a warm room may make you sleepy (Burkle & Marshak, 1989). All your study materials should be left in your study space. The basic premise of a study space is that it facilitates a mind set that you are there to study. When you interrupt study, it is best to leave your materials just as they are. Don't close books or put away notes as you will just have to relocate them, wasting your study time, when you do resume study.

Technique #2:   Define and organize the content. From the test giver, secure an outline or the content parameters which are to be examined. If the test giver's outline is sketchy, develop a more detailed one for yourself using the recommended text as a guideline. Next, identify your available study resources: class notes, old exams, handouts, textbooks, review courses, or study groups. For national standardized exams, such as initial licensing or certification, it is best to identify one or two study resources which cover the content being tested and stick to them.

Attempting to review all available resources is not only mind boggling, but increases anxiety and frustration as well. Make your selections and stay with them.

Technique #3: Conduct a content assessment. Using a simple rating scale of

> 1 = requires no review
> 2 = requires minimal review
> 3 = requires intensive review
> 4 = start from the beginning

Read through the content outline and rate each content area (Dickenson-Hazard, 1990). Table 2 provides a sample exam content assessment. Be honest with your assessment. It is far better to recognize your content weaknesses when you can study and remedy them, rather than thinking during the exam how you wished you had studied more. Likewise with content strengths: if you know the material, don't waste time studying it.

Technique #4: Develop a study plan. Coordinate the content which needs to be studied with the time available (Sides & Cailles, 1989). Prioritize your study needs, starting with weak areas first. Allow for a general review at the end of the study plan. Lastly, establish an overall goal for yourself—something that will motivate you when it is brought to mind.

Table 3 illustrates a study plan developed on the basis of the exam content assessment in Table 2. Conducting an assessment and developing a study plan should require no more than 50 minutes. It is a wise investment of time with potential payoffs of reduced study stress and enhanced exam success.

Technique #5: Begin now and use your time wisely. The smart test taker begins the study process early (Olney, 1989). Sit down, conduct the content assessment and develop a study plan as soon as you know about the exam. DON'T PROCRASTINATE!

Getting Down To Business: The Actual Studying. There is no better way to prepare for an examination than individual study (Dickenson-Hazard, 1989). The responsibility to achieve the goal you set for this exam lies with you alone. The means you employ to achieve this goal do vary and should begin with identifying your peak study times and using techniques to maximize them.

Technique #1: Study in short bursts. Each of us have our own biologic clock which dictates when we are at our peak during the day. If you are a morning person, you are generally active and alert early in the day, slowing down and becoming drowsy by evening. If you are an evening person, you don't completely wake up until late morning and hit your peak in the afternoon and evening. Each person generally has several peaks during the day. It is best to study during those times when your alertness is at its peak (Dickenson-Hazard, 1990).

During our concentration peaks, there are mini peaks, or bursts of alertness (Olney, 1989). These alertness peaks of a concentration peak occur because levels of concentration are at their highest during the first part and last part of a study period. These bursts can vary from ten minutes to one hour depending on the extent of concentration. If studying is sustained for one hour there are only two mini peaks; one at the beginning and one at the end. There are eight mini peaks if that same hour is divided into four, 10-minute intervals. Hence it is more helpful to study in short bursts (Olney, 1989). More can be learned in less time.

Technique #2: Cramming can be useful. Since concentration ability is highly variable, some individuals can sustain their mini-peaks for 15, 20 or even 30 minutes at a time. Pushing your concentration beyond its peak is fruitless and verges on cramming, which in general is a poor study technique. There are, however, times when cramming, a short term memory tool, is useful. Short term memory generally is at its best in the morning. A quick review or cram of content in the morning can be useful the day of the exam (Olney, 1989). Most studying, however, is best accomplished in the afternoon or evening when long term memory functions at its peak.

Technique #3: Give your brain breaks. Regular times during study to rest and absorb the content are needed by the brain. The best approach to breaks is to plan them and give yourself a conscious break (Dickenson-Hazard, 1990). This approach eliminates the ''day dreaming'' or ''wandering thought'' approach to breaks that many of us use. It is better to get up, leave the study area and do something non-study related for longer breaks. For shorter breaks of 5 minutes or so, leave your desk, gaze out the window or do some stretching exercises. When your brain says to give it a rest, accommodate it! You'll learn more with less stress.

Technique #4: Study the correct content. It is easy for all of us to become bogged down in the detail of the content we are studying. However, it is best to focus on the major concepts or the ''state of the art'' content. Leave the details, the suppositions and the experience at the door of your study area. Concentrate on the major textbook facts and concepts which revolve around the subject matter being tested.

Table 2

Sample Content Assessment

Exam Content: Theories & Skills	
Category: Provided by Test Giver	*Rating: Provided by Examinee*
Group dynamics	2
Group process	2
Behavior modification	1
Crisis intervention	4
Reality therapy	3
Communication process	3
Interviewing skills	4
Self-care	3
Decision-making	1
Legal/ethical issues	2
Cognitive techniques	1
Mental status evaluation	2
Problem solving	2
Community resources evaluation	1
Nursing process	4
Nursing theory	4
Role theory	3
Change theory	4
Communication theories	1
Organizational theory	2
Research design	2
Research evaluation	4
Research application	3
Team building	3
Conflict management	1
Teaching/learning skills	2
Supervisory skills	4
Observation skills	3
Evaluation skills	4
Nursing diagnosis	4
DSM IV	1
Grief and loss theory	2
Death and dying	3
Stress management theory	2
Stress management skills	4
Family dynamics	1
Assertiveness training skills	2
Motivation skills	2

Technique #5: Fit your studying to the test type. The best way to prepare for an objective test is to study facts, particularly anything printed in italics or bold. Memory enhancing techniques are particularly useful when preparing for an objective test. If preparing for an essay test, study generalities, examples and concepts. Application techniques are helpful when studying for this type of an exam (Burkle & Marshak, 1989).

Table 3

Sample Study Plan

Goal: Achieve a passing grade on the certification exam. Time available: 2 Months

Objective	Activity	Date Accomplished
Understand elements of milieu therapy	Read section in Chapter 2	Feb. 5 & 6, 1 hour each day
	Read notes from review class and combine with notes taken from text	Feb. 7, 1 hour
	Review combined notes and sample test questions	Feb. 8, 1 hour
Master social/cultural/ethnic factors	Read section in Chapter 2. Take notes on chapter content	Feb. 9 & 10, 1 hour each day
	Read notes from review class and combine with notes taken from text	Feb. 11, 1 hour
	Review combined notes and sample test questions	Feb. 12, 1 hour
Know material contained in Code for Nurses with Interpretive Statements	Read ANA Pub. No. G-56, 1985. Take notes on content	Feb. 13 & 14, 1 hour each day

Technique #6: Use your study plan wisely. Your study plan is meant to be a guide, not a rigid schedule. You should take your time with studying. Don't rush through the content just to remain on schedule. Occasionally study plans need revision. If you take more or less time than planned, readjust the plan for the time gained or lost. The plan can guide you, but you must go at your own pace.

Technique #7: Actively study. Being an active participant in study rather than trying to absorb the printed word is also helpful. Ways to be active include: taking notes on the content as you study; constructing questions and answering them; taking practice tests; or discussing the content with yourself. Also using your individual study quirks is encouraged. Some people stand, others walk around and some play background music. Whatever helps you to concentrate and study better, you should use.

Technique #8: Use study aids. While there is no substitute for individual studying, several resources, if available, are useful in facilitating learning. Review courses are an excellent means for organizing or summarizing your individual study. They generally provide the content parameters and the major concepts of the content which you need to know. Review courses also provide an opportunity to clarify not-well-understood content, as well as to review known material (Dickenson-Hazard, 1990). Study guides are useful for organizing study. They provide detail on the content which is important to the exam. Study groups are an excellent resource for summarizing and refining content. They provide an opportunity for thinking through your knowledge base, with the advantage of hearing another person's point of view. Each of these study aids increases understanding of content and when used correctly, increases effectiveness of knowledge application.

Technique #9: Know when to quit. It is best to stop studying when your concentration ebbs. It is unproductive and frustrating to force yourself to study. It is far better to rest or unwind, then resume at a later point in the day. Avoid studying outside your A.M. or P.M. concentration peaks and focus your study energy on your right time of day or evening.

STRATEGY #4 Become Test-wise

Most nursing examinations are composed of multiple choice questions (MCQs). This type of question requires the examinee to select the best response(s) for a specific circumstance or condition. Successful test taking is dependent not only on content knowledge but on test taking skill as well. If you are unable to impart your knowledge through the vehicle used for its conveyance, i.e., the MCQ, your test taking success is in jeopardy.

Technique #1: Recognize the purpose of a test question. Most test questions are developed to examine knowledge at two separate levels: memory and application. A memory question requires the examinee to recall and comprehend facts from their knowledge base while an application question requires the examinee to use and apply the knowledge (ABP, 1989). Memory questions test recall while application questions test synthesis and problem-solving skills. When taking a test you need to be aware of whether you are being asked a fact or to use that fact.

Technique #2: Recognize the components of a test question. Multiple choice questions may include the basic components of a background statement, a stem and a list of options. The background statement presents information which facilitates the examinee in answering the question. The stem asks or states the intent of the question. The options are 4 to 5 possible responses to the question. The correct option is called the keyed response and all other options are called distractors (ABP, 1989). Knowing the components of a test question helps you sift through the information presented and focus on the question's intent (see Table 4).

Technique #3: Recognize the item types. Basically two styles of MCQs are used for examinations. One requires the examinee to select the one best answer; the other requires selection of multiple correct answers. Among the one best answer styles there are 3 types. The A type requires the selection of the best response among those offered. The B type requires the examinee to match the options with the appropriate statement. The X type asks the examinee to respond either true or false to each option (ABP, 1989). Table 5 illustrates these item types. **Most standardized tests, such as those used for nursing licensure and certification, are composed of four or five option-A type questions.**

Technique #4: Nugent and Vitale (1997) suggest the test taking techniques in Table 6.

Technique #5 Practice, practice, practice. Taking practice tests can improve performance. While they can assist in evaluation of your knowledge, their primary benefit is to assist you with test taking skills. You should use them to evaluate your thinking process, your ability to read, understand and interpret questions, and your skills in completing the mechanics of the test.

STRATEGY #5 Apply Basic Rules of Test Taking

Technique #1: Follow your regular routine the night before a test. Eat familiar foods. Avoid the temptation to cram all night. Go to bed at your regular time (Nugent and Vitale, 1997).

Technique #2: Be prepared for exam day. It is important to familiarize yourself with the test site, the building, the parking and travel route prior to the exam day. If you must travel, arrive early to allow time for this familiarization. It is helpful to make a list of things you need on the exam day: pencils, admission card, watch and a few pieces of hard candy as a quick energy source. On exam day allow yourself plenty of time to arrive at the site. Wear comfortable clothes and have a good breakfast that morning.

Technique #3: Understand all the directions for the test. Know if the test has a penalty for guessing or if you should attempt every question (Nugent and Vitale, 1997).

Table 4

Anatomy Of A Test Question

Background Statement:	A woman brings her 65 year old mother in to see a clinical nurse specialist because she is concerned that it is now a month since her mother was widowed and she continues to be tearful when talking about the loss and wants to visit the grave regularly.	
	Stem:	Which of the following initial approaches would most likely result in compliance with your nursing recommendations?
	Options:	(A) Three or four short questions followed by requesting a psychiatrist to prescribe an antidepressant
		(B) Immediate Reassurance only
		(C) *Careful listening and open-ended questions*
		(D) Refer the mother to a support group

TABLE 5

Item Type Examples

A TYPE

Directions for One Best Choice Items: This item-type requires that you indicate the one best answer from the lettered alternatives offered for each item. After you have decided on the one BEST answer, completely blacken the corresponding lettered circle on the answer sheet.

#1 Sally is a 28 year old client with Schizophrenia. One day she says to the nurse: ''I see you are wearing black shoes today. That means you have it in for me.'' Sally is experiencing:

(A) A delusion
(B) A hallucination
(C) *An idea of reference*
(D) An imaginary fantasy

B TYPE

Directions: Each group of questions below consists of five lettered headings followed by a list of numbered words or statements. For each numbered word or statement, select the one lettered heading that is most closely associated with it and fill in the circle beneath the corresponding letter on the answer sheet. Each lettered heading may be selected once, more than once, or not at all.

#2-4
Laboratory test:

(A) Lithium level
(B) Dexamethasone Suppression Test
(C) MAOI level
(D) Benzodiazepine level

Related to the treatment of:

#2. Depression (B)
#3. Manic Depression (A)
#4. Substance Abuse (D)

X TYPE

#5-9

Directions: Each of the questions or incomplete statements below is followed by five suggested answers or completions. For EACH alternative completely blacken one lettered circle in either column T or F on the answer sheet.

#5 According to Freud, from birth to 18 months the infant is learning muscle control, especially that related to defecation (F)
#6 According to Erikson the task of Adulthood is Generativity vs Stagnation (T)
#7 According to Sullivan the task of late adolescence is developing an enduring relationship with members of the same sex (F)
#8 According to Piaget from ages 7 to 12 the child learns to reason systematically and use abstract thought (T)
#9 According to most theorists, children begin to learn socially acceptable behavior when they can delay gratification and incorporate the demands of significant others (T)

From ''Anatomy of a test question.'' by N. Dickenson-Hazard, 1989, *Pediatric Nursing 15,* p. 396. Copyright 1989 by A. J. Jannetti, Inc. Adapted by permission.

Technique #4:   Read the directions carefully. An exam may have several types of questions. Be on the lookout for changing item types and be sure you understand the directions on how you are to answer before you begin reading the question.

Technique #5:   Use time wisely and effectively. Allow no more than 1 minute per question. Skip difficult questions and return to them later or make an educated guess.

Technique #6:   Read and consider all options. Be systematic and use problem-solving techniques. Relate options to question and balance against each other.

Technique #7:   Check your answers and answer sheet. Reconsider your answers, especially those in which you made an educated guess. You may have gained information from subsequent questions that is helpful in answering previous questions or may be less anxious and more objective by the end of the test. Avoid changing answers without good reason.

STRATEGY #6 Psych Yourself Up: Taking tests is stressful

While a little stress can be productive, too much can incapacitate you in your studying and test taking (Divine & Kylen, 1979). For persons with severe test anxiety, interventions such as Cognitive Therapy, Systematic Desensitization, Study Skills Counseling and Biofeedback have all been used with some success. (Spielberger, 1995) Techniques derived from these approaches can influence the results achieved by changing attitudes and approaches to test taking and thereby reducing anxiety. Psyching yourself up can have a positive affect and make examinations a non-anxiety laden experience (Dickenson-Hazard, 1990). The following techniques are based on the principles of successful test taking as presented by Sides & Cailles (1989). Incorporation of these techniques can improve response and performance in examination situations.

Technique #1:   Adopt an ''I can'' attitude. Believing you can succeed is the key to success. Self belief inspires and gives you the power to achieve your goals. Without a success attitude, the road to your goal is much harder. We all stand an equal chance of success in this world. It is those who believe they can who achieve it. This ''I can'' attitude must permeate all your efforts in test taking, from studying to improving your skills, to actually writing the test.

Technique #2:   Take control. By identifying your goal, deciding how to accomplish it and developing a plan for achieving it, you take control. Do not leave your success to chance; control it through action and attitude.

Table 6

Test Taking Techniques

1. Break the question down into its components.
   Read the stem. What is it asking?
   Don't assume any information not given.
   Look for key words "first," "best," "appropriate," "initially," "most." May want to underline key words.
   Watch for key words that indicate a negative question: "Not," "except," "never," "contraindicated," "least."
   Rank the choices according to priority set by the key words.
   If it is hard to rank them, eliminate the one which is most wrong from the four choices.
   Then eliminate the most wrong answer from the remaining three options.

   > A client who has been taking a tricyclic antidepressant is switched to an MAOI.
   > Which of the following should be of most concern to the nurse before she gives the first dose?
   >
   > a. The client can recite the diet restrictions
   > b. *The client has not received the tricyclic for two weeks*
   > c. The client must be on suicide precautions
   > d. The client cannot leave the unit for two days
   >
   > Which of the following foods should the client be counseled *not* to consume?
   >
   > a. fruits
   > b. vegetables
   > c. salty foods
   > d. *wine*

2. Identify clues in the stem — may have a word or phrase in the stem which is significant, or similar to a word or phrase in the correct answer.

   > According to Maslow's hierarchy, how can the nurse best meet the client in seclusion's *physiological* needs?
   >
   > a. Call the client by name when doing 15 minute checks
   > b. Talk to the client once they have calmed down
   > c. *Offer drinks of water or toilet every two hours*
   > d. Use four point restraints when necessary
   >
   > In working with the schizophrenic client, how can the nurse best enhance the client's *self-esteem?*
   >
   > a. *Encourage the client to perform self-care*
   > b. Escort the client when leaving the unit
   > c. Encourage the client's family to visit
   > d. Keep the client out of bed during the day

3. Identify patient-centered options: choices which put the patient as priority. Eliminate options that deny patient feelings, concerns and needs, are disrespectful or punitive.

   > A mother is depressed due to having lost her baby to SIDS. She is crying and says "I can't bear to go home without him." What is the nurse's best response?
   >
   > a. "But you have two healthy kids at home. They need you."
   > b. *"It must be very hard."*
   > c. "I'm sure your husband will help you."
   > d. "Do you want to stay in the hospital?"

4. Identify answers with words like always, never, all, every, none and only. These terms frequently represent broad generalizations that are usually false and can be eliminated.

   > Which of the following statements is true of Survivors of persons with AIDS?
   >
   > a. *They are at risk for developing pathological grief*
   > b. They would prefer that you not bring up the subject of the loss
   > c. They always require professional counseling
   > d. They feel guilty about the death

   (Continued)

Table 6 (Continued)

Test Taking Techniques

5. Evaluate opposites in options. One of them will be the correct answer or they both may be wrong choices that can be eliminated.

> Persons with AIDS
>
> a. Face a predictable course of illness
> b. May experience hypertension which is exacerbated by HIV
> c. *Are vulnerable to feelings of guilt and rejection*
> d. Are accepted and supported by their employers and communities

6. Identify equally plausible options. These are usually the wrong choice and can be eliminated.

> The best indicator of neurological involvement in AIDS patients is
>
> a. Apathy
> b. Loss of interest in social activities
> c. Impaired memory
> d. *Presence of HIV in cerebrospinal fluid*

7. Options which contain two or more facts per option usually duplicate them in at least two of the four options. If you identify one incorrect fact you can rule out the other option that contains it.

> The two most frequent psychiatric diagnoses in persons with AIDS are
>
> a. AIDS Dementia Complex and Panic Disorder
> b. Bipolar Disorder and AIDS Dementia Complex
> c. *Adjustment Disorder with Depression and AIDS Dementia Complex*
> d. Adjustment Disorder with Depression and Bipolar Disorder

From P.M. Nugent and B.A. Vitale, 1997, *Test Success: Test-Taking Techniques for beginning Nursing Students.* Copyright 1997 by F.A. Davis. Adapted by permission.

Technique #3: Think positively. Examinations are generally based on a standard which is the same for all individuals. Everyone can potentially pass. Performance is influenced not only by knowledge and skill but by attitude as well. Those individuals who regard an exam as an opportunity or challenge will be more successful.

Technique #4: Project a positive self-fulfilling prophecy. While preparing for an examination, project thoughts of the positive outcomes you will experience when you succeed. Self-talk is self-fulfilling. Expect success, not failure, for yourself.

Technique #5: Feel good about yourself. Without feeling a sense of positive self worth, passing an examination is difficult. Recognize your professional contributions and give yourself credit for your accomplishments. Think ''I will pass,'' not ''I suppose I can.''

Technique #6: Know yourself. Focus exam preparation and test taking on your strengths. Try to alter your weaknesses instead of becoming hung up on them. If you tend to overanalyze, study and read test questions at face value. If you're a speed demon when taking a test, slow down and read more carefully.

Technique #7:   Failure is a possibility. We all have failed at something at some point in our lives. Rather than dwelling on the failure, making excuses and believing you'll fail again, recognize your mistakes and remedy them. Failure is a time to begin again; use it as a motivator to do better. It is not the end of the world unless you allow it to be. It is best to deal with the failure and move on, otherwise it interferes with your success.

Technique #8:   Persevere, persevere, persevere! Endurance must underlie all your efforts. Call forth those reserve energies when you've had all you think you can take. Rely upon yourself and your support systems to help you maintain a sense of direction and keep your goal in the forefront.

Technique #9:   Motivation is muscle. Most individuals are motivated by fear or desire. The fear in an exam situation may be one of failure, the unknown or discovery of imperfection. Put your fear into perspective; realize you are not the only one with fear and that all have an equal opportunity for success. Develop strategies to reduce fear and use fear to your advantage by improving the imperfections. Desire is a powerful motivator and you should keep the rewards of your desire foremost in your mind. Whatever motivates you, use it to make you successful. Reward yourself during your exam preparation and once the exam has been completed. You alone hold the key to success; use what you have wisely.

This chapter has provided concepts, strategies and techniques for improving study and test taking skills. Your first task in improvement is to know yourself: how you study and how you take a test. You should use your strengths and remedy the weaknesses. Next you need to develop your thinking skills. Work on techniques to improve memory and reasoning. Now you need to organize your study and concentrate on using your strengths and these new and improved skills to be successful. Create a study space, develop a plan of action, then implement that plan during your periods of peak concentration. Before taking the exam be sure you understand the components of a test question, can identify key words and phrases and have practiced. Apply the test taking rules during the exam process. Finally, believe in yourself, your knowledge and your talent. Believing you can accomplish your goal facilitates the fact that you will.

BIBLIOGRAPHY

American Board of Pediatrics. (1989). *Developing questions and critiques.* Unpublished material.

Burke, M. M., & Walsh, M.B. (1992). *Gerontologic nursing.* St. Louis: Mosby Year Book.

Burkle, C. A., & Marshak, D. (1989). *Study program: Level 1.* Reston, Va: National Association of Secondary School Principals.

Conaway, D. C., Miller, M. D., & West, G. R. (1988). *Geriatrics.* St. Louis: Mosby Year Book.

Dickenson-Hazard, N. (1989). Making the grade as a test taker. *Pediatric Nursing, 15,* 302–304.

Dickenson-Hazard, N. (1989). Anatomy of a test question. *Pediatric Nursing, 15,* 395–399.

Dickenson-Hazard, N. (1990). The psychology of successful test taking. *Pediatric Nursing, 16,* 66–67.

Dickenson-Hazard, N. (1990). Study smart. *Pediatric Nursing, 16,* 314–316.

Dickenson-Hazard, N. (1990). Study effectiveness: Are you 10 a.m. or p.m. scholar? *Pediatric Nursing,* 16, 419–420.

Dickenson-Hazard, N. (1990). Develop your thinking skills for improved test taking. *Pediatric Nursing,* 16, 480–481.

Divine, J. H., & Kylen, D. W. (1979). *How to beat test anxiety.* New York: Barrons Educational Series, Inc.

Millman, J., & Pauk, W. (1969). *How to take tests.* New York: McGraw-Hill Book Co.

Millonig, V. L. (Ed.). (1994). *The adult nurse practitioner certification review guide* (rev. ed). Potomac, MD: Health Leadership Associates.

Nugent, P. M., & Vitale, B. A. (1997). *Test success: Test-taking techniques for beginning nursing students.* Philadelphia: F.A. Davis Co.

Olney, C. W. (1989). *Where there's a will, there's an A.* New Jersey: Chesterbrook Educational Publishers.

Sides, M., & Cailles, N. B. (1989). *Nurse's guide to successful test taking.* Philadelphia: J. B. Lippincott Co.

Sides, M., & Korchek, N. (1994). *Nurse's guide to successful test taking* (2nd ed.). Philadelphia: J. B. Lippincott.

Spielberger, C. D., & Vagg, P. R. (1995). *Test anxiety: Theory, assessment, and treatment.* Washington, DC: Taylor and Francis.

Essentials of Psychiatric Nursing Care

Clare Houseman

Mental Health

- Definition: Traditionally, to both love and work successfully; some definitions also include happiness; involves balance in physical, emotional, social and spiritual spheres

- Components according to Johnson (1997):

  1. Self-governance—autonomy, guidance from values within; functions dependently, interdependently or independently as needed

  2. Growth orientation—strives for self-realization, androgyny,and maximization of capacities

  3. Tolerance of uncertainty—uses faith and hope to face life and death

  4. Self-esteem—built on awareness of abilities and limitations

  5. Environmental mastery—creative and effective in influencing and reacting to surroundings

  6. Reality orientation—tells fact from fantasy and responds accordingly

  7. Stress management—experiences appropriate depression, anxiety, tolerates stress as temporary and can tolerate failure; flexible and copes with crises with help from friends and family

- Hardiness is viewed as a characteristic of mentally healthy people and involves the following:

  1. Control—feel in charge of and able to influence own life

  2. Commitment—feel deeply involved in life and work

  3. Challenge—view change as normal and obstacles as opportunities (Johnson, 1997)

- Absence of mental health may be perceived as uncomfortable to the individual and/or his significant others and result in the perception of a need for change.

Change

- Definition: Process resulting in transformation
- Planned change—deliberate, goal directed effort to solve problems; applicable to any system (individual, family, organization)

- Process involves the following responses according to Huelskoetter and Romano (1991):
    1. Feelings of tension, anxiety, and fear
    2. A sense of need
    3. Feelings of hope
    4. A search
    5. Decision and goal setting
    6. Commitment to goals and change
    7. Creative behavior
    8. Changes in behavior

- Success of change dependent on the change agent's ability to facilitate a helping relationship and collaborate with the individual, group, family, or organization

- Change involves risk and resistance. It cannot be rushed.

- Change is effected by nurses within the nursing process.

The Nursing Process—involves the following:

- Assessment—data are collected in a continuous, comprehensive, accurate, and systematic manner. Interviews are usually conducted with clients and others to complete the nursing history. Relevant data for adult patients include:
    1. Appearance
    2. Presenting problem
    3. Personal and family history
    4. Medical and psychiatric history
    5. Physical status
    6. Mental status
        a. Reaction to interview
        b. Behavior (Speech, ADL, etc)
        c. Level of consciousness
        d. Orientation

       e. Intellect

       f. Thought content and process

       g. Judgment

       h. Affect

       i. Mood

       j. Insight

       k. Memory

       l. Comprehension

7. Sociocultural status

    a. Socioeconomic status

    b. Life values and goals

    c. Social habits—including drinking and drug use

    d. Sexual behavior

    e. Social support network

8. Spiritual status

    a. Philosophy and meaning of life

    b. Sense of oneness or spiritual integrity

    c. Relatedness to God or higher power

    d. Relatedness to people and nature

9. See Chapter 10 for information regarding assessment of children

- Diagnoses are made according to:

  1. North American Nursing Diagnosis Association (NANDA) (See Examples in Clinical Chapters)

  2. Standard classification of mental disorders, i.e., The American Psychiatric Association's Diagnosis and Statistical Manual (DSM IV) or International Classification of Disease (ICD10)

- Planning provides goals and actions that are:

  1. Specific

  2. Individualized

3. Collaborative

- Intervention—treatment according to diagnoses and care plan should be based on scientific theory and includes:

  1. Psychotherapeutic interventions—may be talking, poetry writing, social skills training, cooking, modeling assertiveness, or expression of feelings

  2. Health teaching—about medication, nutrition, sleep hygiene

  3. Self-care activities—e.g., relaxation, exercise, spirituality

  4. Somatic therapies—e.g., nursing care of clients receiving ECT

  5. Therapeutic environment—milieu

  6. Psychotherapy (Clinical Nurse Specialist role)

  7. Interventions can be interdependent (other team members must collaborate) or independent (discussed and determined with client)

- Evaluation of client responses to nursing action is based on client changes in the following:

  1. Cognition

     a. Giving up irrational beliefs

     b. Making positive self-statements

     c. Improving ability to problem solve

  2. Affect

     a. Decreased anxiety

     b. Decreased depression

     c. Decreased loneliness

  3. Behavior

     a. Adaptive responses

     b. Improved coping skills

     c. Improved social skills

- Revisions to plan of care are made as needed and the process continues.

- The nursing process and all nursing interventions occur within the context of the nurse-client relationship.

Nurse-Client Relationship

- Definition: A dynamic, collaborative, therapeutic, interactive process between the nurse and the client

- Purpose—to create a safe climate wherein clients feel free to reveal themselves and their concerns and feel comfortable to try out new ideas and behaviors

- Phases of nurse-client relationship according to Peplau (1952):

  1. Orientation—begin as strangers

     a. Client—seeks or is brought in for help; communicates needs and expectations

     b. Nurse—responds to client; explains parameters of relationship; gathers data; listens and clarifies areas of concern; establishes rapport; negotiates contract which establishes frequency and duration of sessions, specifies type of work to be done, clarifies fees if any, and lays groundwork for termination

  2. Identification

     a. Client—responds to help offered by nurse, explores deeper feelings, identifies with nurse and may be dependent, active, and compliant

     b. Nurse—structures relationship to focus on client and facilitates expression of problems and feelings; avoids fostering unnecessary dependency; encourages self-care

  3. Exploitation—working

     a. Client—more independent in accessing services and working in partnership to interpret behaviors; begins to try out new behaviors

     b. Nurse—supports client and explores feelings and problems at client's pace; deals with resistances, encourages risk taking and facilitates achievement of goals

  4. Resolution—termination

     a. Client—engages in new problem-solving skills and coping behaviors; views self positively and plans for future; may decompensate when anticipating separation

      b. Nurse—reviews goals and accomplishments; shares own feelings and assists client to express feelings about relationship and separation

- Phenomena that occur in nurse-client relationships

  1. Therapeutic use of self—application of nurse's own personality characteristics within the interaction to facilitate healing

  2. Transference—client experiences emotional reaction towards nurse based on unconscious feelings that originated in past relationships. Nursing response is to confront distortions of reality gently in order to facilitate client self-awareness.

  3. Countertransference—nurse responds to client with feelings from own earlier conflicts. Nurse must increase self-awareness and access supervision to assist in dealing with client more effectively.

  4. Resistance—attempts to keep anxiety-provoking thoughts and feelings out of awareness by disrupting the interactional process with avoidance, acting out, forgetting, silence, lateness, etc. Nursing response is to make observations and support client in dealing with anxiety.

  5. Testing behaviors according to McMahon (1992)

     a. Attempting a social relationship

     b. Casting nurse into parental role

     c. Assessing whether nurse trusts them

     d. Attempting to take care of nurse

     e. Avoiding discussion of problems

     f. Asking for personal data

     g. Violating personal space

     h. Seeking attention from nurse

     i. Assessing nurse's commitment

     j. Revealing information to shock nurse

     k. Touching nurse inappropriately

        Nurse must set limits and encourage client to discuss meaning of behavior.

- Psychotherapy—use of relationship and communication to change feelings, attitudes, and behaviors

    1. Supportive—express feelings, explore choices

    2. Re-educative—learn new ways of belief and behavior

    3. Reconstructive—deep emotional and cognitive restructuring

- Clinical Supervision—use of more experienced practitioner or peers to "obtain feedback on interventions and analyze the emotions particular clients generated; this process allows nurses to be objective about their reactions and to decenter emotions" (Delaney & Lettieri-Marks, 1997, p. 134) which may interfere with the nurse-client relationship

Communication

- Definition: Continuous process by which information is transmitted between people and their environment

- Goal—understanding

- Process of communication:

Figure 1: Process of Communication

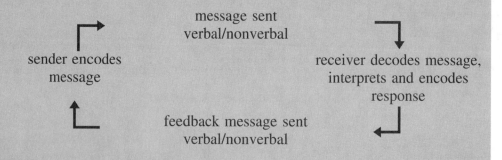

- All behavior communicates some message.

- Verbal messages include the written and spoken word.

- Nonverbal messages are observed by the receiver in four ways:

    1. Kinesics—body motion, i.e., facial expression, posture, position of arms and legs, eye contact, touch

    2. Paralanguage—tone of voice, inflection, emphasis, pauses, sighs, laughter

3. Proxemics—use of personal space, territoriality, i.e., backing away or moving closer, selection of a particular seating arrangement

4. Appearance—personal image, i.e., clothing, makeup, hair, beard

- Nonverbal messages may be congruent with verbal messages or they may conflict with them

- Culture and social class influence perceptions and values which influence how communication is transmitted and received.

- Type of relationship also influences type of communication.

  1. Therapeutic communication takes place between the nurse and client and focuses on the client's thoughts, feelings, behavior, and roles with the expectation that the active listening of the nurse will help the client explore, understand, and change.

  2. Social communication is less goal oriented, more superficial and does not necessarily involve the expectation of help.

- Although nurse-client relationships may involve some social communication, the main component is therapeutic communication.

Therapeutic communication includes:

- Active listening or physical attending skills

  1. Comfortable environment—privacy, low noise, soft light

  2. Facing the other person and leaning towards him/her

  3. Open, relaxed posture

  4. Eye contact

- Attitudes and behaviors which build trust and rapport

  1. Nonjudgmental, positive regard

  2. Punctuality

  3. Honesty

  4. Respect, acceptance and confirmation

  5. Genuineness, empathy

  6. Congruence between verbal and non-verbal behaviors (Johnson, 1997)

  7. Stated purpose of interaction

9. Be unhurried; give undivided attention

10. Be sensitive and responsive to nonverbal communication

11. Listen

12. Be professional but warm, accepting, supportive and objective

13. Recognize and accept culture specific attitudes and behaviors

14. Use understandable and acceptable language

15. Be aware of own feelings and how they affect your behavior

16. Be clear that responsibility for action rests with client

17. Help develop awareness of consequences and alternatives (McMahon, 1997)

- Communication techniques

    1. Using broad openings and open-ended questions

    2. Clarifying content and feelings

    3. Reflecting content and feelings

    4. Confronting content and feelings

    5. Verifying perceptions

    6. Giving information

    7. Providing feedback

    8. Stating observations

    9. Silence

    10. Directing

    11. Focusing

    12. Questioning

    13. Connecting information

    14. Summarizing

- Barriers to therapeutic communication

    1. Advice

    2. Reassurance

    3. Being judgmental

    4. Changing the subject

    5. Excessive questioning/ closed-ended questions

    6. Challenging

    7. Stereotypical comments

    8. Self-focusing behavior

    9. Using emotionally charged words

- Communication with children

    1. Introduce to play materials

    2. Encourage to verbalize at own pace

    3. Ask questions that are relevant to developmental age

- Result of therapeutic communication is enhanced client self-disclosure

- Nurse self-disclosure can enhance or inhibit therapeutic communication depending on its use. Like all interventions, it requires timing and judgment. Its use, according to Auvil and Silver (1984) depends on:

    1. Nurse's theoretical framework—i.e., more likely to occur if working from a humanist perspective than from a psychoanalytic or behaviorist approach

    2. Stage of the relationship:

        a. Orientation—nurse self-disclosure that occurs early in the relationship more likely to meet nurses' needs

        b. Working phase—appropriate if used by the nurse to hasten the therapeutic alliance to help the clients learn about themselves and others, encourage their catharsis of feelings, support their goals and validate their reality (McMahon, 1997)

        c. Termination—expression of feelings about end of relationship to model appropriate behaviors for client

Cultural and Ethnic Factors

- Definitions

    1. Culture—patterns of knowledge, belief, behavior, and custom that are learned by members of a particular society

2. Ethnicity—membership in diverse groups according to race, birth-place, language, culture, or religion

3. Ethnocentric—judging others' behavior by the values of our own culture

4. Culturally relativistic—attempting to understand the behavior of others within the context of their own culture

5. Stereotype—overgeneralizations based on culture or ethnicity; may occur unconsciously

- Impact of culture on mental health nursing

   1. Influences client coping behaviors

   2. Defines what symptoms are labelled as illness

   3. Determines explanations for illnesses e.g., may be personalistic, e.g., caused by purposeful intervention by others

   4. Prescribes taboo topics and behaviors

   5. Determines how mentally ill are perceived

   6. Prescribes health-seeking behaviors and attitudes to health care providers

   7. Determines types of acceptable treatment approaches

   8. Influences behavioral expression of mental illnesses resulting in culture-bound illnesses such as susto, mal ojo (Hispanic), falling out (African American), and voodoo

   9. Determines distribution of illness, e.g., somatic vs depressive symptoms, male vs female

- Cultural differences according to Tripp-Reimer and Lively (1993):

   1. Time—emphasis on present (predominant in African American, Native American and Hispanic culture) vs. future (predominant in U.S. and other highly industrialized nations which also value schedules)

   2. Success—doing: people valued for accomplishments (Predominant U.S.) vs. being: people valued for being themselves (Chinese)

   3. Relational—collectivist: individual goals are subordinate to group goals (African and Native American and Hispanic) vs. individualistic: individual goals are more important than group goals (Predominant U.S.)

4. Nature—people dominant to nature(Middle class U.S.) vs. live in harmony with nature (Native American), vs. subjugated to nature (Moslem cultures)

5. Verbal Communication—volume (Asians speak softly), speed and directness (Asians value indirectness); silence interpreted differently by various cultures

6. Privacy—personal space (arabic:closer vs. U.S.: further); eye contact (Native American prefer less than predominant U.S.)

- Impact of Ethnicity on Mental Health Nursing

    1. Metabolism rates, clinical drug responses and side effects found in research to be significantly different among racial and ethnic populations

    2. Field of ethnic pharmacology developed (Campinha-Bacote, 1997)

- Culturally Competent Nursing Care—''care that is sensitive to issues related to culture, race, gender and sexual orientation; this care is provided by nurses who use cultural nursing theory, models and research principles in identifying and evaluating the care provided within the cultural context of the clients.'' (AAN,1992)

    1. Be aware of one's own cultural beliefs and behaviors

    2. Be culturally aware—have knowledge of cultural differences

    3. Assess the degree to which the client has assimilated the predominant culure; don't assume

    4. Perform a Cultural Assessment to determine from the client and the client's reference group their emic (native) view of what is considered normal and abnormal in both problem definition and expectations for treatment and care. See Table 1.

    5. Intercultural Communication

        a. Adapt activity level, tone of voice, and remarks to the cultural background of the client

        b. Develop listening skills, observe non-verbal behavior and eliminate barriers to communication

        c. Show respect and acceptance to clients in ways they understand

6. Facilitation skills—ability to negotiate interactions that may tend to be inconsistent with the value and belief system of an individual or family from another culture; conflict resolution

7. Flexibility—negotiate a treatment plan that reflects, respects and incorporates both traditional treatment and folk remedies. (Campinha-Bacote, 1997)

8. Design culturally responsive programs which are available, accessible, appropriate, acceptable and adoptable to decrease underutilization of mental health services by ethnic groups

9. Show respect and acceptance to clients in ways <u>they</u> understand.

Table 1

Cultural Assessment Tool

What do you think has caused your problem?
Why do you think it started when it did?
What do you think your sickness does to you?
How severe is your sickness?
What kind of treatment do you think you should receive?
What are the most important results you hope to achieve from these treatments?
What are the chief problems your sickness has caused?
What do you fear the most about your disease?

Note: From "Illness and Care, Clinical Lessons from Anthropologic and Cross-Cultural Research," by Kleinman et al., 1978, *Annals of Internal Medicine,* 88, pp 251-258. Copyright 1978 by the American College of Physicians. Reprinted with permission.

Interdisciplinary Treatment and the Health Care Team

- Components

1. Interdisciplinary treatment utilizes members of different professions who come together to plan and evaluate the treatment of individual clients.

2. Each member is considered to have vital input to the treatment plan based on his/her particular area of expertise.

3. The client is also considered to be a member of the team.

- Goal—targeted interventions, consistently implemented and evaluated by everyone involved with the client

- Attributes of mental health team
  1. Strong team commitment
  2. Shared responsibility, control, and decision making
  3. Common goals and philosophy of intervention
  4. Flattened heirarchy of authority
  5. Decision making by consensus
  6. Open communication
  7. Examination of roles and relationships
  8. Setting limits on own and others' behavior in a nonpunitive way
  9. Flexibility, versatility, creativity, and optimism
- Professions involved with mental health team
  1. Diet therapy—provides culturally relevant, attractive, nourishing foods with awareness of psychological importance of food, conflicts about eating (Eating Disorders) and drug interactions with certain foods (MAO Inhibitors)
  2. Expressive therapies
     a. Art—uses art work of clients to express underlying feelings and conflicts
     b. Music—vicarious listening stimulates the expression of ideas and emotions verbally; active production of music allows for nonverbal expression
     c. Psychodrama—exploration of psychological conflicts through enactment rather than verbalization
  3. Nursing—establishes and maintains milieu; responsible for 24-hour care, activities of daily living and safety; clinical nurse specialists may perform individual, family, or group psychotherapy.
  4. Ministry—assists with spiritual care of client and family; may provide marital therapy or pastoral counseling
  5. Psychiatry—diagnoses and treats conditions amenable to medical treatment; responsible for admission and discharge; may provide individual, group, or family therapy

6. Occupational Therapy—involves clients in meaningful activities and provides vocational rehabilitation if needed

7. Recreational therapy—assists clients to identify appropriate leisure activities

8. Psychology—performs diagnostic testing, and provides plans for treatment based on causative factors; may implement individual, group, or family therapy

9. Social Work—evaluates family, social, and environmental contributions to problem; may provide family, group, or individual psychotherapy

10. Voluntary Agencies—recognized organizations which offer information and support (often provided by peers) to individuals with mental health problems and their families: Recovery Incorporated, Alcoholics Anonymous, National Alliance for the Mentally Ill, National Depressive and Manic Depressive Association; these agencies may vary depending on locality

- Nurses may be case managers for clients or client advocates at all levels within the health care system.

Client Advocacy

- Definition: Interceding on behalf of clients who are unable to speak or act for themselves or are unaware of available options

- Examples

  1. Informing clients about treatment alternatives

  2. Presenting information to the treatment team

  3. Helping clients enter and navigate the health care system

  4. Testifying on behalf of clients in court

  5. Promoting respect for mentally ill in policy and law

- Guidelines for advocacy according to Boyd and Luetje (1991)

  1. Make sure client has need for advocacy.

  2. Check plans with clients and others regarding support system.

  3. Get support and information from others with similar goals.

  4. Present data clearly.

5. Include all pertinent information.

6. Don't use more power than is necessary.

7. Be patient and persistent.

Case Management

- Definition: Assessment for, and coordination of, individualized, culturally appropriate mental health, and other health and social services, for clients and their families or residential care groups

- Goal—improved functioning and empowerment for clients and cost containment and provider accountability for third party payers

- Types

  1. Rehabilitative—refers to time-limited services provided as part of a private benefit plan with emphasis on returning client to productivity

  2. Supportive—refers to services provided to chronically mentally ill clients for as long as necessary

- Outcomes

  1. Enhanced communication, education and participation of clients and families

  2. Discharge planning which begins at start of treatment

  3. Early identification of client problems, possible delays in treatment and barriers to care at both individual and group levels

  4. Increased communication among providers and reduction of duplication or overlapping services (Farnsworth & Biglow, 1997)

- Tools

  1. Interdisciplinary Treatment Plans (ITP)—integrates the care of all health care team members; directed by case manager

  2. Critical Pathways—essential treatment interventions that must be performed each day to meet the expected time specific client outcomes; usually reflects a specific DRG (Farnsworth & Biglow, 1997)

  3. Nursing Care Plans—more detailed than ITPs and more individualized than critical pathways; uses NANDA nursing diagnoses and interventions derived from individual assessment of the client

    4.   Research Based Practice Protocols

       a.   Agency for Health Care Policy and Research (ACHPR) guidelines for depression

       b.   Nursing Intervention Classification (NIC) (Farnsworth & Biglow, 1997).

Psychiatric Liason Nursing

- Clinical Nurse Specialist, as member of the health care team, provides direct care, including psychotherapy, to individuals, groups, and families as well as consultation to nursing and other hospital staff, around client, unit, or institutional issues.

- Liason nurses use knowledge about "systems, change, organizations, problem solving, stress, crisis, interpersonal relationships, communication, and sociocultural concepts" (Walker & Price-Hoskins, 1992, p. 267). See Chapter 11 for more information.

Milieu

- Definitions

  1. Therapeutic environment—physical and psychosocial surroundings as an integrated, interrelated whole are seen as the treatment agent in a variety of settings (Watson, 1992)

  2. Milieu therapy—scientific planning of the social and physical environment so that every interaction and activity is therapeutic

  3. Therapeutic community—a structured environment with an established philosophy of care

  4. Token community—therapeutic community drawn from behavior modification theory; uses tokens to reinforce adaptive behavioral responses; clients can then exchange tokens for privileges.

- Structured aspects of milieu

  1. Community meetings

  2. Daily schedule

  3. Physical environment

  4. Rules and regulations

    5.   Classes, activities, and groups

- Unstructured aspects of milieu

    1.   Daily interactions among clients

    2.   Interactions between clients and staff

- Characteristics of successful milieu

    1.   Effective interaction between and among staff and clients

    2.   Norms which provide predictability and security

    3.   Patient government using democratic process

    4.   Patient's active responsibility for own treatment and for treatment of others

    5.   Fosters growth in direction of increased recognition of strengths and personal empowerment

    6.   Encourages self awareness, risk taking, and change

    7.   Confronts misperceptions, destructive behavior, and poor judgment

    8.   Links with client's family and significant others

    9.   Links with community

- Nurses' role in milieu

    1.   Creation and maintenance of milieu

    2.   Physical care and assurance of safety

        a.   Assess, reinforce and promote client's ability to perform activities of daily living (ADLs)—eating, bathing, dressing etc.

        b.   Assess for physical illness or reactions to medications

        c.   Assess for detoxification reactions in chemically dependent

        d.   Assess for self or other destructive behavior

            (1)   Provide for surveillance—observations every 15 minutes

            (2)   Ensure safety in physical environment (Greene, 1997)

    3.   Medication administration and education

    4.   Attitude therapy—active friendliness, passive friendliness, kind firmness, no demand

5. Model healthy behavior as participant in community

6. Intervene to influence attitudes, behaviors, and relationships in therapeutic way as described by Greene (1993):

   a. Clarify and correct perceptions of current stressors

   b. Identify thoughts and feelings evoked by stressors

   c. Examine how thoughts and feelings influence behavior

   d. Evaluate the extent to which coping behaviors are adaptive or effective

   e. Identify alternative adaptive coping strategies

   f. Test identified alternative coping stragegies in milieu

Group dynamics and group process theory

- Background

   1. Groups are complex human systems whose whole is greater than the sum of their parts.

   2. Individuals can learn, grow, and change more in groups due to opportunities for feedback and consensual validation.

   3. Nurses who participate in groups or Clinical Nurse Specialists who serve as group therapists are aware of the powerful forces harnessed by group work.

- Curative factors of groups (Yalom, 1995)

   1. Instillation of hope

   2. Universality

   3. Imparting information

   4. Altruism

   5. Corrective recapitulation of primary family group

   6. Development of socializing techniques

   7. Imitative behaviors

   8. Interpersonal learning

   9. Group cohesiveness

10. Catharsis

11. Existential factors

- Descriptors of groups

    1. Homogeneous—members chosen for preselected criteria, i.e., sexually abused women

    2. Heterogeneous—mix of individuals regarding diagnosis, sex, age, etc.

    3. Mixed—share essential feature, i.e., same diagnosis but vary sex, age, etc.

    4. Closed—after group begins, no new members are added

    5. Open—members and leaders change

- Types of groups

    1. Task—emphasis on accomplishing what needs to be done

    2. Teaching—impart information, i.e., orient to unit

    3. Supportive/therapeutic—help others who share same experience cope with stress and overcome dysfunction, i.e., bereavement, weight loss.

    4. Psychotherapy—emphasis is on person reducing intrapsychic stress, changing behavior, ideas, etc. may follow a variety of theoretical frameworks, i.e, Psychoanalytic, Transactional Analysis, Rational Emotive, Rogerian, Gestalt, Interpersonal, Bion; Clinical Nurse Specialist role

    5. Psychoeducational—structured group involving teaching, with member disclosure of related thinking and behavioral problems, and homework to put learned information and skills into practice, e.g., groups for family members of the chronically mentally ill and assertiveness training groups

    6. Peer support group—share stresses related to common situation, e.g., hospice nurses

    7. Multiple family—teach about disease process and utilize group process to understand mental health issues; may also refer to a group modality in which the therapist works with one family while other families watch and learn vicariously

- Basic Roles of Therapist (Yalom, 1995)
  1. Technical Expert
  2. Model Setting Participant
- Group dynamic issues according to Long and McMahon (1992)
  1. Rank—position member holds in relation to other members of the group; members who participate frequently and actively usually rank high in the group and thus have greater influence on group behavior
  2. Status—prestige given to certain positions or individuals in a group; members vie for status in group; may be due to member characteristics or behavior
  3. Group content—what is said in a group, i.e., information discussed
  4. Group process—activities in a group, i.e., how interactions occur among members, timing of interactions, roles of members, seating arrangements, tone of voice of members, and nonverbal behaviors
  5. Sociogram—method of recording group process
- Group process issues
  1. Style of leader
     a. Autocratic—leader is in charge and controls
     b. Democratic—leader shares responsibility with members
     c. Laissez Faire—leader is nondirective
  2. Roles of members
     a. Building or maintenance roles—contribute to group process and functioning, e.g., encourager, gatekeeper, harmonizer.
     b. Task roles—emphasize completing the task, e.g., initiator, opinion giver, evaluator, energizer, information seeker
     c. Individual roles—not related to group tasks or maintenance and may inhibit group, e.g., aggressor, dominator, help-seeker, playboy, special-interest pleader, blocker.
- Therapeutic Group Norms (Yalom, 1995)
  1. Self-Monitoring—asssumes responsibility for own functioning
  2. Self-Disclosure

3. Procedural Norms—spontaneous, interactive

4. Group important to members

5. Members are agents of help

6. Support

7. Working in the here and now

- Group development stages (Tuckman, 1965)

    1. Forming—(orientation)—group leader more directive and active, members look to leader for structure and approval. Leader describes group contract (i.e., goals, confidentiality, and communication rules), encourages interaction among group, and maintains working level of anxiety. Members develop initial roles.

    2. Storming—conflict regarding control, power, and authority. Anxiety increases and resistance may occur as evidenced by client absence, shared silence, excessive dependency on leader, scapegoating, excessive hostility toward the leader, forming subgroups and acting out. Leader encourages healthy expression of anger.

    3. Norming—(cohesiveness stage)—members express positive feelings toward one another and feel strongly attracted to the group. Self-disclosure occurs and new roles are adopted.

    4. Performing—(working phase)—leader's activity decreases and usually consists of keeping the group on course or dealing with resistance of group and individuals within. Responsibility for group is more equally shared. Anxiety of group is decreased and energy is channeled to completing tasks.

    5. Mourning—(termination)—begins during first phase but is most acutely felt in closed group when it approaches end and in open group when members or leaders leave. Leaders encourage discussion of ending and expression of pain and loss experienced in grieving process. Members may try to avoid, experience anxiety, anger, or regression; they should also be encouraged to reminisce, evaluate, and experience sense of accomplishment and give feedback to one another (Lasalle & Lasalle, 1991).

- Transference and countertransference also occur in groups and may be dealt with by group members as well as leaders.

Family Therapy

- Background

    1. Treatment modality which theorizes that the presenting problem displayed by the client with psychiatric symptoms (identified patient) is of the result of pathology throughout the entire family system.

    2. This family dysfunction is due to imbalances in the system, generally caused by conflict between the marital partners. This conflict is expressed unconsciously by the following behaviors:

        a. Triangling—another family member is brought in, in order to stabilize the emotional process.

        b. Scapegoating—another family member is blamed.

    3. Result of these behaviors is psychiatric symptoms.

- Therapeutic goals

    1. Assist family members to identify and express their thoughts and feelings.

    2. Resolve conflict between marital partners to decrease need for triangling and scapegoating.

    3. Assist parents to work together and strengthen their parental authority.

    4. Clarify family expectations and roles.

    5. Practice different, more constructive methods of interacting.

- Techniques used in family therapy according to Hogarth (1993)

    1. Joining—finding similarities and matching family's behaviors; respecting their values and hierarchies

    2. The family history

        a. Data are gathered beginning with the parents' initial relationship and include each family member in chronological order.

        b. Information may be recorded in a genogram which maps out significant events and relationships over three generations of the family.

        c. History taking takes focus off identified patient and emphasizes the family as a whole.

3. Encouraging interactions and relationships

    a. The family, or specific family members, are instructed to discuss a pertinent issue.

    b. Therapist clarifies and interprets the family's communication.

    c. Individuals required to speak for themselves in expressing feelings and concerns rather than allowing others to speak for them

    d. Family members asked to share responsibility for resolution of problems instead of laying blame

4. Experiential activities

    a. Homework—tasks assigned by the therapist, which when enacted by the family members further the therapeutic process; completion or failure to complete the task is discussed at the next session.

    b. Paradoxical prescription—instructions to perform the opposite of what is intended in order to produce change

    c. Sculpting—enactment of an experience with words omitted that when ''frozen'' is a symbolic representation of the family members' relationships; by asking a family member to rearrange the ''sculpture,'' change is modeled.

5. Results in family therapy are measured by the degree to which families are moved from dysfunctional to functional patterns. Optimal family functioning according to Hogarth (1993) includes:

    a. Open systems orientation

    b. Clear boundaries

    c. Positive links to society

    d. Contextual clarity

    e. Clear and congruent communication

    f. Strong parental coalition

    g. Appropriate power distribution

    h. Autonomous persons

    i. Warm, caring affective tone

    j. High self-esteem of members

    k. Efficient negotiation and task performance

    l. Transcendent values of hope and altruism

Ethical Aspects

- Ethics—branch of philosophy that deals with morality

- Ethical theories or perspectives according to Sellin (1991):

    1. Egoism—the right act is the one best for oneself

    2. Utilitarianism—the right act promotes the greatest good for the greatest number

    3. Deontology or formalism—the right act is established by use of ethical principles as follows:

        a. Autonomy—individuals are respected for themselves and should have control over their own choices whether or not these are in their best interest or agree with our opinions. If someone decides what is best for another it is termed paternalism. Children, the mentally retarded, and the mentally ill are often thought not to be competent enough to be autonomous.

        b. Beneficence—promoting the good of others and preventing them from harm

        c. Nonmaleficence—responsibility to do no harm; many suggest that it is more important to avoid harm than to do good. Some interpret it as a person's duty to prevent someone else from harming a third person.

        d. Justice—distribution of resources, benefits and burdens fairly among members of a society

        e. Ethical principles may conflict with one another so that it is difficult to determine which act produces the most good

        f. From ethical principles client rights have been specified

- Right—a just claim that is due an individual or group; rights may be established by policies and/or protected by laws. Important patient rights in psychiatric nursing include:

- Right to privacy

    1. Confidentiality—no information shared about client, including fact of hospitalization or whether in therapy

2. Privileged communication—in five states court may not legally mandate nurses to give information obtained in a professional capacity (Stuart & Sundeen, 1991); does not apply to patient records

3. Exceptions:

   a. Tarasoff—therapist reasonably certain that a client is going to harm someone, must breach confidentiality and inform potential victim

   b. Possible child abuse—many states mandate that cases be reported to authorities

   c. Guardianship or involuntary commitment hearings—clinical information must be shared.

- Right to treatment—patients cannot be held against their will without an individualized treatment plan and certain other standards of care specified by law

- Right to treatment in least restrictive setting

  1. Clients who are not dangerous cannot be hospitalized against their will.

  2. Clients capable of functioning on an open ward should not be held in a locked ward.

  3. Clients can wear their own clothes and keep their own personal effects excluding dangerous objects and valuables that cannot be protected.

  4. Clients who with support can live in the community should be discharged to outpatient care.

  5. Seclusion and restraint can only be utilized when therapeutically necessary and all other methods have failed to control violent behavior to self or others.

- Right to informed consent

  1. Voluntary permission given by a competent client after procedures to be performed have been explained and are understood

  2. Clients often sign forms on admission which cover psychiatric treatment.

  3. Commitment procedure gives hospital the right to treat involuntary patients.

4. Written consent for ECT and experimental drugs

- Right to refuse treatment

    1. Clients, including committed patients in nonemergencies, may not be forcibly medicated.

    2. Guardians can give permission or a court order can be sought for incompetent clients.

    3. If patient is violent to self or others and all less restrictive methods have failed, patients (including those who have been voluntarily admitted) may be forcibly medicated.

    4. Nurses must know the laws in their state and assure adequate written documentation.

- Right to habeas corpus—committed clients may at any time petition the court for release on the grounds that they are sane.

- Right to independent psychiatric examination—clients may demand evaluation by physician of own choice and must be released if determined to be not mentally ill.

- Right to outside communication

    1. Clients may have visitors, write and receive letters, make and receive phone calls, including those to judges and lawyers.

    2. The hospital can limit times for phone and visitors and deny access when they could cause harm to clients or staff.

- Right to be employed if possible—clients cannot be forced to work, and if they choose to as part of therapy, must be paid minimum wage.

Mental Health Education

- Definition: Imparting of knowledge to clients and families

- Goals according to Walker and Price-Hoskins (1992)

    1. Offering information about the illness and interventions

    2. Helping people recognize symptoms

    3. Teaching people when and how to intervene for themselves

    4. Offering relief from blame and guilt

    5. Clarifying family expectations

6. Instilling confidence that change can occur

7. Developing an objective perspective and balance

- Methods of Learning

    1. Lecture

    2. Discussion

    3. Modeling

    4. Observation

    5. Experiential

        a. Role playing

        b. Behavioral rehearsal

    6. Coaching

    7. Audio or videotaped presentation

    8. Self-instruction

        a. Keeping a diary

        b. Monitoring thoughts, feelings, and behaviors

- Guidelines for teaching adult learners

    1. Assess knowledge base

    2. Increase awareness of need for learning

    3. Encourage self-direction

    4. Encourage learners to apply material to what they already know

    5. Use mode of learning most useful to the learner, i.e., auditory, visual, or kinesthetic

    6. Repeat as often as necessary changing and combining methods and modes as required

    7. Accommodate teaching to the client's capacity for learning and attention span both of which may be affected by illness

QUESTIONS
select the best answer

1. According to traditional definitions of mental health, which of the following would the nurse be most likely to describe as mentally healthy?

    a. Jerry Jones, a VietNam veteran with no family ties, who has been unemployed for 10 years
    b. Tom Sarris, a CEO, who spends 14 hours at work each day and is too tired to do anything with his family on weekends
    c. George Connors, a shoe salesman who delights in playing affectionately with his children but has been unable to hold a steady job since they were born
    d. Sam Thomas, a restaurateur who loves his work, but sets limits on the hours he spends there in order to enjoy his family and friends

2. Which of the following would be described as a component of mental health according to Johnson?

    a. Refusing to be involved in any relationship that limits independence
    b. Absence of anxiety under any circumstances
    c. Dependence on friends and family to assist with crises
    d. Ignoring cues from the environment when deciding what to do

3. In helping a client change, the nurse should:

    a. Encourage the client to move rapidly to avoid delay
    b. Realize that the problems the client is facing will make him or her eager to change
    c. Encourage feelings of hope
    d. Understand that change is a natural process which never involves anxiety and fear

4. In facilitating change the nurse should:

    a. Avoid deliberate goal-directed activity since this will inhibit the process
    b. Restrict clients to few choices to avoid overwhelming them
    c. Give up if resistance is encountered
    d. Form a helping relationship and collaborate with clients

5. John Korman is a 36-year-old male recently admitted to a psychiatric unit. The nurse taking his history observes that his speech is slurred, and he states that he cannot remember where he has been for the past 12 hours, but the police

who brought him in stated that he was arrested driving the wrong way on a one-way street. Which of the following items on the mental status exam would the nurse NOT mark "impaired"?

    a. Behavior
    b. Judgment
    c. Memory
    d. Affect

6. Which of the following is NOT necessary for the nurse to make a spiritual assessment?

    a. Assure that the client has a religious affiliation
    b. Determine if client believes in a higher power
    c. Evaluate the client's relationship to others
    d. Determine the client's philosophy of life

7. Which of the following interventions would be labeled as an independent nursing intervention on a psychiatric unit?

    a. Giving medications
    b. Making discharge plans
    c. Deciding privileges
    d. Assuring safety

8. The staff of a day treatment program have determined that all clients must participate in a group outing to a local museum because all of the staff want to see the exhibit. Two women clients in the group voice their opposition to visiting the museum because they do not wish to risk being identified as psychiatric clients by others in the community. The staff refuse to listen to their concerns and insist that they go on the trip, but do not describe any particular reason. Which adjective describes the type of goal planning evident in this situation?

    a. Specific
    b. Individualized
    c. Collaborative
    d. Authoritarian

9. Which of the following behaviors would indicate a good client response to a nursing action?

    a. The client's body is noticably less tense and he or she has stopped pacing.

b. The client stops interacting with others on the unit.

c. The client states "If I don't do what people want they won't like me."

d. The client refuses to listen to feedback from other members of the community.

10. A nurse brings a client the Clozapine medication that she has been taking. The client doesn't look well and complains of a sore throat. The nurse notes that her temperature is elevated and concludes that the client has an upper respiratory infection. After giving the client the medication, she states that she will ask the doctor for a PRN aspirin order. The doctor orders a CBC and determines that the client has agranulocytosis. At which step of the Nursing Process did this nurse's problem begin?

a. Diagnosis

b. Planning

c. Intervention

d. Revision of plan

11. Which of the following is NOT true of the Resolution or Termination Phase of the Nurse-Client relationship?

a. Preliminaries for this phase are introduced in the Orientation phase

b. Talk about the impending separation should be avoided so that the client does not decompensate

c. The client should be encouraged to review his progress and goals

d. The nurse should model appropriate expression of feelings

12. Which of the following statements would the nurse NOT make in negotiating a contract with the client within the Nurse-Client Relationship?

a. "I would like to meet with you on a once a week basis while we are trying to resolve this crisis."

b. "We need about 10 sessions to work on this problem."

c. "I have malpractice insurance in case there is any problem."

d. "We will not be exploring your past, but only looking at things that are going on now."

13. In a session with the nurse, the client begins to whine about his inability to complete his assigned task from the previous session. The nurse responds by scolding him for his failure. This is an example of:

a. Transference

b. Countertransference

c. Transference and Countertransference

d. Goal setting

14. Sarah has been at least 10 minutes late for each of her previous sessions. To-day she arrives 20 minutes late. The nurse should:

    a. Express anger towards Sarah
    b. Confront Sarah firmly and set limits on her behavior
    c. Discuss terminating their sessions if she continues this pattern
    d. Comment on her observations and assist Sarah to understand her behavior

15. Jim, a 14-year-old client, is discussing his drug abuse problem with his nurse. When she asks him to clarify the types of substances he routinely uses, he responds by saying "How about you, have you ever used Marijuana?" How should the nurse respond?

    a. "That's none of your business, Jim, now let's get back to your problem."
    b. "Why, yes I have, but I was older and more responsible."
    c. "As you recall, Jim, we agreed to work on your problems with drugs in our sessions. I wonder what concerns you about whether I have used drugs."
    d. "That's an inappropriate question. I don't have to answer that and wonder why you'd even ask it."

16. According to the Communication Process, at the end of the feedback loop, the sender becomes the receiver

    a. True
    b. False

17. Which of the following statements is true concerning communication?

    a. Some behavior is random and does not communicate a message
    b. The message sent by the sender is obvious and does not have to be interpreted by the receiver
    c. The main goal of communication is understanding
    d. The only real form of communication is the verbal message, either written or spoken

18. Sobbing and grunting would be forms of what kind of nonverbal messages?

    a. Kinesics
    b. Paralanguage
    c. Proxemics

    d. Appearance

19. Terry Barr is describing to the nurse that he sees himself as extremely patient and laid back. As he speaks, he drums his fingers on the arm of the chair. What can the nurse infer from this communication?

    a. Terry is obviously lying and trying to fool the nurse
    b. Terry's verbal and non-verbal communications are not congruent
    c. Terry is in touch with his feelings and expressing them openly and honestly
    d. Terry's culture is interfering with his ability to communicate

20. As they are walking down the hall the nurse and client are discussing their favorite movies. This is an example of:

    a. Social communication
    b. Therapeutic communication
    c. Inappropriate communication
    d. Lack of communication

21. Which of the following would be the best example of an open ended question?

    a. How did you come to be in the hospital?
    b. Did your husband bring you over to the hospital?
    c. Who brought you to the hospital?
    d. When did you come into the hospital?

22. Adrienne has just finished describing how devastated she was at the recent loss of her mother. Which of the following responses by the nurse would NOT be a barrier to therapeutic communication?

    a. "I know how you feel. I lost my mother recently too."
    b. "Well, it's better to have loved and lost, if you know what I mean."
    c. "When did she die? Of what? Does anyone else in your family have that problem?"
    d. "It sounds like it's been a really tough period for you."

23. Timmy, a six-year-old, is accompanying his parents to a family therapy session to deal with his school phobia. Which of the following behaviors by the nurse would NOT constitute therapeutic communication skills with a child?

    a. "Let's pick out some toys from the closet to play with while I talk to your Mom and Dad?"
    b. "What do you like best about school, Timmy? What do you like least?"

    c. "Tell me about the picture you drew of your family."
    d. "Is there something that makes you anxious about going to school, Timmy?"

24. In a peer supervision group a nurse is discussing a recent self-disclosure to a client. The group is most likely to question the appropriateness of the behavior if:

    a. The nurse has been using a humanistic theoretical approach
    b. The nurse/client relationship was in the termination phase
    c. The nurse/client relationship was in the working phase
    d. The nurse/client relationship was in the orientation phase

25. Susan, a new graduate, has recently joined the staff of an inner-city Mental Health Clinic. She is shocked at some of the parenting behaviors of her initial client and tells other clinicians that she thinks her client should know better. How could her attitude be labeled?

    a. Stereotyping
    b. Culturally relativistic
    c. Ethnocentric
    d. Culturally deprived

26. Susan finds herself frustrated when her client uses some money she receives to buy winter coats for her nephews instead of saving it to buy a car so she could commute to a better job. Susan's client is demonstrating which cultural values?

    a. Present oriented, individualistic
    b. Future oriented, individualistic
    c. Present oriented, collectivist
    d. Future oriented, collectivist

27. A Middle Eastern client comes to the nurses station and stands face to face less than a foot away from the nurse. The nurse should be aware that:

    a. The client is becoming aggressive and trying to intimidate the nurse.
    b. The client has a different sense of personal space than the predominant American culture.
    c. The client is testing the nurse and needs to be confronted.
    d. The client is being seductive with the nurse.

28. An Asian American client arrives for her first session with the nurse. She speaks softly and avoids discussion of her problem directly. The nurse should:

    a. Understand that she has low self-esteem and suggest that they work on this problem

    b. Realize that this behavior is due to extreme guilt and shame and indicates a secret that needs disclosing

    c. Be aware that this is defensive behavior and probably foreshadows a great deal of resistance

    d. Understand that this is culturally appropriate behavior and should be respected and mirrored

29. In a well functioning mental health team who is the most important member?

    a. The doctor
    b. The nurse
    c. The psychologist
    d. The client

30. Which of the following characteristics are most indicative of success in a mental health team?

    a. A team leader with a decisive authoritarian approach
    b. A set of firm rules and regulations to cover most situations that could arise
    c. Many diverse philosophies of treatment
    d. Open communication

31. The goal of Art Therapy and Music Therapy is:

    a. To assist clients in passing time in the hospital productively
    b. To teach clients a new skill or hobby
    c. To evaluate clients for possible job training
    d. To stimulate the expression of feelings

32. Which of the following is not a responsibility of the generalist nurse?

    a. Psychotherapy
    b. 24 hour care
    c. Milieu management
    d. Safety

33. Which of the following is most true about a Clinical Nurse Specialist who testifies in court on behalf of a child who has been sexually abused?

    a. The nurse is functioning as an advocate for the child
    b. The nurse is functioning as a case manager for the child

c. The nurse is exceeding her capabilities as a Clinical Nurse Specialist
d. The nurse is functioning as a Psychiatric Liason Nurse

34. Of the following advocacy guidelines which is true?

a. All clients are in need of advocacy as provided by the nurse
b. Joining forces with other groups with similar goals should be avoided since this leads to a large group which is difficult to handle
c. The maximum power possible should be brought to the task to ensure the maximum benefit
d. Patience and persistence are important characteristics of successful client advocates

35. Jerry Coleman is a 46-year-old client with Bipolar Disorder who has recently had an exacerbation of his Manic symptoms. He has been referred for appropriate services to a Clinical Nurse Specialist by his disability insurance company. What kind of services might he expect to receive from his case manager?

a. A thorough evaluation of his case and coordination of all services
b. Referral for medication evaluation and maintenance
c. Referral for vocational rehabilitation if necessary
d. Weekly reports to his boss concerning the details of his disability

36. Sharon Getty has been admitted to a neurological unit with a complaint of chronic pain. She has been referred to the Clinical Nurse Specialist who functions as the Psychiatric Liason Nurse for that unit. Which might be a response of the Liason Nurse?

a. Discussion with R.N.s on the unit about the need for them not to talk with the client about the emotional components of her pain
b. Avoid talking with the client's family because they will probably be upset to learn that they might be contributing to the client's problems with pain
c. Realize that individual psychotherapy with the client is the role of the psychiatrist
d. Referring the client to occupational therapy if appropriate

37. Which of the following is NOT true?

a. Milieu therapy implies that all activity is therapeutic
b. A therapeutic environment cannot exist without community meetings
c. Token communities use privileges to reward appropriate behavior
d. The physical environment is an important part of the Milieu

38. To which of the following values would the nurse working within the therapeutic milieu probably NOT subscribe?

    a. The need for accessible team members and cooperative working relationships
    b. Empowerment of clients and staff to make decisions that affect the group
    c. Emphasis on the individual at the expense of the group
    d. Encouragement of risk taking and growth

39. Carmine d'Angelo is a 29-year-old client with a diagnosis of Schizophrenia, Paranoid Type. When he is denied off unit privileges at a community meeting he becomes hostile and accuses certain community members of "having it in for him." What would be the most appropriate response of the nurse?

    a. Ignore the behavior because it is inappropriate
    b. Confront Mr. D'Angelo with his inappropriate behavior and put him in seclusion
    c. Meet with him at their usual time and clarify his misperceptions
    d. Ask the community members that he accused to have nothing more to do with him

40. What types of things would the nurse NOT work on with Mr. d'Angelo over the next few sessions?

    a. How his thoughts and feelings influence his behavior
    b. Whether or not his behavior at the previous community meeting achieved his purpose
    c. What other coping strategies might be more effective
    d. Who seems to be "most out" to get him

41. In a therapy group, a client makes inappropriate demands of the Clinical Nurse Specialist who is the group therapist. The Clinical Nurse Specialist responds assertively and effectively resolves the problem to the satisfaction of all concerned. What curative factor, according to Yalom does this situation exemplify?

    a. Altruism
    b. Catharsis
    c. Interpersonal Learning
    d. Universality

42. Mrs. C.S. is an extremely shy individual who was admitted to the hospital with

a Depressive Disorder. What characteristics of therapy groups will best serve her needs?

   a. The realization that no one else in the group has anything like the problem she has
   b. The fact that two members of the group are talking constantly without interuption will protect her from feeling like she must participate
   c. The experience of being left alone by other group members will protect her autonomy and decrease her performance anxiety
   d. The fact that others support one another in learning to change will encourage her to take the risks needed to grow.

43. A Clinical Nurse Specialist is called in as a consultant to a nursing home seeking to enhance the morale of its residents. The Clinical Nurse Specialist decides to begin an ongoing Resocialization Group since many of the clients have been pretty much isolated from others in their previous living situations. How would such a group be classified?

   a. Homogeneous, closed ended
   b. Heterogeneous, open ended
   c. Open ended, task
   d. Closed ended, psychotherapy

44. Ann and John lose their first child to Sudden Infant Death Syndrome. They decide to attend a hospital-sponsored group for people who have had this experience. What type of group will they be attending?

   a. Teaching group
   b. Psychotherapy group
   c. Task group
   d. Supportive/Therapeutic group

45. A Clinical Nurse Specialist working as a group psychotherapist makes observations about the effective way members handled a participant who was acting out in the group. What type of leadership style does this nurse exhibit?

   a. Autocratic
   b. Democratic
   c. Laissez Faire
   d. Materialistic

46. After a particularly difficult community meeting, the staff of a unit sit down

and begin to talk about which clients were seated in close proximity and who agreed with whom on the issues that came up. What is the staff discussing?

a. Gossip
b. Rank and Status
c. Group Content
d. Group Process

47. A nursing group has convened to make decisions about renovation plans for a psychiatric unit. One of the members is discussing how little the hospital ever pays attention to input from nursing staff. Which member role is this participant exhibiting?

a. Maintenance role
b. Task role
c. Individual role
d. Gatekeeper role

48. A Clinical Nurse Specialist has had several meetings with a therapy group. On this particular occasion it is noted that members seem angry with the nurse and each other. They seem to be competing with each other to see who can refrain from breaking the silence longest. Which stage of group development do these behaviors signify?

a. Storming
b. Norming
c. Performing
d. Mourning

49. A Clinical Nurse Specialist notes that members of her therapy group have become most supportive of one another and very attached to the group. Which stage of group development do these behaviors signify?

a. Forming
b. Storming
c. Norming
d. Performing

50. Whose responsibility is it to deal with transference issues in group therapy?

a. The nurse
b. The group members
c. The nurse and the group members
d. The group member who is involved in the transference

51. How should a member terminating be handled in groups?

    a. Little attention should be paid to it since this person is now ready to leave and other members are more in need of assistance
    b. Members may discuss it if they wish, but should be allowed to avoid it if it causes anxiety
    c. Members should be encouraged to focus only on the positive aspects of the leaving so that negative feelings don't arise
    d. Members should be encouraged to express whatever feelings arise in the process of leaving

52. Which of the following best summarizes the family therapist's position on how mental illness occurs?

    a. The symptomatic person is the innocent victim of other members of the family.
    b. If other family members are given education and support, they can help the symptomatic person.
    c. The symptomatic person is the result of pathology throughout the entire family system.
    d. If other family members set limits and confront the symptomatic person with reality, they can help him or her.

53. A Clinical Nurse Specialist is the family therapist for a family whose youngest child is the identified patient. The child has been brought in for therapy because he has been doing poorly and acting out at school. How will the nurse begin the initial session with the family?

    a. By asking the child why he is doing poorly in school
    b. By asking the parents why they think he is doing poorly at school
    c. By asking each family member how they did in school
    d. By asking questions about the family in general

54. In working with the family, the nurse finds that the child is waking many times during the night and climbing into the parents' bed. Which of the following would the nurse probably NOT use as an intervention in this situation?

    a. Suggesting that one of the parents sleep in the child's room so everyone can get a good night's sleep
    b. Encouraging the parents to work together to set limits on the child's sleeping in their bed
    c. Asking the parents to talk together about how they will handle the situation when the child wakes up in the night

   d. Encouraging each member of the family to talk about his/her feelings in the matter

55. The nurse suggests that if the child can't sleep that he/she play a cassette tape on his recorder and try to listen to as many cassettes as he can, making sure that he gets out of bed, so that he doesn't fall asleep in the process. This intervention is known as:

   a. Homework
   b. Paradoxical prescription
   c. Sculpting
   d. Triangling

56. The nurse also asks the parents to keep a record of the number of nights the child stays in his own room and to reward him with a treat if he can do it three nights in a row. This intervention is known as:

   a. Homework
   b. Paradoxical prescription
   c. Sculpting
   d. Triangling

57. A family with extremely rigid boundaries will probably NOT have:

   a. Positive links to society
   b. Clear boundaries
   c. Strong parental coalition
   d. Efficient negotiation and task performance

58. Members of a therapeutic community decide at a community meeting that it is not right for two extremely demanding clients to determine the activities for the entire group. This decision can best be classified under which ethical perspective?

   a. Egoism
   b. Utilitarianism
   c. Deontology
   d. Formalism

59. When the nurse asks potentially suicidal clients to relinquish any sharp objects they have in their possession, which ethical principle is being utilized?

   a. Autonomy
   b. Beneficence

    c. Nonmaleficence

    d. Justice

60. A government agency doing a security check on an individual calls a Clinical Nurse Specialist seeking information about any mental health problems that the individual might have. What initial response is the best for the Clinical Nurse Specialist?

    a. Turn all written records over to the investigators

    b. Submit a treatment summary describing the client's problems

    c. Write a report that describes the client's problems in the least damaging way possible

    d. Refuse to acknowledge that the client is in therapy until a release of information form is signed by the client

61. A Clinical Nurse Specialist has been treating a client for several months. Recently the client has become increasingly agitated and expressed a great deal of hostility towards his ex-wife. At their last session, the client described a detailed plan to kill her and kidnap his children. What is the Clinical Nurse Specialist's response?

    a. Call the client's ex-wife and inform her that she may be in danger

    b. Call the police and discuss the case with them

    c. Consult a lawyer about the case

    d. Preserve the client's right to confidentiality

62. A mother brings her adolescent son in to be seen by a Clinical Nurse Specialist. The mother wishes to hospitalize the boy. She indicates that she can no longer control his behavior and that he is dating girls of whom she does not approve and staying out past his curfew. Based on the boy's right to treatment in the least restrictive setting, what is the Clinical Nurse Specialist's best response?

    a. Determine the most secure facility to hospitalize the child because he is probably a "run risk"

    b. Seek a Day Treatment Program since the child's behavior is not dangerous.

    c. Offer to work with the mother and son in regard to appropriate expectations and discipline.

    d. Tell the mother that all adolescents act that way and that she is wrong to be upset about this normal behavior.

63. Leroy Jones was committed to an inpatient psychiatric unit because of hallucinations which have not been controlled by oral medications prescribed on an outpatient basis. In the hospital, Mr. Jones has been prescribed I.M. Prolixin. When the nurse brings the first injection, Mr. Jones refuses the medication. What is the nurse's best immediate response in this situation?

    a. Talk with Mr. Jones about his objections to the medication
    b. Tell Mr. Jones that he cannot refuse the medication since it is necessary for his treatment
    c. Call his doctor and tell him/her that Mr. Jones has refused the medication
    d. Call an emergency team to restrain Mr. Jones while the medication is being given

64. Which of the following is NOT an accurate statement regarding client rights?

    a. Committed clients may petition the courts for release
    b. Committed clients may demand an evaluation by any physician
    c. Committed clients may not have letters restricted
    d. Committed clients may not be hospitalized involuntarily

65. A nurse who is unaware of standards of care and fails to provide care which results in harm to the client is not subject to being charged with Malpractice.

    a. True
    b. False

66. The parents of an autistic child consult a Clinical Nurse Specialist about their failure to relate to their child. The nurse decides that some education would be helpful to this family in dealing with the problem. What could the family NOT expect to receive as a result of the nurse's teaching intervention?

    a. An objective perspective
    b. Decreased blame and guilt
    c. Clarification of expectations
    d. A solution to their problems

67. In an assertiveness group, a nurse encourages a client to role play a distressing interaction she has had repeatedly with her mother-in-law. The nurse has the client play herself while the nurse plays the mother-in-law. Which methods of learning are exemplified in this situation?

    a. Lecture
    b. Experiential
    c. Self-instruction

    d. Audio presentation

68. Alice Walsh is a 46-year-old admitted to a psychiatric unit with a Major Depressive Disorder. Her doctor prescribes an MAO inhibitor which she will be taking when she leaves the hospital in four days. Her nurse wants to teach her about the side effects of her medication, particularly the dietary restrictions. She prepares a 45-minute presentation which covers everything about the medication. Afterwards Mrs. Walsh seems confused and still cannot relate several essential facts about the medication. What is the best nursing response to the situation?

    a. Phone the doctor and suggest that Mrs. Walsh be placed on another medication with fewer restrictions

    b. Realize that Mrs. Walsh will probably not be able to understand the essentials regarding her medication and teach a relative instead

    c. Realize that Mrs. Walsh's depression is probably inhibiting her ability to learn and repeat the presentation in a few days when she is a little better

    d. Break down the essential facts into a few brief sessions that can be repeated over the next several days and assess Mrs. Walsh's knowledge of the previous session before proceeding

ANSWERS

1. d	25. c	49. c
2. c	26. c	50. c
3. c	27. b	51. d
4. d	28. d	52. c
5. d	29. d	53. d
6. a	30. d	54. a
7. d	31. d	55. b
8. d	32. a	56. a
9. a	33. a	57. a
10. b	34. d	58. b
11. b	35. d	59. b
12. c	36. d	60. d
13. c	37. b	61. a
14. d	38. c	62. c
15. c	39. c	63. a
16. a	40. d	64. d
17. c	41. c	65. b
18. b	42. d	66. d
19. b	43. b	67. b
20. a	44. d	68. d
21. a	45. b	
22. d	46. d	
23. d	47. c	
24. d	48. a	

BIBLIOGRAPHY

American Academy of Nursing Expert Panel Report. (1992). Culturally competent nursing care. *Nursing Outlook, 40*(6), 277–283.

Auvil, C. A., & Silver, B. W. (1984). Therapist self-disclosure: When is it appropriate? *Perspectives in Psychiatric Care, 22*(2), 57–64.

Boyd, M. A., & Luetje, V. M. (1991). Nursing advocacy in mental health settings. In R. B. Murray & M. M Huelskoetter (Eds.) *Psychiatric mental health nursing: Giving emotional care* (pp. 731–748). Norwalk, CT: Appleton and Lange.

Campinha-Bacote, J. (1997). Understanding the influence of culture. In J. Haber, B Krainovich-Miller, A. L. McMahon, & P. Price-Hopkins (Eds.) *Comprehensive psychiatric nursing* (pp. 75–90). St. Louis: Mosby.

Delaney, K. R., & Lettieri-Marks, D. (1997). Planning intervention and evaluation. In B. S. Johnson (Ed.), *Psychiatric mental health nursing: Adaptation and growth* (pp 123–139). Philadelphia: J. B. Lippincott.

Farnsworth, B. J., & Biglow, A. (1997). Psychiatric case management. In J. Haber, B. Krainovich-Miller, A. L. McMohn, & P. Price Hoskins (Eds.), *Comprehensive psychiatric nursing* (pp. 318–331). St. Louis: Mosby.

Greene, J. A. (1997). Milieu therapy. In B. S. Johnson (Ed.), *Psychiatric and mental healh nursing: Adaptation and growth* (pp. 221–231). Philadelphia: J. B. Lippincott.

Greene, J. (1993). Milieu therapy. In B. S. Johnson (Ed.), *Psychiatric-mental health nursing: Adaptation and growth* (183–193). Philadelphia: J. B. Lippincott.

Hogarth, C. R. (1993). Families and family therapy. In B. S. Johnson (Ed.), *Psychiatric-mental Health Nursing: Adaptation and Growth* (pp. 233–256). Philadelphia: J. B. Lippincott.

Huelskoetter, M. M. & Romano, E. (1991). The change process. In R. B. Murray & M. M. Huelskoetter (Eds.) *Psychiatric mental health nursing: Giving Emotional care* (pp. 191–204). Norwalk, CT: Appleton and Lange.

Johnson, B. S. (1997). Mental health promotion. In B. S. Johnson (Ed.), *Psychiatric and mental health nursing: Adaptation and Growth* (pp. 21–28). Philadelphia: J. B. Lippincott.

Lasalle, P. C. & Lasalle, A. J. (1991). Small groups and their therapeutic forces. In G. W. Stuart & S. J. Sundeen (Eds.), *Principles and practice of psychiatric nursing* (pp. 809–826). St. Louis: Mosby Year Book.

Long, P., & McMahon, A. L. (1992). Working with groups. In J. Haber, A.

McMahon, P. Price-Hoskins & B. Siedeleau (Eds.), *Comprehensive psychiatric nursing* (pp. 324–346). New York: Mosby-Year Book.

McMahon, A. L. (1997). The nurse-client relationship. In J. Haber, B. Krainovich-Miller, A. L. McMahon, & P. Price-Hopkins (Eds.), *Comprehensive psychiatric nursing* (pp. 143–159). St. Louis: Mosby.

Peplau, H. (1952). *Interpersonal relations in nursing.* New York: G. P. Putnam.

Sellin, S. R. (1991). Ethical issues in psychiatric mental health nursing. In G. K. McFarland & M. D. Thomas (Eds.), *Psychiatric mental health nursing* (pp. 943–949). Philadelphia: J. B. Lippincott.

Shanks, S. R. (1991). Legal issues in psychiatric mental healh nursing. In G. K. McFarland & M. D. Thomas (Eds.), *Psychiatric mental health nursing* (p. 933–942). Philadelphia: J. B. Lippincott.

Stuart, G. W., & Sundeen, S. J. (1991). Legal and ethical aspects of psychiatric care. In G. W. Stuart & S. J. Sundeen (Eds.), *Principles and practice of psychiatric nursing* (pp. 205–236). St. Louis: Mosby Year Book.

Tripp-Reimer, T., & Lively, S. H. (1993). Cultural considerations in mental health-psychiatric nursing. In R. P. Rawlins, S. R. Williams, & C. K. Beck (Eds.), Mental health-psychiatric nursing: *A holistic life-cycle approach* (pp. 166–179). New York: Mosby-Year Book.

Tuckman, B. W. (1965). Developmental sequences in small groups. *Psychology Bulletin, 63,* 384–389.

Walker, M., & Price-Hoskins, P. (1992). Role of the nurse in psychiatric settings. In J. Haber, A. McMahon, P. Price-Hoskins and B. Siedeleau (Eds.), *Comprehensive Psychiatric Nursing* (pp. 267–287). New York: Mosby Year Book.

Watson, J. (1992). Maintenance of therapeutic community principles in an age of biopharmacology and economic restraints. *Archives of Psychiatric Nursing, 6*(3), 183–188.

Yalom, I. D. (1995). *The theory and practice of group psychotherapy.* New York: Basic Books.

Major Theoretical Frameworks for Psychiatric Nursing

Clare Houseman
Joan Donovan

Theory

- Definition: A set of concepts, definitions, and propositions, used to describe, explain, predict, or control a phenomenon
- Characteristics
  1. Can interrelate concepts in such a way as to create a different way of looking at a phenomenon
  2. Must be logical in nature
  3. Should be relatively simple, yet generalizable
  4. Can be the basis for hypotheses that can be tested
  5. Contribute to and assist in increasing the general body of knowledge within the discipline through the research implemented to validate them
  6. Can be utilized by the practitioners to guide and improve their practice
  7. Must be consistent with other validated theories, laws and principles, but will leave open unanswered questions that need to be investigated (George, 1990)

Theory and Research

1. Theory is constructed through deductive or inductive approaches:
   a. Deductive theory construction proceeds from the general to the specific. The theorist or investigator borrows concepts from other bodies of knowledge and tests the concepts and relationships in nursing practice. An example is Rogers' Theory of Nursing.
   b. Inductive theory construction proceeds from the specific to the general. The theorist or investigator immerses himself/herself in the data and attempts to generate theoretical statements. An example is Orem's theory of Self Care (Riehl & Roy, 1980).
2. Theory serves to:
   a. Guide research—the theory sets limits on questions to ask and methods to pursue in research.
   b. Guide practice—after validation from research, theory can give direction to practice.

c. Provide a common language between practitioners and re-searchers.

d. Enhance professional autonomy and accountability—theory, supported by research, allows nurse to predict consequences of care, contributing to autonomous nursing practice (Meleis, 1985).

Research

Systematic method of gathering data which provides means of developing and testing theories as well as measuring outcomes of nursing interventions in the clinical area. Participation in research is an ANA Psychiatric Mental Health Standard of Practice.

- Researcher Roles for Nurses
    1. Principal investigator
    2. Coinvestigator
    3. Member of research team
    4. Data collector
    5. Client advocate
    6. Critique of research findings
    7. User of research outcomes
    8. Problem area identifier
- Research Process
    1. Determine problem.
    2. Review relevant literature.
    3. Identify a theoretical framework.
    4. Determine the research variables.
    5. Formulate hypothesi(e)s.
    6. Select research instruments.
    7. Collect data.
    8. Analyze data.
    9. Determine results and conclusions.

- Types of Research

  1. Experimental—experimenter uses random sampling, manipulates the independent variable and uses control and experimental groups.

  2. Quasi-experimental—variable may be manipulated but subjects not assigned randomly to control and treatment groups.

  3. Non-experimental—researcher measures variables as they occur naturally; uses correlations to determine nature and extent of relationship between and among variables; includes prospective and retrospective.

  4. Qualitative—researcher makes observations or interviews participants. Data used to describe process or phenomena—most common forms are Phenomenological and Ethnographic.

  5. Case Study—researcher describes and analyzes one or a small number of cases.

- Research Instruments—may measure physical or psychological characteristics. Often questionnaires are used which must be evaluated for

  1. Reliability—ability to measure the same trait repeatedly

  2. Validity—ability to measure what it is supposed to be measuring

- Statistical Data Analysis (Polit and Hungler, 1991)

  1. Descriptive—Means, Medians, Modes, Standard deviation

  2. Inferential Statistics—used to test hypotheses and decide if relationship between variables is supported

     a. Testing differences between two group means

        (1) t-Tests for independent samples

        (2) Paired t-Tests

     b. Testing differences between three or more groups

        (1) ANOVA

        (2) Kruskal-Wallace test

        (3) Mann Whitney U

        (4) Friedman test

     c. Comparing differences between cases that fall into categories—Chi Square Test

    d. Testing the relationshp between two variables

        (1) Pearson product moment correlation (r)

        (2) Spearman's rho

        (3) Kendall's tau

    e. Multivariate statistics

        (1) Multiple regression analysis—used to understand the effects of two or more independent variable on a dependent measure

        (2) Stepwise multiple regression—all potential predictors considered simultaneously to determine the combination of variables providing the most predictive power

        (3) Analysis of Covariance—used statistically to control one or more extraneous variables; useful to adjust for initial differences in situations where random assignment is impossible

        (4) Factor Analysis—reduces a large set of variables into a smaller set of related variables

  3. Level of Significance—describes the probability of a particular result occurring by chance

- Protection of Human Subjects

  1. Right to Informed Consent—may be more complicated with psychiatric clients due to nature of illness

  2. Right to Confidentiality (privacy of data) and Anonymity (privacy of source of information)

  3. Right to Refuse to Participate or Withdraw at Anytime

Nursing Theoretical Models

Developed around four core concepts:

- Individual—the person or client in need of nursing care

- Environment—the combination of all forces that affect an individual

- Health—a state of well being

> • Nursing—the discipline and practice of assisting others to maintain or recover health (George, 1990; Fawcett, 1984)

Nursing Theories

- The Theory of Self-Care (Dorothea Orem)

    1. Self-care—an individual's activities to maintain life, health, and well being. Self-care requisites are actions directed toward the provision of self-care. The three categories of self-care requisites are:

        a. Universal—activities of daily living

        b. Developmental—specialized activities related to a developmental task or an event

        c. Health deviation—activities required by illness, injury, or disease

    2. Self-care deficit—the inability to provide complete self-care; the need for nursing care. Nursing care includes the following:

        a. Entering into and maintaining nurse-patient relationships

        b. Assessing how patients can be helped

        c. Responding to patients' requests and needs

        d. Prescribing, providing, and regulating direct help

        e. Coordinating and integrating nursing with other services

    3. Nursing systems refer to the amount of nursing care a patient requires. Categories are as follows:

        a. Wholly compensatory—the nurse provides all care.

        b. Partly compensatory—the nurse and patient provide care.

        c. Supportive-educative—the patient provides care. The nurse promotes the patient as a self-care agent (Foster & Janssens, 1990).

- Theory of Goal Attainment (Imogene King)

    King describes her theory of goal attainment within an open systems framework.

    1. The three systems in the framework are as follows:

        a. Personal systems—each individual is a personal system.

   b.   Interpersonal systems—the interaction among human beings

   c.   Social systems—an organized boundary system of roles, behaviors, and practices

2.   The theory of goal attainment states that people come together to help and be helped to maintain health. Concepts of the theory are as follows:

   a.   Interaction—goal-directed communication

   b.   Perception—organizing, processing, storing, and exporting information

   c.   Communication—information is given from one person to another.

   d.   Transaction—observable behaviors of people interacting with their environment

   e.   Role—set of behaviors expected of a person occupying a certain position

   f.   Stress—an energy response to a stressor

   g.   Growth and development—continuous changes that take place in life

   h.   Time—a sequence of events moving to the future

   i.   Space—physical area; territory (George, 1990)

- Theory of Nursing (Martha Rogers)

1.   The phenomenon central to nursing is the life process of human beings.

2.   Assumptions of Rogers' Theory:

   a.   The human being is a unified whole possessing his/her own integrity and manifesting characteristics that are more than and different from the sum of his/her parts.

   b.   The person and environment are continually exchanging matter and energy with each other.

   c.   The life process revolves irreversibly and unidirectionally along the space-time continuum.

   d.   Pattern and organization identify individuals and reflect their wholeness.

    e. The human being is characterized by the capacity for abstraction and imagery, language and thought, sensation and emotion.

3. Building blocks of Rogers':

    a. Energy field—an electrical field in a continuous state of flux

    b. Openness—energy fields are open to exchange with other energy fields.

    c. Pattern—energy fields have patterns that change as required.

    d. Four dimensionality—energy fields are embedded in a four-dimensional space-time matrix.

4. Principles of homeodynamics are built upon the five assumptions and four building blocks.

    a. Integrality—the continuous, mutual, simultaneous interaction between human and environmental fields

    b. Resonancy—the identification of human and environmental fields by changing wave patterns

    c. Helicy—the evolving innovative repatterning growing out of the mutual interaction of man and environment (Rogers, 1983; Falco & Lobo, 1990)

- The Adaptation Model (Sister Callista Roy)

  There are five essential elements of the model:

  1. Each person is an adaptive system with input, internal processes, adaptive modes, and output.

      a. Input—internal or external stimuli

      b. Internal processes—coping mechanisms

          (1) Regulator subsystem—chemical, neural, and endocrine transmitters

          (2) Cognator subsystem—perception, information processing, judgment, emotion

      c. Adaptive modes or system effectors

          (1) Physiological function mode—identifies patterns of physical functioning

(2) Self-concept mode—identifies patterns of values, beliefs, and emotions

(3) Role function mode—identifies patterns of social interactions

(4) Interdependence mode—identifies patterns of human value, affection, love, and affirmation

   d. Output:

(1) Adaptive response, or

(2) Ineffective response

2. The goal of nursing—the promotion of adaptive responses in relation to the adaptive modes

3. Health—a process of being and becoming an integrated person

4. Environment—conditions, circumstances, and influences affecting the growth and the behavior of a person

5. The Nursing Process:

   a. First-level assessment—behavioral assessment; assessment of four adaptive modes

   b. Second-level assessment:

(1) Identification of focal, contextual, and residual stimuli

(2) Identification of ineffective responses

   c. Identification of nursing diagnosis

   d. Goal setting with the client

   e. Implementation—manipulating focal, contextual, or residual stimuli

   f. Evaluation—assessment of goal behaviors and possible readjustment of goals and interventions (Galbreath, 1990)

- Theory of Culture Care Diversity and Universality (Madeleine Leininger)

1. The main tenet of the theory is that "care is the essence of nursing and the central, dominant, and unifying focus" (Leininger, 1991, p. 35).

2. Other concepts include:

   a. Culture—the learned, shared, and transmitted values, beliefs, norms, and lifeways of a group that guide their actions and decisions

b. Cultural care diversity—differences in meanings, patterns, values, or symbols of care, within or between collectivities related to human care expressions

c. Cultural care universality—uniform meanings, patterns, or symbols that are manifest in many cultures and reflect ways to help people

d. Cultural and social structure dimensions—patterns of structural and organizational factors of a particular culture, including:

(1) Religious factors

(2) Social and kinship factors

(3) Political and legal factors

(4) Economic factors

(5) Educational factors

(6) Technological factors

(7) Cultural values

(8) Ethnohistorical factors

e. Ethnohistory—past facts, events, and experiences of individuals, groups, cultures, or institutions which are people-centered and which describe, explain, and interpret human lifeways within a certain culture

f. Cultural care preservation or maintainance—actions and decisions that help people retain relevant cultural care values to maintain well-being, recover from illness, and face handicaps or death

g. Cultural care accommodation or negotiation—actions and decisions to help people of a designated culture negotiate for a beneficial outcome with health caregivers

h. Cultural care repatterning or restructuring—actions and decisions to help clients modify their lifeways for beneficial health care, while respecting their cultural values and beliefs

     i. Cultural congruent nursing care—actions and decisions tailored to fit cultural values and beliefs (Leininger, 1991)

- Peplau—See chapter 2

Personality Theories (Object Relations)

- Psychoanalytic/Psychodynamic (Sigmund Freud)

  Concepts in the theory of Freud include the following:

  1. Levels of awareness

     a. Conscious—thoughts, feelings, and desires a person is aware of and able to control

     b. Preconscious—thoughts, feelings, and desires that are not in immediate awareness but can be recalled to consciousness

     c. Unconscious—thoughts, feelings, and desires that are not available to the conscious mind

  2. Stages of development—according to Freud, each person passes through the following stages of psychosexual development. A person can get stuck in any stage.

     a. Oral—the focus is on sucking and swallowing, gratification of oral needs

     b. Anal—focus on spontaneous bowel movements, control over impulses

     c. Phallic—focus on genital region, identification with parent of the same gender

     d. Latency—sexual impulses are dormant; focus is on coping with the environment.

     e. Genital—focus on erotic and genital behavior, developing mature sexual and emotional relationships

  3. Personality structure—the personality has three main components:

     a. Id—the pleasure principle; unconscious; desire for immediate and complete satisfaction; disregard for others

     b. Ego—the reality principle; rational and conscious; weighs actions and consequences

     c. Superego—the censoring force of the personality; conscious and unconscious; evaluates and judges behavior (Scroggs, 1985)

4. Several terms common to psychiatric nursing originated with Freud, including:

    a. Oedipus Complex or Electra Conflict—at the age of four or five, the child falls in love with the parent of the opposite sex and feels hostility toward the parent of the same sex.

    b. Defense mechanisms—conscious or unconscious actions or thoughts to protect the ego from anxiety (See Table 1).

    c. Freudian slips—also known as parapraxes—overt actions with unconscious meanings

    d. Free association—a method for discovering the contents of the unconscious by associating words with other words or emotions

    e. Transference—feelings, attitudes, and wishes linked with a significant figure in one's early life are projected onto others in one's current life

    f. Countertransference—feelings and attitudes of the therapist are projected onto the patient inappropriately

    g. Resistance—anything that prohibits a person from producing material from the unconscious

    h. Fixation—getting stuck in one stage of development (Scroggs, 1985; Drapela, 1987)

5. Treatment—psychoanalysis:

    a. Daily therapy sessions for several years

    b. The patient reveals thoughts, feelings, dreams, etc.

    c. The therapist reveals no personal information, functioning primarily as a shadow figure. The therapist interprets the patient's behavior for him or her.

- Psychoanalysis (Carl Jung)

    The major concepts of Jung's theory are as follows:

    1. Archetype—unconscious, intangible collective idea, image, or concept; Scroggs (1985) defines the main archetypes identified by Jung:

Table 1

Defense Mechanisms

Type	Definition	Example
Compensation	An individual makes up for a felt lack in one area by emphasizing strengths in another	A student who feels devoid of athletic ability becomes an outstanding member of the debating team
Denial	Failure to acknowledge the reality of an anxiety-producing situation	A woman ignores behavior changes in her husband that would indicate to others that he is having an affair
Displacement	Shifting of feelings from an emotionally charged person or object to a substitute, less threatening, person or object	A nurse becomes angry with a second nurse, later, the second nurse berates a family member for asking too many questions
Dissociation	Temporary but drastic modification of character or sense of personal identity to avoid emotional distress	A soldier, fearful of leading his patrol into enemy territory and not wanting to acknowledge cowardice,
Fantasy	Symbolic wish fulfillment with nonrational thought	A young boy, unable to protect his mother from his father's abuse, daydreams of singlehandedly killing a herd of wild animals that surround his home, thereby saving the family
Identification	Internalizing the characteristics of an idealized person	A young woman has high regard for her aunt and chooses to become a nurse just like her
Intellectualization	Reasoning or logic is used in an attempt to avoid confrontation with an objectionable impulse or affect	A man deals with intellectual formulations about the nature of death and the thoughts of various philosophers and scientists on the subject rather than the personally relevant feelings about his father's recent death
Introjection	Taking on another person's ego and becoming like that other person	A young child incorporates the personality of an adult and actually behaves like one
Isolation	Splitting of affect from the rest of a person's thinking	When a man who had been angry with his father (yet also loved him) hears of his father's death, he acknowledges the death, but deals with it in a mechanical way—he prevents himself from having feelings about the event
Projection	False attribution of the person's own undesirable feelings, thoughts, and impulses to others	A client states that a coworker does not like her, as a projection of her own dislike for the coworker
Rationalization	Finding logical or acceptable, but incorrect, reasons or excuses for behavior that is unacceptable to one's self-image	A college student who has low grades because of careless study habits rationalizes that he could have good grades if he had different instructors
Reaction formation	Substitution of behavior, thoughts and feelings diametrically opposed to unacceptable ones	A man who finds his sexual impulses unacceptable adopts puritanical beliefs and totally devotes himself to fighting pornography
Regression	Return to an earlier, more comfortable level of development	A child upset by the arrival of a new sibling may return to thumb-sucking or bed-wetting
Repression	Involuntary exclusion from consciousness of those ideas, feelings, and situation that are unacceptable to the self	After a painful interpersonal experience, the individual involved cannot recall his part in the interaction
Sublimation	Establishment of a secondary goal that an individual can satisfy in place of a primary goal that is socially unacceptable or physically impossible	A teenager with strong aggressive tendencies gains social acceptance through sports
Suppression	Voluntary exclusion from level of thought those feelings and situations that produce discomfort and some anxiety	A student with a poor report card "forgets" to give it to his parents for their signature
Undoing	A person symbolically acts out in reverse something unacceptable that has already been done	A man, raised to believe sex is immoral and dirty, relieves his sexual desires from time to time by masturbating; afterward, feeling tremendous guilt, he tries to undo the way he has fouled his hands (by touching his genitals) and develops a compulsion to wash his hands over and over

Note. From ''Defensive Coping'' by M. I. Fitch and L. L. O'Brien-Pallas in G. K. McFarland and M. O. Thomas, 1991, *Psychiatric Mental Health Nursing,* (p. 202), Philadelphia: J. B. Lippincott. Copyright 1991 by J. B. Lippincott Company. Reprinted by permission.

    a. The Way—the image of a journey or voyage through life

    b. The Self—the aspect of mind that unifies and orders experience

    c. Animus and Anima—the image of gender

    d. Rebirth—the concept of being reborn, resurrected, or reincarnated

    e. Persona—the role or mask one shows to others

    f. Shadow—the dark side of one's personality

    g. Stock characters—dramatic roles that appear over and over in folktales

        (1) Hero—the character who vanquishes evil and rescues the downtrodden

        (2) Trickster—the character who plays pranks or works magic spells

        (3) Sage—the wise old person

    h. Power—symbol, such as the eagle or the sword

    i. Number—certain numbers reappear throughout history and across cultures.

2. Psychological types—Jung described two attitudinal and four functional types of personalities:

    a. Attitudinal types

        (1) Introvert—one oriented toward the inner, subjective world

        (2) Extrovert—one oriented toward the outer, external world

    b. Functional types

        (1) Thinking—intellectual process involving ideas

        (2) Feeling—evaluative function involving value or worth

        (3) Sensing—function involving recognition that something exists, without categorizing or evaluating it

        (4) Intuiting—function involving creative inspiration, knowing without having the facts (Scroggs, 1985)

3. Collective unconscious

- Theory of Individual Psychology (Alfred Adler)

  Adler saw individuals in a social context; he is considered a social -interpersonal theorist by some. Key ideas include:

  1. Inferiority feelings are the source of all human strivings.

  2. Personal growth results from the attempts to compensate for inferiority.

  3. Complexes:

     a. Inferiority complex—an inability to solve life's problems

     b. Superiority complex—an exaggerated opinion of one's abilites and accomplishments, a result of the attempt to overcompensate for an inferiority complex

  4. The goal of life—to strive for superiority

  5. Lifestyle—the unique set of behaviors created by each individual to compensate for inferiority and achieve superiority

  6. The influence of birth order:

     a. First-born—happy and secure, the center of attention, until dethroned by the second child; develops interest in authority and organization

     b. Second-born—born into a more relaxed atmosphere; has the first-born as a model, or a threat to compete with; develops interest in competition

     c. Youngest child—pet of the family; may retain dependency (Schultz, 1987; Adler, 1983)

- Theory of Basic Anxiety (Karen Horney)

  Because of her focus on family, some consider Horney a social/interpersonal theorist. Concepts include:

  1. A child has two basic needs—safety and satisfaction.

  2. When those needs are not met, the child feels hostility.

  3. The child represses the hostility, and this leads to basic anxiety.

  4. Basic anxiety—a pervasive feeling of being lonely or helpless in a hostile world

5. Protective mechanisms against basic anxiety in relationships:

   a. Moving toward people

   b. Moving against people

   c. Moving away from people

6. Neurosis—compulsive and unconscious extension of maladaptive childhood mechanisms (Scroggs, 1985; Wilson & Kneisl, 1992)

Theories of Growth and Development

- Theory of Psychosocial Development (Erik Homburger Erikson)

1. The term used in naming each stage identifies the conflict to be resolved during that stage.

2. In each stage, the individual has a particular focus and a task, which result in adaptive or maladaptive characteristics.

   a. Infant (0-2 years)

     Trust—focus on oral needs, acquisition of hope vs Mistrust—withdrawal (schizoid or depressive)

   b. Toddler (1.5-3 years)

     Autonomy—focus on anal needs, acquisition of skill vs Shame and Doubt—low self esteem, secretiveness, persecution

   c. Preschooler (3-6 years)

     Initiative—focus on genital needs, purpose, task-oriented vs Guilt—denial, inhibition, showing off, self-righteous psychosomatic disease

   d. School-age (6-12 years)

     Industry—focus on socialization, competence, perserverance vs Inferiority—inadequacy, self-restriction, conformity

   e. Adolescent (13+ years)

     Identity—focus on search for self, idealistic, confidence vs Identity diffusion—delinquency, psychosis, overidentifies with heroes, cliques

   f. Young Adult

     Intimacy—focus on human closeness, sexual fulfillment,

love vs Isolation—distancing behaviors, self-absorption, character problems

g. Middle Aged Adult

Generativity—focus on productivity, creativity, guiding next generation vs Stagnation—lack of faith, obsessive need for pseudointimacy, early invalidism

h. Older Adult

Integrity—emotional and spiritual integration, fellowship with others, leadership vs Despair—disgust, fear of death (Erikson,1963; Whiting,1997)

- Theory of Cognitive Development (Jean Piaget)

  Piaget's stages of development are:

  1. Sensory-Motor Period—0 to 2 years

     a. Stage I—0 to 1 month—no distinction between self and outer reality; characterized by reflexive, uncoordinated body movements

     b. Stage II—1 to 4 months—response patterns begin to be formed; the baby's fist finds its way into his or her mouth.

     c. Stage III—4 to 8 months—response patterns are coordinated and repeated intentionally.

     d. Stage IV—8 to 12 months—more coordinated responses ensue; child pushes obstacles aside, searches for vanished objects.

     e. Stage V—12 to 18 months—behavior patterns are deliberately varied, as if to observe different results; groping toward a goal emerges.

     f. Stage VI—18 months to 2 years—behavior patterns are internalized; symbolic representation emerges.

  2. Pre-operational Period—2 to 7 years—characterized by egocentric thinking expressed in artificialism, realism, and magic omnipotence

     a. Pre-conceptual Stage—2 to 4 years—conceptualization begins to emerge, represented in language, drawings, dreams, and play.

    b. Perceptual or Intuitive Stage—4 to 7 years—prelogical reasoning appears, based on appearances; trial and error may lead to discovery of correct relationships.

3. Concrete Operations Period—7 to 11 years—characterized by thought that is logical and reversible; the child understands classes, relationships, and part-whole relationships dealing with concrete things.

4. Formal Operations Period—11 years to adulthood—characterized by the development of logic and reasoning and second-order thoughts, that is, thinking about thoughts (Pulaski, 1971).

- Theory of Moral Development (Lawrence Kohlberg)

   The stages of moral development are:

   1. Level I—external standards

       a. Stage 1—avoidance of punishment; the punishment or power of others determines what is right and wrong.

       b. Stage 2—desire for reward or benefit; action is based on getting something in return, in satisfying gratification. There is a sense of fairness and reciprocity, but not a sense of loyalty, gratitude, or justice.

   2. Level II—conventional order.

       a. Stage 3—anticipation of disapproval of others, or ''good boy-nice girl'' orientation; there is conformity to expectations of appropriate behavior, seeking approval.

       b. Stage 4—anticipation of dishonor; behavior is oriented toward respecting authority, maintaining social order, and obeying social rules for their own goodness.

   3. Level III—Principled Morality.

       a. Stage 5—social contract, legalistic orientation; behavior is oriented toward the belief that justice flows from a social contract that assures equality for all. Behavior is geared toward rules and legalities.

       b. Stage 6—universal ethical principles orientation. Behavior is oriented toward universal, ethical abstract principles (Kohlberg, 1984).

- Theory of Moral Development (Carol Gilligan)

    Moral development of women is based more upon an ethic of caring and attachment (Gilligan, 1982). Gilligan has not yet described stages of development in females.

Personality Theories (Social/Interpersonal)

- Theory of Interpersonal Development—Harry Stack Sullivan

    Sullivan focuses on behavior as interpersonal. Major concepts include:

    1. Self-system—a construct built from the child's experience, made up of reflected appraisals from the approval or disapproval of significant others

    2. Two basic drives that underlie behavior:

        a. The drive for satisfaction—basic physiological drives, e.g., hunger

        b. The drive for security—a sense of well being and belonging

    3. Anxiety—any painful feeling or emotion that arises from social insecurity or blocks to satisfaction; characteristics of anxiety are:

        a. Interpersonal

        b. Can be described; can be observed in behavior

        c. Individuals try to reduce anxiety.

    4. Security operations—measures taken by individuals to reduce anxiety, e.g., selective inattention

    5. Mental illness—self-system interferes with ability to attend to basic drives.

    6. Therapy is based upon the belief that by experiencing a healthy relationship with the therapist, the patient can learn to build better relationships. Therapy is an active partnership based on trust (Sullivan, 1953).

Personality Theories (Existential/Humanistic)

The theorists focus on experience in the here and now, with little attention to the past.

- Client Centered Therapy (Carl Rogers)

   The key concept is that people can become fully functioning persons when they are unconditionally valued. Rogers described:

   1. The attributes of the therapist:

      a. Congruence—inner feelings match outer actions.

      b. Unconditional positive regard—the therapist sees the client as a person of intrinsic worth, likes the client, and treats the client non-judgmentally.

      c. Empathic understanding—the therapist is an empathetic, sensitive listener.

   2. The goal of therapy is to help the client become a fully functioning person. The client reaches this goal by:

      a. Relinquishing facades

      b. Banishing "oughts"

      c. Moving away from cultural expectations and becoming non-conformist

      d. Pleasing oneself, as opposed to pleasing others; being self directed

      e. Opening up and dropping defenses

      f. Trusting his or her inner self, his or her intuition

      g. Becoming willing to be a complex process

      h. Accepting others (Rogers, 1961; Scroggs, 1985)

- Gestalt (Frederick (Fritz) Perls)

   1. Here-and-now therapy of immediate experiencing, attained by removing masks and facades

   2. Involves a creative interaction between therapist and client to gain ongoing awareness of what is being felt, sensed, and thought

   3. Describes boundary disturbance—lack of awareness of the immediate environment, which takes the following forms:

      a. Projection—fantasy about what another person is experiencing

      b. Introjection—accepting the beliefs and opinions of others without question

    c. Retroflection—turning back on oneself that which is meant for someone else

    d. Confluence—merging with the environment

    e. Deflection—a method of interfering with contact, used by receivers and senders of messages

4. Goal of therapy—integration of self and world awareness

5. Techniques of therapy include:

    a. Playing the projection—taking and experiencing the role of another

    b. Making the rounds—speaking or doing something to other group members to experiment with new behavior

    c. Sentence completion—e.g., ''I take responsibility for. . . .''

    d. Exaggeration of a feeling or action

    e. Empty chair dialogue—having an interaction with an imaginary provocateur

    f. Dream work—describing and playing parts of a dream (Hardy, 1991)

- Humanistic/Holistic (Abraham Maslow)

1. When basic needs are met, health and growth will naturally follow.

2. Best known for his description of a heirarchy of basic needs:

    a. Physiological needs

    b. Safety needs

    c. Love and belongingness needs

    d. Self esteem needs

    e. Self-actualization needs (Drapela, 1987; Scroggs, 1985)

- Rational Emotive Therapy (Albert Ellis)

Some consider this an existential theory while others refer to it as a ''cognitive'' theory, because the focus is on changing thinking, rather than on feeling or experiencing. Assumptions and key concepts include:

1. People largely control their own destinies.

2. People act on their basic values and beliefs.

3. People interpret events according to their basic values or beliefs and the interpretation can change.

4. A-B-C of therapy:

   a. Activating event

   b. Belief

   c. Consequences—emotional and/or behavioral

5. Irrational beliefs have four basic forms:

   a. Something should, ought, or must be different.

   b. Something is awful, terrible, or horrible.

   c. One cannot bear, stand, or tolerate something.

   d. Something or someone is damned, as a louse, rotten person, etc.

6. "Musturbatory" ideologies have three forms:

   a. I must do well and win approval or I am a rotten person.

   b. You must act kindly and justly toward me or you are a rotten person.

   c. My life must remain comfortable and easy or the world is damnable and life hardly seems worth living.

7. Therapy consists of detecting and eradicating irrational beliefs and musturbatory ideologies by:

   a. Disputing—detecting irrationalities, debating against them, discriminating between logical and illogical thinking, and defining what helps to create new beliefs

   b. Debating—questioning and disputing the irrational beliefs

   c. Discriminating—distinguishing between wants and needs, desires and demands, and rational and irrational ideas

   d. Defining—define words and re-define beliefs

Personality theories (Behavioral)

The behavioral theories are generally not concerned with thoughts, feelings, or unconscious phenomena, except to view them as "behaviors." The focus of behavioral therapy is on replacing maladaptive behaviors with more effective behaviors.

- Behavior Therapy (Burrhas Frederic Skinner)

  All behavior is determined by contingencies of reinforcement (Scroggs, 1985). Important concepts include:

  1. Operant conditioning (also called instrumental learning)—the individual performs a behavior which leads to a positive or negative reinforcement, making it either more or less likely that the behavior will be repeated.

  2. Schedules of reinforcement—Skinner found that different schedules of reinforcement had different effects on supporting or extinguishing particular behaviors.

     a. Fixed ratio schedule—behaviors are rewarded or reinforced every time they are repeated.

     b. Variable ratio schedule—behaviors are rewarded randomly.

     c. Fixed interval schedule—behaviors are rewarded at specific time intervals.

     e. Random interval schedule—behaviors are rewarded at random time intervals (Skinner, 1974; Scroggs, 1985).

- Reciprocal Inhibition (Joseph Wolpe)

  A "process of relearning whereby in the presence of a stimulus a non-anxiety producing response is continually repeated until it extinguishes the old, undesirable reponse" (Wolpe, 1969, p. 91). Types of reciprocal inhibition include:

  1. Systematic desensitization—used primarily in the treatment of phobias—the following steps comprise the most common mode of systematic desensitization:

     a. Training in deep muscle relaxation

     b. Listing examples of phobic reactions; arranging them in descending order of intensity

     c. Desensitization:

        (1) Fantasy desensitization—while the client relaxes as deeply as possible, the examples are presented to his or her imagination. They are repeated until the anxiety is eliminated.

> (2) In vivo desensitization—in addition to fantasy desensitization, the client actually faces the feared object or situation.
>
> 2. Avoidance (aversive) conditioning is the application of the reciprocal inhibition principle to overcome undesirable responses. An example of avoidance conditioning is the use of the drug antabuse to overcome an alcoholic's undesirable response of drinking (Wolpe, 1968).

- Reality Therapy (William Glasser)

   Focuses on changing present behavior—the basic premise is that everyone who seeks psychiatric treatment is unable to fulfill his or her basic needs and is denying the reality of the world around him or her. Major concepts include:

   1. Each person has two basic needs:

      a. The need to love and be loved—each person needs to be involved with at least one other person who is in touch with reality and able to fulfill his/her own basic needs.

      b. The need to feel worthwhile to himself and others—to be worthwhile, one must maintain a satisfactory standard of behavior.

   2. Responsibility—the ability to fulfill one's needs in a way that does not deprive others of the ability to fulfill their needs; the cause of all psychiatric problems is irresponsibility.

   3. Role of the therapist:

      a. Become so involved with the patient that the patient can face reality.

      b. Reject the behavior which is unrealistic while accepting the patient and maintaining involvement.

      c. Teach the patient better ways to fulfill his needs.

      d. Emphasize behavior, not attitude or emotions.

      e. Emphasize responsibility and planning to change inappropriate behavior.

Cognitive Theories

- Cognitive Therapy (Aaron Beck)

  While practicing psychoanalysis, Beck discovered that, in addition to the thoughts verbalized during "free association," his patients had a concurrent, second set of thoughts. He called these "automatic thoughts." Automatic thoughts were those that labelled, interpreted, and evaluated, according to a personal set of rules. Beck called dysfunctional automatic thoughts "cognitive distortions." Concepts in cognitive therapy include:

  1. The relationship between therapist and client:

     a. The relationship is a collaborative partnership.

     b. Therapist and client determine the goal of therapy together.

     c. The therapist encourages the client to verbalize disagreement with the therapist when appropriate.

  2. The process of therapy:

     a. The therapist explains to the client that:

        (1) Perception of reality is not reality.

        (2) Interpretation of sensory input depends on cognitive processes.

     b. Recognize maladaptive ideation—the client is trained to observe his cognitive and emotional reactions to events, identifying:

        (1) The observable behavior

        (2) The underlying motivation

        (3) His thoughts and beliefs

     c. Distance and decenter—the client practices distancing the maladaptive thoughts.

     d. Authenticate conclusions—the client explores his conclusions and tests them against reality.

     e. Change the rules.

        (1) The client makes the rules less absolute and extreme.

        (2) The client drops false rules from the repertoire and substitutes adaptive rules.

- Social Learning Theory (Albert Bandura)

    Combines cognitive and behavioral theories—the key concept of the theory is modeling, also called imitating or learning by observation. Other concepts include:

    1. Retention process—verbally encoding an observed behavior

    2. Motor Reproduction Process—practicing the motor skills of the observed behavior

    3. Reinforcement and Motivational Process—receiving reward or reinforcement for the behavior (Scroggs, 1985)

Theories of Communication

Theories of communication focus upon the process of verbal and nonverbal communication between and among people.

- Neurolinguistic Programming (NLP) (Richard Bandler & John Grinder)

    The assumption behind NLP is that we all create personal models or maps of the world and use language to represent our models. People ''get stuck,'' not by their situation, but by the choices they perceive are available to them because of their maps. Concepts include:

    1. Representational Systems—sensory modalities through which people access information

        a. Auditory

        b. Visual

        c. Kinesthetic

    2. Cues to representational systems—patterns that are associated with representational systems and can be heard or observed

        a. Preferred predicates—e.g., the word ''view'' suggests a visual system.

        b. Eye-Accessing cues—e.g., looking upward suggests a visual system.

        c. Gross hand movements—e.g., pointing toward the ear suggests an auditory system.

        d. Breathing patterns—e.g., deep abdominal breathing suggests a kinesthetic system.

    e.   Speech pattern and voice tone—e.g., quick bursts of high pitched words suggest a visual system.

3. Language structure

    a.   Surface structure—the sentences that native speakers of a language speak and write

    b.   Deep structure—the full linguistic representation from which the surface structures of a language are derived

    c.   Ambiguity—a surface structure may represent more than one deep structure

4. Human modeling—the process of representing something, e.g., the world of experience is represented in language. Modeling involves the following processes:

    a.   Generalization—a specific experience comes to represent the entire category of which it is a member.

    b.   Deletion—selected portions of the world are excluded from the representation created by an individual.

    c.   Distortion—the relationships among the parts of the model differ from the relationships they are supposed to represent (Bandler & Grinder, 1975, 1976; Wilson & Kneisl, 1992).

- Transactional Analysis (TA) Eric Berne

    The focus is on the interaction between persons. Concepts include:

1. Ego State—frame of mind

    a.   Parent—exhibits feelings and behaviors learned from parents and authorities; the parent may be nurturing or critical.

    b.   Adult—exhibits feelings and behaviors of a mature adult, e.g., analysis, perception, and sociability

    c.   Child—exhibits feelings and behaviors natural to children under seven years old; the child may be natural or adapted. The adapted child is acting under parental influence.

2. Transaction—verbal and non-verbal communication between two people

    a.   Complementary transactions

      (1)   A message sent *from* the ego state of Person A is responded to in that ego state.

      (2)   A message sent *to* an ego state in Person B is responded to from that ego state.

   b. Crossed transactions

      (1)   A message sent *from* the ego state of Person A is responded to in another ego state.

      (2)   A message sent *to* an ego state in Person B is responded to from another ego state.

   c. Ulterior transactions—messages that occur on two levels

      (1)   The social or overt level

      (2)   The hidden or psychological level

3.   Games—recurring sets of ulterior transactions with a concealed motive, e.g., ''Why don't you . . . Yes, but.''

4.   Script—an unconscious life plan

5.   Therapy using TA may be done in conjunction with other modes of therapy, e.g., psychoanalysis. Therapy consists of:

   a. Explaining TA to the client

   b. Structural analysis of the client's ego states

   c. Transactional analysis of the client's interactions

   d. Game analysis

   e. Script analysis (Berne, 1961, 1964; Wilson & Kneisl, 1992)

Theories of Group Behavior and Therapy

Many theories already described in this chapter have been applied to group behavior and group therapy, including theories of psychoanalysis, personality and communication. The theory considered basic to all groups is systems theory.

- Systems Theory (Von Bertalanffy)

    According to Von Bertalanffy (1934) the world consists of entities called "systems." The theory has frequently been used to explain group behavior. Selected concepts include:

1. All systems are hierarchically arrayed.

    a. Suprasystem

    b. System

    c. Subsystem

2. A system has three functions:

    a. Meet its purpose

    b. Self maintainance

    c. Adaptation

3. The whole is more than the sum of the parts.

4. A change in one part affects other parts and/or the whole system.

5. There is feedback or input and output:

    a. Within the system

    b. Between the system and the environment (Von Bertalanffy, 1934; Van Servellen, 1984)

- Group Theories—See Yalom citations, chapter 2

- Psychodrama (J. L. Moreno)

    Psychodrama is a here-and-now action psychotherapy, a therapeutic drama, used primarily in group settings. The therapist functions as the "Director" of the drama chosen by the client. Psychodrama consists of a three-part process:

    1. Warm up—the protaganist chooses the time, place, scene, and auxiliary egos for his production.

    2. Action—the issue or conflict is acted out or re-lived.

    3. Post-action Sharing—group members discuss their identification with the subject (Moreno, 1964)

Family Theories (Natural Systems Theory)

Family therapies focus on the family as a whole. The family member who has a problem to be dealt with in therapy is known as the "identified patient."

- Family Systems Theory (Murray Bowen)

Bowen applied systems theory to the treatment of dysfunctional families, developing a "transgenerational" therapy. The main concepts of the theory are:

1. Differentiation of self—the lower the level of self-differentiation, the less adaptive one is under stress. There are two types of differentiation of self:

    a. Differentiating thought from emotion

    b. Differentiating oneself from one's "family ego mass"

2. Triangles—when a two-member alliance, or dyad, becomes emotionally stressed, the members pull in a third member to reduce anxiety. Bowen considers a triangle the basic building block of any emotional system.

3. Nuclear family emotional system—patterns of emotional interaction among family members

4. Multigenerational transmission process—relationship patterns and anxiety about specific issues that have been transmitted through the generations

5. Family projection process—assignment of characteristics to certain family members

6. Sibling position—birth order and gender

7. Emotional cutoff—distancing to deal with intense unresolved emotional issues

8. Therapy—consists of role modeling and guiding family members to:

    a. Increase differentiation of self from a "pseudoself" consisting of beliefs and values acquired in the family to a highly differentiated self

    b. Detriangle—observe one's own effect and control one's participation in the triangle, while maintaining emotional contact (Bowen, 1978; Stuart & Sundeen, 1991; Kerr & Bowen, 1988)

- Structural Family Therapy (Salvador Minuchin)

    In this theory, the therapist joins the family and works to modify the family structure. Concepts in Structural Family Therapy include:

1. The family in transition—the family is considered a social system in transformation that must maintain its continuity and adapt to internal and external stressor.

2. Stages of family development—each stage requires restructuring. The stages are:

    a. Courtship period—when the young person reaches adulthood and seeks a mate

    b. Marriage—when one member moves from the family of origin to create a new family

    c. Middle years of marriage—when parents must wean themselves from their children

    d. Retirement and old age—one spouse may die; adult children may assume care provider role.

3. Family structure, which consists of:

    a. Power and influence—the hierarchy of power and authority; parental authority is advocated.

    b. Subsystems—sets of relationships or dyads formed by generation, gender, interest, or function

    c. Boundaries—rules of who participates with whom—boundary problems include:

        (1) Enmeshment—weak or absent boundaries between individuals and/or subsystems; perceptions of self and others are poorly differentiated.

        (2) Disengagement—rigid boundaries between individuals and/or subsystems; communication and contact is minimal.

4. Tasks of the therapist include:

    a. Joining and accommodation—tasks include:

        (1) Maintainance—e.g., join the family and maintain family strengths by pointing them out.

        (2) Assessment—e.g., assess the family structure and transaction patterns.

    b.   Restructuring

        (1)   Actualize family transactional patterns—e.g., re-create communication channels.

        (2)   Mark boundaries—delineate individual and subsystem boundaries.

        (3)   Escalate stress—e.g., block transactional patterns.

        (4)   Assign tasks within and between sessions.

        (5)   Utilize symptoms—e.g., exaggerate, de-emphasize or re-label symptoms; move to new symptoms.

        (6)   Support, educate, and guide (Minuchin and Nichols, 1993; Helm, 1991).

- Strategic Family Therapy (Madanes and Haley)

Strategic Family Therapy, also known as Problem Solving Therapy, is brief therapy that focuses on solving the presenting problem(s) (Haley, 1987; Madanes, 1981). Concepts include:

1. Symptom—a behavior that analogically or metaphorically expresses a family problem

2. Problem—part of a sequence of acts between people; the way one person communicates with another

3. Focus of therapy—changing analogies and metaphors

4. Goal—prevent repetition of problem sequences; introduce more complexity and alternatives

5. Hierarchy—parents are considered responsible for and in charge of children.

6. Interventions:

    a.   Decide which family members are involved.

    b.   Design and implement a strategy to shift the family organization so the present problems are not necessary.

    c.   Directives—the therapist tells the family members to do something. Directives may be:

        (1)   Straightforward—e.g., the mother is directed to assume a parental role.

(2) Paradoxical, e.g.—a spouse is directed to encourage the other spouse to have the "symptom" more frequently.

   d. Changes are planned in stages so that changes in one situation or relationship will lead to changes in another. The therapist may even create another problem and shift to another abnormal hierarchy before shifting to a normal hierarchy.

   e. If the strategy does not work within a few weeks, the therapist plans and implements another strategy (Madanes, 1981; Haley, 1987).

Neurobiological Theories

The 90s have been termed "The Decade of the Brain" by the National Institutes of Mental Health as more and more theories have been developed and tested in this area. Neurobiological theories are based on the following general statements:

1. Cognitive and emotional dysfunctions result from multiple causes, such as genetic influences, nutrition, infectious processes and other pathological conditions that contribute to neurotransmitter imbalances in the brain (Sanford, 1995)

2. Neurotransmitters are chemical substances, found at the synapses between neurons in the Central Nervous System which influence cognitive, emotional and behavioral functioning by carrying messages from the axon of one neuron to the receptor sites on the postsynaptic neuron. See Table 2

3. At the end of the process, neurotransmitters are either inactivated by enzymatic degradation or taken back into the presynaptic neuron (reuptake)

4. There are thought to be more than a 100 different transmitters and many neurons that release more than one neurotransmitter (Harris & McMahon, 1997, p. 224)

5. "Psychotherapeutic drugs are prescribed to manipulate the processes of neurotransmitter production and absorption to reestablish 'normal' neurochemical balance." (Sanford, 1995, p. 31)

Table 2
Neurotransmitters and effects on Mental Health

Acetylcholine	Underactivity implicated in Alzheimer's disease (Harris & McMahon, 1997)
Dopamine	Overactivity implicated in schizophrenia and mania (Sanford, 1995)
	Antipsychotic medications provide dopamine post synaptic receptor blockade and cause extrapyramidal side effects (Harris & McMahon, 1997)
Norepinephrine Epinephrine	Underactivity implicated in depresssion
	Antidepressants increase functional activity
	Depleted in dementia of the Alzheimer's type (DAT) and Korsakoff's syndrome (Harris & McMahon, 1997)
	Transmission and uptake impaired in anxiety and addiction (Sanford, 1995)
Serotonin (5-HT)	Underactivity implicated in depression and obsessive-compulsive disorder (OCD) (Harris & McMahon, 1997)
	Dysregulation implicated in anxiety, violence and schizoaffective disorder and personality disorders (Sanford, 1995)
	Tricyclic and SSRI antidepressants increase functional activity by blocking reuptake
Gamma-aminobutyric acid (GABA) Glutamate, (amino acids)	Person with low levels or fewer GABA receptors more susceptible to anxiety disorders (Sanford, 1995)
	Activity increased by antianxiety Aspartate and Glycine medications
	Transmitter-receptor action destroyed by chronic use of alcohol
Substance P Endorphins and Enkephalins (Peptides)	Activation and regulation of response to stress and injury
	Involved in pain perceptions and reflex actions
	Morphine and heroin are opioid endorphins

6. Neuroendocrinology—According to Harris and McMahon (1997), brain biochemicals, by way of the hypothalamus, stimulate the pituitary gland which affects the endocrine glands along the following three brain endocrine axes (cascades):

Axis	Response
Hypothalamic-pituitary thyroid axis (HPTA)	Blunted TSH response to thyrotropin releasing hormone (TRH) in depression
Hypothalamic-pituitary adrenal axis (HPPA)	Hyperactive in depression and some anxiety
	Nonsuppression of cortisol by dexa-methasone suppression test in depression
	Elevated cortisol levels in depression
	Elevated corticotropin-releasing hormone (CRH) levels in depression
Hypothalamic-pituitary gonadal axis	Blunted prolactin response in exogenous obesity
	Reduces testosterone levels in depression

Miscellaneous

- Solution Focused Therapy (de Shazer & O'Hanlon, 1985)

  1. Assumption that complaints are maintained by client belief that their response to the original difficulty was the only right thing to do (de Shazer, 1985)

  2. Therapist reframes the beliefs and puts them in a different perspective which allows symptoms to be transformed into part of a mutually developed solution.

  3. Focus on the present and future rather than the past.

     a. Only information about past success is sought

     b. Emphasizes strengths of client; "Tell me how you dealt with a similar situation in the past" (Cline & Davidson, 1997).

  4. Emphasis on outcomes with expectations of rapid change:

     a. "When you are not feeling depressed what will you be feeling instead?" (Cline & Davidson, 1997)

     b. "How will you know when the problem is solved?"

  5. Help clients to reformulate goals to a reachable level, i.e. "having a more calm approach" instead of "stop yelling" (de Shazer, 1985).

6. Compliment clients on what they are doing right

7. Use exceptions: ''What do you do when you overcome the urge to yell?'' (deShazer, 1985)

8. Formulate solution around reframed belief and way clients describe life after ''problem'' no longer occurs.

   a. Have client leave with beginning step toward solution.

   b. Goals or tasks may be assigned: ''Between now and the next time we meet I would like you to notice what happens in your relationship that you would like to continue to have happen.'' (de Shazer, 1997).

9. Evaluate at next session.

   a. If ''problem'' is better, warn of relapse: ''These things rarely resolve without some recurrences. You will probably have a big fight in the next few weeks.''

   b. If problem is the same: ''You must be doing something right or it would be worse.''

   c. If worse: ''May have to go from bad to worse before it gets better.'' '' Is this the bottom or do things need to go from worse to worst before getting better?''(de Shazer, 1985)

10. Average number of sessions is usually 5 or 6 with clients choosing time between sessions to allow for a comfortable rate of change as determined by the client.

- Crisis Intervention (Donna Aguilera)

   1. Types of crises:

      a. Situational—external events that cause unusual stresses, e.g., hospitalization or divorce

      b. Maturational—normal processes of growth and development in which there is difficulty with maturation, e.g., adolescence and adulthood

      c. Adventitious—accidental, uncommon, and unexpected events, e.g., fire, earthquake, or flood (Aguilera, 1990)

   2. Phases of crisis intervention:

a. Assessment—assessing the precipitating event and the client's perceptions of the event

b. Planning of the intervention—evaluating strengths, coping skills, support systems, and alternative methods of coping

c. Intervention—treatment lasting one to six weeks, with the goal of returning the individual to his previous level of functioning

   (1) Helping the person gain an intellectual understanding of the crisis

   (2) Helping the person express feelings

   (3) Exploring coping mechanisms

   (4) Reopening the social world

d. Resolution and anticipatory planning—reinforcing adaptive mechanisms, summarizing the process of intervention and planning for future coping (Aguilera, 1990)

- Theory of Self-Concept (John Hattie)

   The attributes of self-concept include:

   1. A cognitive appraisal consisting of beliefs about self

   2. Three aspects of self-concept are:

      a. Expectations from self and others—high expectations in a dimension or a task can lead to low self concept and vice-versa. For example, if an average high school athlete expects to become a professional basketball star, his or her high expectation may lead to low self-concept.

      b. Descriptions of oneself which are:

         (1) Hierarchical—from a description of a simple, isolated characteristic to a general, all-inclusive description of self

         (2) Multi-faceted—having numerous dimensions

      c. Prescriptions—standards of correctness

   3. Integrated across various dimensions by means of

      a. Self-verification—soliciting feedback to confirm the view of self

    b.   Self-consistency—internal harmony among opinions, attitudes, and values

    c.   Self-complexity—viewing self as complex and multi-faceted

    d.   Self-enhancement—viewing self's positive qualities as more important than self's negative qualities

4.   Subject to confirmation from self and others

5.   Implicit and culturally bound (Hattie, 1991)

- Theory of Self-disclosure (Richard L. Archer)

Summarizing the research and definitions of self-disclosure, Archer (1987) focused on the orientations and functions of self-disclosure which are as follows:

1.   The self-orientation—disclosures are concerned with exploring the nature and contents of oneself, for oneself.

2.   The self-to-other orientation—disclosures are concerned with locating oneself in relation to others by getting feedback.

3.   The other-to-self orientation—disclosures are used as a means of social control or of obtaining benefits from others.

4.   The other orientation—disclosure is geared toward obtaining reciprocal disclosure.

5.   The self-and-other orientation—disclosure is concerned with interdependence of participants in a relationship (Archer, 1987).

- Stress Theory (Hans Selye)

Selye developed a theory of the physical response to stress called the General Adaptation Syndrome (GAS). The stages of the GAS are as follows:

1.   Alarm stage—a threat is perceived, and the endocrine system and the immune system respond, creating physical and mental alertness.

2.   Resistance Stage—the threat continues, and attempts are made to adapt.

3.   Exhaustion Stage—if the threat continues, the adaptive hormones are depleted and the body succumbs to illness (Selye, 1976; Wilson & Kneisl, 1992).

- Coping (Monat & Lazrus, 1991)

  According to Monat and Lazarus (1991) Coping 'refers to a person's efforts to master demands (conditions of harm, threat, or challenge) that are appraised (or perceived) as exceeding or taxing a person's resources'

  1. Problem Focused Coping

     a. Define the problem

     b. Generate alternative solutions

     c. Weigh alternatives re cost and benefits

     d. Choose alternatives

     e. Implement

  2. Emotion Focused Coping

     a. Cognitive reappraisal to alter the meaning of situation without changing objective facts

     b. Behavioral strategies such as physical exercise, meditation or talking to friends

  3. Defense mechanisms (see chapter 2) can be viewed as unconscious coping methods.

- Role Theory (Hardy & Conway)

  According to Hardy and Conway (1988, p. 63), Role Theory ''represents a collection of concepts and a variety of hypothetical formulations that predict how actors will perform in a given role, or under what circumstances certain types of behavior can be expected''. Concepts include:

  1. Approach to studying roles:

     a. Structural approach—roles are fixed positions with certain expectations and demands, enforced by societal sanctions.

     b. Symbolic Interactionist approach—behavior is a response to the symbolic acts (primarily gestures and speech) of others.

  2. Role making—a process of modifying a role; phases of role making include:

     a. Initiator behavior

     b. Other response

    c. Interpretation

    d. Altered response

    e. Role validation

3. Role taking—the proces of imagining oneself in the place of another

4. Socialization—the process of learning the social roles, skills, and knowledge that prepare one for role performance

5. Role stress—a condition in which role obligations are unclear, conflicting or impossible to meet

6. Role strain—a subjective state of frustration or distress in meeting role expectations

7. Stratification—a hierarchical ranking of people according to wealth, status, power, or occupation (Hardy & Conway, 1988)

QUESTIONS
Select the best answer

1. The purpose of a theory is to:

   a. Describe, explain, predict or control a phenomenon
   b. Encourage the development of more research
   c. Prove that there can be one way to describe a phenomenon
   d. Prove that a phenomenon exists

2. Characteristics of theories include:

   a. They provide laws by which to govern practice.
   b. They have little in common with practice.
   c. They can guide and improve practice.
   d. They need not be logical.

3. Inductive theory construction:

   a. Consists largely of concepts borrowed from other disciplines
   b. Validates deductive theory construction
   c. Proceeds from the general to the specific
   d. Proceeds from the specific to the general

4. Which of the following do theories *NOT* do?

   a. Guide practice
   b. Guide research
   c. Provide a common language for practitioners and researchers
   d. Limit autonomy of practice

5. The concepts central to nursing theoretical models are:

   a. Self-care, self-care deficit, and nursing systems
   b. Caring and curing
   c. Assessment, diagnosis, intervention, and evaluation
   d. Person, environment, health, and nursing

6. Dorothea Orem's theory of nursing is also called the theory of:

   a. Behavioral systems
   b. Self-care
   c. The environment
   d. Adaptation

7. In Orem's theory, Nursing Systems are described as:

    a. Desciptions of a variety of ideal hospital staffing models
    b. The theories that she drew from
    c. Simple, complex, and combined
    d. Wholly compensatory, partly compensatory, and supportive-educative

8. Nurse A, who utilizes Orem's theory, is caring for Patient B. Patient B requires a complete bed bath. When charting, Nurse A will describe the Patient B's inability to provide complete self-care as:

    a. A health deviation
    b. Illness
    c. A self-care deficit
    d. A diagnostic indication

9. Imogene King's theory of nursing is:

    a. A theory of personal systems
    b. A theory of goal attainment
    c. A theory of adaptation
    d. A behavioral systems theory

10. In King's theory, a set of behaviors expected of a person occupying a certain position is called a:

    a. Role
    b. Perception
    c. Transaction
    d. Developmental position

11. One of the basic assumptions in the theory of Martha Rogers is:

    a. People come together to help and be helped to maintain health.
    b. The universe is a continuously expanding, evolving, growing field of energy.
    c. The person and environment are continually exchanging matter and energy with each other.
    d. Energy fields are four dimensional, unidirectional expanding sources of knowledge.

12. According to Rogers, which of the following do *NOT* describe the human being?

    a. Characterized by the capacity for abstraction and imagery
    b. Characterized by the capacity for reversibility and multidirectionality
    c. Characterized by the capacity for language and thought
    d. Characterized by the capacity for sensation and emotion

13. The building blocks of Rogers' theory are:

    a. Energy, openness, pattern and four-dimensionality
    b. Person, life process, pattern and organization, energy
    c. Person, environment, health, nursing
    d. Openess, environment, pattern and energy

14. Sister Callista Roy's theory of nursing is:

    a. The Interpersonal Relations Model
    b. The Problem Solving Model
    c. The Communication Model
    d. The Adaptation Model

15. Roy's adaptive modes are:

    a. Physiological function, self-concept, role function, and interdependence
    b. Regulator, cognator, external, and informational
    c. Value, belief, thought, and emotion
    d. Adaptive response, ineffective response, output

16. The nurse who utilizes Roy's model in providing nursing care would first:

    a. Identify focal stimuli
    b. Manipulate focal stimuli
    c. Identify input and internal processes
    d. Conduct a first-level assessment

17. The nurse who utilizes Roy's model in providing nursing care will include in the second-level assessment:

    a. Identification of ineffective responses
    b. Identification of nursing diagnosis
    c. Identification of goals
    d. Patterns of physical functioning

18. The main concept in Leininger's Theory of Culture Care Diversity and Universality is that:

    a. Culture is the learned, shared, and transmitted values, beliefs, norms, and lifeways of a group

    b. Care is the essence of nursing

    c. There is diversity and universality in every culture

    d. Nurses should seek to know the universality of Transcultural nursing

19. According to Leininger, the important factors to study in cultural care include:

    a. Religious factors

    b. Nutritional factors

    c. Rest patterns

    d. Prenatal care

20. Cultural care accommodation refers to:

    a. Actions and decisions to help people of a given culture negotiate for a beneficial outcome with health caregivers

    b. Actions and decisions to help a client modify their lifeways for beneficial health care, while respecting their cultural values and beliefs

    c. Actions and decisions that help people retain relevant cultural care values

    d. Actions and decisions that are based on universal cultural care

21. The two most famous psychoanalytic theorists are:

    a. Horney and Adler

    b. Freud and Jung

    c. Kohlberg and Gilligan

    d. Adler and Sullivan

22. According to Freudian theory, unconscious actions or thoughts to protect the ego from anxiety are called:

    a. Freudian slips

    b. Unconscious motivation

    c. Defense mechanisms

    d. Transference

23. According to Freudian theory, thoughts, feelings, and desires that are not in immediate awareness, but can be recalled to consciousness, are considered:

    a. Conscious

    b. Preconscious

    c. Subconscious

    d. Unconscious

24. According to Freudian theory, the personality has three main components. The component characterized by the desire for immediate and complete satisfaction is the:

    a. Reality principle
    b. Id
    c. Ego
    d. Superego

25. Freud suggests that children of four or five fall in love with the parent of the oppostie sex. This is known as:

    a. Projection
    b. Transference
    c. The pleasure principle
    d. The oedipus complex

26. According to Freud, whatever inhibits a person from producing material from the unconscious is considered:

    a. Resistance
    b. Transference
    c. Counter-transference
    d. Fixation

27. In Jungian theory, the unconscious collective intangible idea, image, or concept is the:

    a. Persona
    b. Shadow
    c. Archetype
    d. Rebirth

28. Jung's archetypes do *NOT* include:

    a. The animus
    b. The shadow
    c. Stock characters
    d. The id

29. The functional types described by Jung include:

    a. Extrovert and introvert
    b. The hero, the trickster, and the sage

    c. Thinking, feeling, sensing, intuiting

    d. Animus and anima

30. Adler developed the Theory of Individual Psychology. The main concern of Adler's theory is:

    a. The individual going through the stages of development

    b. Personal growth through compensating for inferiority

    c. Providing client-centered therapy

    d. The effect of relationships on unconscious behaviors

31. Adler identified effects of the birth order of siblings. According to his theory, the child most likely to be interested in authority and organization is:

    a. The first-born

    b. The second-born

    c. The middle child in a large family

    d. The youngest child

32. The key concept in the personality theory of Horney is:

    a. Neurosis

    b. Hostility

    c. Basic anxiety

    d. Satisfaction of needs

33. According to Horney, which of the following is *NOT* a way by which people protect themselves:

    a. Moving toward other people

    b. Moving against other people

    c. Moving away from other people

    d. Moving in accord with other people

34. Erikson identified eight stages of growth and development. The stage characterized by a focus on genital needs and the acquisition of a purpose is:

    a. Trust vs. mistrust

    b. Autonomy vs. shame

    c. Initiative vs. guilt

    d. Industry vs. inferiority

35. If a child's activities are primarily social interaction, doing homework and practicing basketball, then according to Erikson, he is in the following stage of development:

    a. Trust vs. mistrust
    b. Autonomy vs. shame
    c. Initiative vs. guilt
    d. Industry vs. inferiority

36. According to Erikson, the stage of development characterized by the acquisition of wisdom is:

    a. Identity vs. identity diffusion
    b. Intimacy vs. isolation
    c. Generativity vs. stagnation
    d. Integrity vs. despair

37. Jean Piaget developed a theory of:

    a. Psychosexual development
    b. Cognitive development
    c. Moral development
    d. Social development

38. In the developmental theory of Piaget, the period characterized by egocentric thinking, expressed in artificialism, realism and magical thinking is the:

    a. Sensory motor period
    b. Pre-operational period
    c. Concrete operations period
    d. Formal operations period

39. In the developmental theory of Piaget, the period characterized by the development of logic and reasoning, and second-order thoughts, that is, "thinking about thoughts," is

    a. Sensory motor period
    b. Pre-operational period
    c. Concrete operations period
    d. Formal operations Period

40. The nurse is working with Mrs. L. who has been sexually promiscuous and manipulative with her family. While developing a treatment plan for Mrs. L, the

nurse recognizes that her behavior is consistent with the behavior in Stage 2 of Kohlberg's theory of moral development. Mrs. L. will be motivated by:

    a. Avoidance of punishment
    b. Desire for reward or benefit
    c. Anticipation of disapproval of others
    d. Anticipation of dishonor

41. If Mrs. L.'s behavior was consistent with the behavior of Stage 4 of Kohlberg's theory of moral development, she would be motivated by:

    a. Anticipation of disapproval of others
    b. Anticipation of dishonor
    c. A legalistic orientation
    d. Belief in universal ethical principles

42. In Kohlberg's theory of moral development, behavior in Stage 6 is motivated by:

    a. Anticipation of disapproval of others
    b. Anticipation of dishonor
    c. A legalistic orientation
    d. Belief in universal ethical principles

43. According to the work of Gilligan on moral development:

    a. In applying Kohlberg's theory, women are generally more moral than men.
    b. Most women achieve the moral reasoning in Stage 6 of Kohlberg's theory.
    c. Women and men have the same moral reasoning.
    d. The moral development of women is based on different motivations than that of men.

44. The main focus of the social-interpersonal theories of personality is:

    a. Neurosis
    b. Anxiety about relationships
    c. The effects of interactions with others
    d. Inferiority and superiority feelings

45. In the interpersonal theory of Harry Stack Sullivan, the "self-system" is:

    a. The part of the personality that satisfies the drive for security,

   b. A construct to describe the narcissism inherent in all interpersonal relationships

   c. A construct built from the child's experience, made up of reflected ap-
praisals by significant others

   d. The part of the personality that satisfies the drive for satisfaction

46. According to Sullivan, the basic drives that underlie human behavior are:

   a. The drive to reduce anxiety and the drive to avoid fear

   b. The drive for satisfaction and the drive for security

   c. The drive to fulfill basic physical needs and the drive to fulfill sexual
needs

   d. The drive for love and work

47. The existential theories of personality focus on:

   a. The meaning of life for the individual

   b. Present experience, with little attention to the past

   c. One's philosophy of life

   d. Conforming to societal demands

48. According to Carl Rogers, the important attributes of the therapist are:

   a. Congruence, unconditional positive regard and empathetic understanding

   b. Knowledge of Rogers' theory, patience, and ability to interpret dreams

   c. Knowledge of Rogers' theory, congruence, and interest in human development

   d. Willingness to drop facades, openness to individual meanings, and com-
passion

49. According to Monat and Lazarus which of the following would be considered
as part of emotion focused coping?

   a. Defining the problem

   b. Physical exercise

   c. Generate alternative solutions

   d. Weigh alternatives re cost and benefits

50. The therapist utilizing Gestalt therapy recognizes that introjection is:

   a. A fantasy about what another person is experiencing

   b. Accepting the beliefs and opinions of others without question

   c. Turning back on oneself that which is meant for someone else

   d. Merging with the environment

51. The main goal of Gestalt Therapy is;

    a. Dropping facades
    b. Differentiating between self and others
    c. Integration of self and world awareness
    d. Resolving conflicts from past

52. Techniques in Gestalt therapy do *NOT* include:

    a. Playing the projection
    b. Making the rounds
    c. Exaggeration of a feeling or action
    d. Paradoxical prescription

53. Maslow's hierarchy of basic needs include:

    a. Safety and satisfaction, health and growth
    b. Physiological needs, safety, love and belongingness, self esteem, and self-actualization
    c. Physical, biological, psychological, sociological, and spiritual needs
    d. Food, fluid, activity, meaning and purpose, and self-actualization

54. The A-B-Cs of Ellis's Rational Emotive Therapy are:

    a. Action, behavior, congruence
    b. Anticipation, belief, consequence
    c. Acceptance, behavior, caring
    d. Activating behavior, belief, consequence

55. According to Ellis's Rational Emotive Therapy, a basic form of irrational beliefs is that:

    a. One cannot meet one's goals.
    b. Life is difficult.
    c. Something is awful, terrible, or horrible.
    d. Behavior has meaning

56. For the nurse who uses Rational Emotive Therapy in practice, the focus of treatment is on:

    a. Behavior rather than beliefs
    b. Accepting the beliefs of others
    c. Disputing, debating, discriminating, and defining
    d. Anticipating, acting, and accepting

57. Behavioral theories of personality are concerned with:

    a. Unconscious phenomena
    b. Cognition
    c. Emotions
    d. Reinforcement

58. One concept of Skinner's theory is that an individual performs a behavior which leads to a positive or negative reinforcement, making it either more or less likely that the behavior will be repeated. This is called:

    a. A schedule of reinforcement
    b. A fixed ratio
    c. A variable interval
    d. Operant conditioning

59. In a variable ratio schedule of reinforcement, behaviors are rewarded:

    a. Each time they are performed
    b. Every time they are repeated
    c. At specific times of performance
    d. At random times of performance

60. Mrs. J. seeks treatment for her fear of automobiles. After the initial assessment, the nurse decides to use systematic desensitization. The first step in systematic desensitization is to:

    a. Help Mrs. J. get a prescription for valium and take her for an automobile ride
    b. Explore other means of transportation
    c. Train Mrs. J. in deep muscle relaxation
    d. Show Mrs. J. a picture of an automobile and ask how she feels

61. The two types of systematic desensitization are:

    a. Automatic desensitization and standard desensitization
    b. Fantasy desensitization and in vivo desensitization
    c. Desensitization with medication and desensitization without medication
    d. Reciprocal inhibition and aversive conditioning

62. According to the Reality Therapy of William Glasser, each person has the following two basic needs:

    a. Psychological needs and spiritual needs

b. Physiological needs and psychological needs
c. The need to love and be loved, and the need to be productive
d. The need to love and be loved, and the need to feel worthwhile

63. According to Glasser, the cause of all psychiatric problems is:

a. Neurosis
b. Irresponsibility
c. Childhood training
d. Irrational beliefs

64. The therapist who is utilizing Glasser's therapy will emphasize:

a. Unconscious motivation
b. Dream interpretation
c. Changing behavior
d. Re-experiencing traumatic childhood events

65. Aaron Beck developed a theory of cognitive therapy after he discovered that his clients had "automatic thoughts." The automatic thoughts:

a. Came from too much free association
b. Labelled, interpreted, and evaluated situations according to a personal set of rules
c. Indicated to the client that he should not trust the therapist
d. Warned clients of any physiological needs

66. The therapist who utilizes Beck's therapy will warn the client:

a. To try to ignore or suppress his automatic thoughts
b. That emotionally healthy individuals do not have automatic thoughts
c. That automatic thoughts are deeply imbedded and cannot be changed
d. That a perception of reality is not necessarily reality

67. The therapist utilizing Beck's therapy will help the client to:

a. Recognize and change his automatic thoughts
b. See reality as the therapist sees it
c. Change his reality by changing his environment
d. Recognize and accept that automatic thoughts suggest delusional thinking

68. In the Social Learning Theory of Alfred Bandura, the key concept is:

a. Modeling

b. Encoding a behavior
c. Rewarding behavior appropriately
d. Rewarding behavior on a ratio interval scale

69. In the Neurolinguistic Programming (NLP) of Bandler and Grinder, the "representational systems" are:

    a. Auditory, visual and kinesthetic
    b. Methods of analyzing communication
    c. Right brain and left brain
    d. Parent, adult and child

70. An assumption behind NLP is that:

    a. We all have irrational beliefs
    b. We all create models of the world, and use language to represent them
    c. We are all philosophers
    d. Verbal and non-verbal communication is important in nursing

71. In NLP, the sentences which native speakers of a language speak and write are called:

    a. Deep structure
    b. Surface structure
    c. Multi-model sentences
    d. Cues to beliefs

72. In NLP, human modeling does *NOT* involve:

    a. Generalization
    b. Deletion
    c. Distortion
    d. Disintegration

73. In Transactional Analysis (TA), the theory by Eric Berne, ego states include:

    a. Sane, neurotic, and psychotic
    b. Rational and irrational
    c. Parent, adult, and child
    d. Manic, depressive, and schizophrenic

74. In TA, when a message is sent from an ego state of Person A and is responded to in that ego state, there is a:

    a. Crossed transaction
    b. Ulterior transaction
    c. Complementary transaction
    d. Confused transaction

75. In TA, a message that occurs on two levels is:

    a. A crossed transaction
    b. An ulterior transaction
    c. A complementary transaction
    d. A game

76. Concepts in Systems theory include:

    a. Systems are designed to serve people
    b. Systems are by nature complex
    c. All systems are hierarchically arrayed
    d. All systems have five functions

77. According to Systems Theory, the functions of a system include:

    a. Cooperation
    b. Conflict
    c. Adaptation
    d. Accommodation

78. The originator of Psychodrama was:

    a. Moreno
    b. Minuchin
    c. Beck
    d. Adler

79. In Psychodrama, the therapist functions as a:

    a. Protagonist
    b. Auxiliary ego
    c. Director
    d. Partner

80. The nurse utilizing Bowen's theory in family therapy will observe the patterns of emotional interaction within a family. Bowen calls these patterns:

    a. Triangles

b. The family projection process
c. The nuclear family emotional system
d. The family differentiation process

81. In Bowen's Family Systems Therapy, the multigenerational family transmission process refers to:

    a. Genetic traits
    b. Relationship patterns and anxiety about specific issues that have been transmitted through the generations
    c. Relationships between grandparents and grandchildren
    d. Hereditary disorders

82. The nurse practicing Bowen's Family Systems Therapy will guide family members to:

    a. Use their sibling position to their advantage
    b. Periodically cut off other family members emotionally
    c. Create specific triangles
    d. Increase differentiation of self

83. When the nurse using Minuchin's Structural Family Therapy observes that a mother holds a 7-year-old child in her lap, answers questions for the child, and describes protecting the child from siblings and neighbors, the nurse will suspect.

    a. Accommodation
    b. Enmeshment
    c. Disengagement
    d. An unusual transaction

84. In Minuchin's Structural Family Therapy, the main tasks of the therapist are:

    a. Joining and restructuring
    b. Clarifying the family structure and explaining it
    c. Identifying family communication patterns and maintaining family strengths
    d. Enacting the family structure and delineating boundaries

85. A therapist who utilizes Minuchin's Structural Family Therapy will probably:

    a. Point out family strengths
    b. Identify multigenerational transactions
    c. Maintain his position of authority

d. Decrease stress

86. In the Structural Family Therapy of Minuchin, when the therapist blocks the usual transactional patterns or emphasizes differences among family members, he is probably trying to:

    a. Accommodate the family
    b. Identify the true patient
    c. Escalate stress
    d. Identify the executive subsystem

87. A therapist who utilizes the Structural Family Therapy of Minuchin would *NOT* utilize symptoms by:

    a. Moving to new symptoms
    b. De-emphasizing symptoms
    c. Exaggerating symptoms
    d. Rewarding symptoms

88. The focus of Strategic Family Therapy is to:

    a. Emphasize symptoms
    b. Change analogies and metaphors in the family
    c. Help the family to be more democratic
    d. Identify and solve all family problems

89. After identifying the symptom and the problem, the nurse who is practicing Strategic Family Therapy will:

    a. Identify the family structure
    b. Work to detriangle all family members
    c. Design a strategy to shift the family organization
    d. Mark subsystem boundaries

90. In a depressed client which of the following neurobiological explanations can the nurse expect?

    a. Overactivity of Serotonin (5-HT)
    b. Underactivity of Norepinephrine/Epinephrine
    c. Overactivity of Dopamine
    d. Underactivity of Acetylcholine

91. A client seeks treatment from a Solution Focused Therapist for somatic complaints. What would the therapist's question to her most likely be?

a. Can you tell me what happened in your childhood?
b. Tell me about the surgeries you have had?
c. When you aren't in terrible pain, or visiting your doctor, what will you be doing instead?
d. What was going on in your life when the pain started?

92. According to the Crisis Intervention Theory of Aquilera, types of crises are:

    a. Familial, academic, and social
    b. Major disasters and daily events
    c. Situational, maturational, and adventitious
    d. Growth inducing and growth hindering

93. Crisis Intervention Therapy usually lasts:

    a. From one to six weeks
    b. From one to six months
    c. From three months to one year
    d. More than one year

94. The main goal of Crisis Intervention is to:

    a. Assist the client in identifying his strengths
    b. Assist the client to gain insight as to why he reacted as he did
    c. Help the client to return to his previous level of functioning
    d. Help the client to prevent another crisis

95. According to the Self-Concept Theory of Hattie, the first attribute of self-concept is:

    a. A cognitive appraisal of oneself
    b. A feeling of wholeness
    c. Determined completely by one's environment
    d. Un-defined

96. In the Self-Concept Theory of Hattie, internal harmony among opinions, values, and attitudes is called:

    a. Self-complexity
    b. Self-verification
    c. Self-consistency
    d. Self-regulation

97. Self-concept is:

   a. Subject to confirmation from others
   b. Culturally bound
   c. Multi-faceted
   d. Fixed at birth

98. Purposes of self-disclosure include:

   a. Exploring oneself
   b. Locating oneself in relation to others
   c. Social control
   d. Cutting off feedback

99. The General Adaptation Syndrome, as identified by Hans Selye, has the following stages:

   a. Surprise, alertness, reaction
   b. Inflexibility, adaptation, engulfment
   c. Alarm, resistance, exhaustion
   d. Openness, closedness, paranoia

100. In the structural approach to role theory, roles are considered:

   a. Subject to change depending on immediate circumstances
   b. Fixed positions with certain expectations and demands
   c. Responses to a number of things in the environment
   d. Synonymous with job descriptions

101. Role taking refers to:

   a. Socialization into a role
   b. The process of moving into a role that was previously held by another person
   c. The process of imagining oneself in the place of another
   d. Being taken by surprise by the expectations of a certain role

ANSWERS

1. a	35. d	69. a
2. c	36. d	70. b
3. d	37. b	71. b
4. d	38. b	72. d
5. d	39. d	73. c
6. b	40. b	74. c
7. d	41. b	75. b
8. c	42. d	76. c
9. b	43. d	77. c
10. a	44. c	78. a
11. c	45. c	79. c
12. b	46. b	80. c
13. a	47. b	81. b
14. d	48. a	82. d
15. a	49. b	83. b
16. d	50. b	84. a
17. a	51. c	85. a
18. b	52. d	86. c
19. a	53. b	87. d
20. a	54. d	88. b
21. b	55. c	89. c
22. c	56. c	90. b
23. b	57. d	91. c
24. b	58. d	92. c
25. d	59. d	93. a
26. a	60. c	94. c
27. c	61. b	95. a
28. d	62. d	96. c
29. c	63. b	97. d
30. b	64. c	98. d
31. a	65. b	99. c
32. c	66. d	100. b
33. d	67. a	101. c
34. c	68. a	

Bibliography

Adler, A. (1983). *The practice and theory of individual psychology.* Totowa, NJ: Helix Books.

Archer, R. L. (1987). Commentary: Self-disclosure, a very useful behavior. In V. J. Derlega & J. H. Berg (Eds.), *Self-disclosure: Theory, research and therapy* (pp. 329–341). NY: Plenum Press.

Aguilera, D. (1990). *Crisis intervention: Theory and methodology* (6th ed.). St. Louis: C. V. Mosby.

Bandler, R., & Grinder, J. (1975). *The structure of magic I.* Palo Alto: Science and Behavior Books.

Bandler, R., & Grinder, J. (1976). *The structure of magic II.* Palo Alto: Science and Behavior Books.

Berne, E. (1961). *Transactional analysis in psychotherapy.* NY: Ballantine.

Berne, E. (1964). *Games people play.* New York: Grove press.

Bowen, M. (1971). Family therapy and family group therapy. In H. Kaplan & B. Sadok (Eds.), *Comprehensive group psychotherapy* (pp. 384–421). Baltimore: Williams & Wilkins.

Bowen, M. (1978). *Family therapy in clinical practice.* NY: Jason Aronson.

Carter, B., & McGoldrick, M. (1988). *The changing family life cycle: A framework for family therapy.* New York: Garden Press.

Clements, I. W., & Buchanan, D. M. (1982). *Family therapy: A nursing perspective.* NY: John Wiley & Sons.

Cline, J. L., & Davidson, J. R. (1997). Individual psychotherapy. In B. S. Johnson (Ed.). (9th ed.). *Psychiatric and mental health nursing: Adaptation and growth* (pp. 233-255). Philadelphia: J. B. Lippincott.

de Shazer, S. (1985). *Keys to solution in brief therapy.* New York: W. W. Norton and Company

Dollard, J., & Miller, N. E. (1950). *Personality and psychotherapy: An analysis in terms of learning, thinking and culture.* NY: McGraw-Hill.

Drapela, V. J. (1987). *A review of personality theories.* Springfield, IL: Charles C. Thomas.

Ellis, A. (1977). The basic clinical theory of rational-emotive therapy. In A. Ellis & R. Grieger (Eds.), *Handbook of rational-emotive therapy* (pp. 3–34). NY: Springer.

Erikson, E. (1963). *Childhood and society* (2nd ed.). NY: W.W. Norton & Co. Inc.

Falco, S. M., & Lobo, M. L. (1990). Martha E. Rogers. In J. George (Ed.), *Nursing theories: The base for professional practice.* Norwalk, CT: Appleton & Lange.

Fawcett, J. (1984). *Analysis and evaluation of conceptual models of nursing.* Philadelphia: F. A. Davis.

Foster, P. C., & Janssens, N. P. (1990). Dorothea E. Orem. In J. George (Ed.), *Nursing theories: The base for professional nursing practice.* Norwalk, CT: Appleton & Lange.

Galbreath, J. G. (1990). Sister Callista Roy. In J. George (Ed.), *Nursing theories: The base for professional nursing practice.* Norwalk, CT: Appleton & Lange.

George, J. B. (Ed.). (1990). *Nursing theories: The base for professional nursing practice* (3rd ed.). Norwalk, CT: Appleton & Lange.

Gilligan, C. (1982). *In a different voice.* Cambridge, MA: Harvard University Press.

Glasser, W. (1975). *Reality therapy: A new approach to psychiatry.* NY: Harper & Rowe.

Haley, J. (1987). *Problem-solving therapy,* (2nd. ed.). San Francisco: Jossey Bass Publishers.

Hardy M. E., & Conway, M. E. (1988). *Role theory: Perspectives for health professionals* (2nd ed.). Norwalk, CT: Appleton & Lange.

Hardy, R. E. (1991). *Gestalt psychotherapy: Concepts and demonstrations in stress, relationships, hypnosis and addiction.* Springfield, IL: Charles C. Thomas.

Harris, B., & McMahon, A. L.,(1997). Psychobiology. In J. Haber, B. Krainovich-Miller, A. L. McMahon, & P. Price Hoskins, (Eds.), *Comprehensive psychiatric nursing* (pp. 219-238). St. Louis: Mosby.

Hattie, J. (1991). *Self-concept.* Hillsdale, NJ: Lawrence Erlbaum Associates.

Helm, P. (1991). Family therapy. In G. W. Stuart & S. J. Sundeen (Eds.), *Principles and practice of psychiatric nursing* (pp. 827–851). St. Louis: Mosby.

Horney, K. (1945). *Our inner conflicts: A constructive theory of neurosis.* NY: W. W. Norton & Company.

Kerr, M., & Bowen, M. (1988). *Family evaluation: An approach based on Bowen's Theory.* NY: W. W. Norton.

Kohlberg, L. (1984). *The psychology of moral development.* San Francisco: Harper & Row.

Leininger, M. (1991). *Culture care diversity and universality: A theory of nursing.* NY: National League for Nursing Press.

Madanes, C. (1981). *Strategic family therapy.* San Francisco: Jossey Bass Publishers.

Maslow, A. H. (1987). *Motivation and personality* (2nd. ed.). NY: Harper & Row.

Meleis, A. I. (1985). *Theoretical nursing: Development and progress.* Philadelphia: J. B. Lippincott.

Minuchin, S., & Nichols, M. (1993). *Family healing.* NY: The Free Press.

Monat, A., & Lazarus, R. S. (1991). *Stress and coping.* New York: Columbia University Press.

Moreno, J. L. (1946). *Psychodrama: Volume I.* Boston, MA: Beacon Press.

Perls, F. S., Hefferline, R. F., & Goodman, P. (1977). *Gestalt therapy.* NY: Bantam Books.

Piaget, J. (1967). *The child's conception of the world.* London: Routledge & Kegan Paul Ltd.

Polit, D. F., & Hungler, B. P. (1991). *Nursing research principles and methods.* Philadelphia: J. B. Lippincott.

Pulaski, M. A. (1971). *Understanding Piaget.* NY: Harper & Row.

Riehl, J. P., & Roy, S. C. (1980). *Conceptual models for nursing practice* (2nd ed.). NY: Appleton-Century Crofts.

Rogers, C. (1961). *On becoming a person.* Boston: Houghton Mifflin.

Rogers, M. (1983). *The theoretical basis of nursing.* Philadelphia: F. A. Davis.

Sanford, M. (1995). Concepts of psychiatric care: Therapeutic models. In D. Antai-Otong (Ed.), Psychiatric nursing: Biological & behavioral concepts (pp. 17-45). Philadelphia: W. B. Saunders.

Satir, V. (1967). *Conjoint family therapy* (Rev. ed.). NY: Science and Behavior Books.

Schultz, D. (1987) *Theories of personality.* Monterey, CA: Brooks/Cole.

Scroggs, J. R. (1985). *Key ideas in personality theory.* NY: West Publishing Company.

Skinner, B. F. (1974). *About behaviorism.* NY: Alfred A. Knopf.

Stuart, G. W., & Sundeen, S. J. (1991). *Principles and practice of psychiatric nursing.* St. Louis: C. V. Mosby.

Sullivan, H. S. (1953). *The interpersonal theory of psychiatry* NY: W. W. Norton.

Van Servellen, G. M. (1984). *Group and family therapy.* St. Louis: C. V. Mosby.

Von Bertalanffy, L. V. (1934). *Modern theories of development: An introduction to theoretical biology.* London: Oxford University Press.

Whiting, S. A. (1997). Development of the person. In B. S. Johnson (Ed.), *Psychiatric and mental health nursing: Adaptation and growth* (pp.357-373). Philadelphia: J. B. Lippinicott.

Wilson, H. S., & Kneisl, C. R. (1992). *Psychiatric nursing* (4th ed.). Menlo Park, CA: Addison-Wesley.

Wolpe, J. (1969). *The practice of behavior therapy.* New York: Pergammon Press.

Yalom, I. D. (1983). *Inpatient group psychotherapy.* NY: Basic Books.

Yalom, I. D. (1985). *Theory and practice of group psychotherapy* (3rd ed.). NY: Basic Books.

Zuckerman, M. (1991). *Psychobiology of personality.* NY: Cambridge University Press.

Mental Disorders Due to Substance Abuse

Therese K. Killeen

Psychoactive Substance Use Disorders

- Definition

    1. A primary, chronic disease with genetic, psychosocial, and environmental factors influencing its development and manifestations

    2. Progressive and fatal

    3. Characterized by continuous or periodic:

        a. Impaired control over substance use

        b. Preoccupation with the drug

        c. Use of the drug despite adverse consequences

        d. Distortions in thinking, most notably denial (ASAM/NCAdd committee,1990)

    4. Recent results from the 1995 National Household Survey on Drug Abuse found that 6.1% of the population 12 years or older reported past month illicit drug use. About 15.8% of the population 12 years and older engaged in past month binge drinking (5 or more drinks on one occasion) and 5.5% of the population 12 years and older reported past month heavy drinking (5 or more drinks on the same occasion on at least 5 days). Rates of illicit drug use in the 12 to 17 age group has increased between 1994 and 1995 (cocaine, 0.3% to 0.8%; hallucinogens, 1.1% to 1.7%; marijuana, 6% to 8.2%). In addition, the rate of new users of alcohol in 12 to 17 year olds has increased from 125 per 1000 person years in 1991 to 172 in 1993.

- Signs and Symptoms

    1. Criteria established by the Diagnostic and Statistical Manual for Mental Disorders (DSM-IV) for psychoactive substance **dependence** include the occurrence of at least three of the following within the same 12-month period (American Psychiatric Association, 1994):

        a. Use of amounts greater than intended

        b. Attempts at control

        c. Excessive time spent in obtaining, using, recovering

        d. Use despite social obligations or hazards

        e. Use despite recurrent problems

      f.   Presence of *tolerance*—needing increasing amounts of substance to produce desired effect or markedly diminished effect with continued use of same amount of substance

      g.   Presence of *withdrawal* or use to avoid or relieve withdrawal symptoms—pathophysiological state of disequilibrium brought on by an abrupt discontinuation, or rapid decrease in, dosage of a psychoactive substance

  2. Criteria for psychoactive substance abuse (PSA) include:

      a.   Recurrent use resulting in a failure to fulfill major role obligations

      b.   Continued use despite having persistent or recurrent social or interpersonal problems caused or exacerbated by the effects of the substance

      c.   Recurrent use in hazardous situations

      d.   Recurrent substance-related legal problems

  3. Psychoactive substances with abuse potential include: alcohol, sedative/hypnotics, amphetamines, cocaine, cannabis, hallucinogens, narcotics, phencyclidine, inhalants, caffeine, nicotine.

- Differential Diagnosis

  1. DSM IV Disorders with similar symptoms/presentations

      a.   Mood/Depressive Disorders

      b.   Anxiety

      c.   Psychotic Disorders

      d.   Personality Disorders

      e.   Impulse Control Disorders

      f.   Adjustment Disorders

      g.   Sleep Disorders

      h.   Sexual Dysfunction Disorders

      i.   Amnesia, Dementia and Delirium Disorders

  2. Evidence that symptoms are better accounted for by a disorder that is not substance induced include:

      a.   Symptoms precede onset of the substance abuse/dependence

    b. Symptoms persist for a substantial period of time after the cessation of acute withdrawal or severe intoxication

    c. Symptoms substantially in excess of what would be expected given the character, duration or amount of the substance used

    d. Other evidence suggesting the existence of an independent non-substance induced disorder (history of recurrent non-substance related episodes)

- Diagnostic Studies/Tests

    1. Common laboratory values associated with Substance Use Disorders (SUD)

        a. Liver enzymes increased in alcohol dependence—gamma-glutamyltransferase (GGT), aspartate aminotransferase (AST) and alanine aminotransferase (ALT). Other increased values include mean corpuscular volume (MCV), high density lipoprotein cholesterol and carbohydrate deficient transferrin (CDT).

        b. Breathalyzer—represents blood alcohol concentration (BAC); legal intoxification level is 0.1% (100 mg/100 ml); levels above 0.1% without associated behavioral symptoms indicate possible tolerance

    2. Screening Instruments

        a. CAGE questionnaire

        b. Self Administered Alcohol Screening Test (SAAST)

        c. Brief Drug Abuse Screening Test (B-DAST)

        d. Addiction Severity Index (ASI)

    3. Urine drug screening (UDS) detects presence of drug in the urine—diagnostic limitations include:

        a. Short "window" of detection of metabolites

        b. Intermittent use patterns of abusers

        c. Issues of civil liberties

- Assessment—involves careful interview skills, focused on presenting symptoms and problems in major areas of functioning; interview is goal directed, adapted to age and ethnic culture of client, and client's current cognitive ability

1. Interview

   a. Drug and/or drink of choice—include amount, frequency of use, duration of use, route of administration, time and amount of last use

   b. Other substances used

   c. Past history of and response to withdrawal

   d. History of delirium tremens, seizures, falls , blackouts or alcoholic amnesia, injury to self or others

   e. Changes in mood and behavior (anger, apathy, anxiety, depression, labile mood, irritable, low or high energy, impulsivity, isolation, change in peer group, secretive, guardedness or paranoia)

   f. Sleep pattern and eating habits

   g. Problems with interpersonal and social relationships, finances, occupation, school, family, legal system, medical disorders, psychiatric disorders

   h. Family history of alcohol, drug and/or psychiatric illness

   i. Access and availability of substances

   j. Context of substance use (solitary vs. social consumption)

   k. Previous treatments and longest periods of sobriety

   l. Presence of defense mechanisms such as denial, minimization and rationalization warrants collateral interview from family members or significant others

   m. Assess motivation and stage of change (Prochaska, DiClemente & Norcross, 1992)

      (1) Precontemplation—personal realization and decreased defensiveness and rationalization through social pressure, dramatic experience, media, consequences and social norms

      (2) Contemplation—shifting decisional balance, making a commitment to a change attempt and resolving ambivalence

      (3) Preparation—commitment, plan and concrete strategies

(4) Action—daily implementation of plan, coping with withdrawal and desire to use, behavioral coping activities

(5) Maintenance—lifestyle changes, shifts in social network, behavioral coping activities

2. Physical and mental status examination—system by system assessment for presence and stage of physical withdrawal as well as medical complications

a. Vital signs

b. Urine/blood drug screens, breathalyzer

c. Assess for trauma—broken bones, bruises, lacerations, edema

d. Assess for dehydration and malnutrition, weight loss

e. Assess for masses and lesions

f. Evaluate respiratory, cardiac and gastrointestinal status

g. Evaluate neurologic status

(1) Orientation to time, place, person, date, day of the week

(2) Assess cognitive functioning for confusion or delirium, concentration and attention, recent and remote memory, abstract reasoning, problem solving ability, thought disturbances and sensory perceptual distortions

(3) Pupil size

(4) Check reflexes for hyperreflexia

(5) Assess for numbness and tingling in extremities

- Medical Complications associated with SUD

1. Hepatic Complications—alcoholic fatty liver, alcoholic hepatitis, alcoholic cirrhosis

2. Gastrointestinal Complications—esophagitis, gastritis, pancreatitis associated with alcohol

3. Cardiovascular Complications—cardiomyopathy, hypertension, arrhythmias associated with alcohol and cocaine

4. Neurological Complications

a. Stroke, seizures associated with alcohol and cocaine

b. Polyneuropathy, alcoholic dementia, Wernicke-Korsakoff Syndrome (thiamine deficiency) associated with alcohol

5. Nutritional complications—vitamin and iron deficiency, malnutrition associated with alcohol

6. Pulmonary damage associated with smoking crack, cannabis and nicotine

7. Infectious disease—increased chance of hepatitis, HIV, sexually transmitted diseases, cellulitis, endocarditis associated with high risk addiction behaviors

   a. Unprotected sexual promiscuity and prostitution

   b. Intravenous route of administration

8. Obstetrical complications

   a. Noncompliance with prenatal care is associated with SUD in pregnancy

   b. Premature labor and delivery, spontaneous abortion, abruptio placenta associated with cocaine and crack addiction

   c. Hypertension, spontaneous abortion, abruptio placenta, premature delivery and postpartum hemorrhage associated with heroin addiction

   d. Miscarriage and spontaneous abortion associated with alcohol

   e. Earlier menopause, osteoporosis, reduced fertility and increased risk of strokes when taking oral contraceptives associated with tobacco addiction; spontaneous abortion, unexplained vaginal bleeding, abruptio placenta and placenta previa associated with tobacco addiction

9. Teratogenic complications

   a. Low birth weight, prematurity, small head circumference, anomalies associated with cocaine, cannabis, nicotine

   b. Neonatal abstinence syndrome related to withdrawal from narcotics occurs anytime between birth to the sixth day of life

      (1) Irritability, shrill or persistent cry, inability to self-regulate state, more sensitive to external stimuli, sleep-wake pattern disturbance

(2) Disturbed feeding problems, gastrointestinal disturbances such as vomiting and diarrhea, respiratory depression and hypoxia

(3) Frequent yawning, nasal flaring and sneezing

(4) Jitteriness, increased muscle tone, tremors, depressed normal neurological reflexes, temperature instability, seizures

   c. Fetal alcohol syndrome (FAS) characterized by:

(1) Growth retardation

(2) Central nervous involvement—developmental delay, neurological or intellectual impairment

(3) Facial dysmorphology

- Mental status variations and clinical manifestations

   1. Acute alcohol, sedative/hypnotic intoxication

     a. Disinhibition and increased confidence

     b. Slurred speech

     c. Impaired insight, judgement and memory

     d. Decreased concentration

     e. Altered motor skills and sensory perception

     f. Mood swings

   2. Acute cocaine/crack (stimulant) intoxication—crack cocaine became popular around 1985. Cocaine hydrochloride powder is converted into crack by cooking it with an alkaloid such as baking soda and water in a procedure known as "freebasing." After heat drying, a hard substance is formed that can be broken down into "rocks" for smoking. It is a much more potent form of cocaine that produces an intense, immediate, euphoric high that lasts about 5 minutes. This rapid absorption, along with crack's inexpense and availability, increase its abuse liability and dependence potential. It has become a drug of choice for lower socioeconomic, inner city populations and is associated with crime, poverty, child neglect and homelessness.

     a. Euphoria

     b. Grandiosity

    c.   Psychomotor agitation

    d.   Hypervigilance

    e.   Impaired judgement

    f.   Elevated blood pressure, tachycardia

    g.   Visual/tactile hallucinations

3. Marijuana intoxication

    a.   Excitement and dissociation of ideas

    b.   Distortions of time and space

    c.   Diminished attention span and memory

    d.   Deterioration of motor skills

    e.   Increased appetite

    f.   Dry mouth

    g.   Tachycardia

4. Acute hallucinogen intoxication—''tripping''

    a.   Anxiety and feeling loss of control

    b.   Paranoid ideation/suspiciousness

    c.   Delusions and hallucinations

    d.   Confusion and delirium

    e.   Distortion of time, place, distance

    f.   Impaired judgement

5. Acute narcotic intoxication

    a.   Euphoria and sense of well being

    b.   Analgesia, sedation and somnolence

    c.   Lethargy and apathy

    d.   Pupillary constriction

    e.   Decreased respirations and hypotension

6. Alcohol withdrawal syndrome—usually appears 6 hours after a substantial fall in blood alcohol concentration, peaks at about 24-36 hours and subsides after 48 hours

    a. Tremulousness

    b. Malaise

    c. Anorexia, nausea, vomiting

    d. Hyperreflexia

    e. Tachycardia, increased blood pressure

    f. Irritability

    g. Insomnia

    h. Diaphoresis

    i. Perceptual distortions

    j. Possible seizures

7. Delirium tremens (5% incidence) most severe manifestation of alcohol withdrawal; onset between 72-96 hours after cessation of drinking

    a. Gross tremors and agitation

    b. Disorientation

    c. Confusion

    d. Hallucinations

    e. Hyperpyrexia

    f. Increased psychomotor and autonomic nervous system activity

    g. Seizures

8. Cocaine/Crack (stimulant) withdrawal—variable due to typical binge pattern of abuse but symptoms can occur 9 to 96 hours after last use

    a. Fatigue

    b. Depression

    c. Insomnia/hypersomnia

    d. Psychomotor agitation

    e. Intense cravings or desire to use

9. Narcotic withdrawal—onset depends on drug's half life and chronicity of use, peaks between 36-72 hours, subsides by 5-8 days

    a.   Anorexia

    b.   Stomach cramps and diarrhea

    c.   Lacrimation and rhinorrhea

    d.   Muscle aches

    e.   Mild elevations in temperature, respiratory rate, pulse and blood pressure

    f.   Profuse sweating

    g.   Insomnia

    h.   Irritability and restlessness

10.   Sedative hypnotics/benzodiazepines withdrawal—onset with short acting drugs 12 to 24 hours, long acting drugs 5 to 8 days

    a.   Seizures

    b.   Insomnia and nightmares

    c.   Nausea and vomiting

    d.   Confusion, delirium, memory problems, hallucinations (tactile)

    e.   Restlessness, anxiety, tremors, diaphoresis, hyperpyrexia, muscle spasms

    f.   Tachycardia, palpitations

11.   Nicotine withdrawal—peak onset in 24 hours

    a.   Irritability, anxiety, restlessness, short attention span, diaphoresis

    b.   Depression, fatigue, sleep problems

    c.   Lightheadedness, hunger, tightness in chest, tingling in limbs

12.   Dual diagnosis—concomitant existence of a substance use and psychiatric disorder; many co-occurring psychiatric symptoms remit with 2 to 4 weeks abstinence from substances; the most common co-occurring psychiatric disorders include antisocial personality, affective and anxiety disorders

- Nursing diagnosis—see Table 1

Table 1
Multidimensional Assessment

Medical Problem Areas	Nursing Diagnosis
I. Intoxification/withdrawal	Comfort, alteration in Injury, potential for Violence, potential for
II. Biochemical conditions/ complications	Health maintenance alteration Tissue integrity, impaired Nutrition, alteration in Sleep pattern disturbance Infection, potential for
III. Emotional/behavioral conditions/complications	Anxiety Coping, ineffective individual Thought processes, altered Sensory-perceptual alterations Self-esteem disturbance Social interaction, impaired Impaired communication Personal identity disturbance Powerlessness Anticipatory grieving
IV. Treatment acceptance/ resistance	Denial, ineffective Fear Knowledge deficit Non-compliance
V. Relapse potential	Adjustment, impaired Decisional conflict Diversional activity, altered Role performance, altered Spiritual distress
VI. Recovery environment	Coping, ineffective family Home maintenance, altered Altered parenting

- Genetic/biological origins

    1. Children of alcoholics are three to four times more likely to experience alcohol and/or drug problems; family history positive individuals have less sensitivity to effects of alcohol (high tolerance)

    2. Certain individuals have a genetic inactivity of enzyme, aldehyde dehydrogenase, which results in a build up of toxic alcohol metabolite,

acetaldehyde, causing symptoms of flushing, headaches, tachycardia and discomfort.

3. Chemical imbalance in neurotransmitter levels leads to self medication with substances of abuse in an attempt to correct imbalance; pharmacotherapy interventions act on depleted neurotransmitter levels

- Biochemical interventions—act on depleted neurotransmitter systems (serotonin, dopamine, opiate, (GABA)

    1. Agents to treat withdrawal (detoxification)

        a. Alcohol, sedative/hypnotics

            (1) Benzodiazepines—short acting lorazepam (ativan) 1 to 3 mg or oxazepam (serax) 15 to 60 mg every 6 hours initially with dosage tapered on subsequent days (15% to 25% per day); adverse effects include memory disruption, lethargy, motor impairment, disinhibition and high abuse potential

            (2) Carbamazepine (tegretol) 200 to 1000 mg daily—anticonvulsant that has an antikindling effect, (kindling occurs when repeated subthreshold stimulation to the brain raises the seizure threshold); inadequately treated withdrawals could have a cumulative effect, thereby producing future withdrawals of increased severity

            (3) Clonidine (catapres)—an alpha adrenergic agonist and propranolol (inderal), a beta adrenergic blocker decreases hyperactivity of the sympathetic nervous system (decreases blood pressure, tachycardia, diaphoresis and tremors); both drugs are nonaddicting and do not cause as much sedation and mental clouding; do not block the development of seizures or delirium

        b. Opiates/Narcotics

            (1) Clonidine—0.1 mg to 0.3 mg tid sublingual or transdermal patch 0.4 to 0.6 per day reduces excessive noradrenergic activity in the locus ceruleus of the brain; has no effect on craving, insomnia or muscle aches or pains; adverse effects include hypotension, sedation, dry mouth and dizziness

        (2)   Buprenorphine—4 to 8 mg per day, opioid partial ago-
nist antagonist, reduces heroin craving, use of opiates
and other illicit drugs such as cocaine thereby retaining
clients in treatment longer; adverse effects include constipation and symptoms of opiate withdrawal

2.   Agents to decrease craving—used with psychosocial therapy

   a.   Alcohol

      (1)   Naltrexone (ReVia) 50 mg per day—opioid antagonist
reduces the reinforcement value of alcohol by decreasing the activity of the opioid system which is activated
by alcohol; side effects include increased liver enzymes,
nausea, abdominal distress, joint and muscle pain, early
insomnia and anxiety

   b.   Cocaine/Crack

      (1)   Bromocriptine—2.5-10 mg daily, amantadine 200-400
mg daily, pergolide 1 mg tid, dopamine agonists are
more effective in acute phases of treatment replenishing
the depleted neurotransmitter, dopamine; side effects include dizziness, lightheadedness, headache, nausea, GI
distress dyskinesia, somnolence and orthostatic hypotension

      (2)   Carbamazepine—200 to 1000 mg daily blocks the devel-
opment of cocaine-induced kindling and dopamine receptor sensitivity caused by chronic cocaine use; adverse effects include initial sedation, dizziness, nausea and
vomiting, hepatotoxicity, agranulocytosis, platelet dysfunction, thrombocytopenia, hand tremor and ataxia at
high doses

      (3)   Desipramine—tricyclic antidepressant, 2.5 mg per kg
daily to reverse the cocaine induced-neurochemical damage associated with anhedonia and depression; adverse
effects include cardiac toxicity, arrhythmias, insomnia,
anxiety, dry mouth, blurred vision, constipation, urinary
retention, nausea and vomiting; additive cardiotoxicity
when taken with cocaine; delayed onset of action is a
drawback

3.   Maintenance Agents—used with psychosocial therapies

    a.   Opioids/Narcotics

        (1)   Methadone—opioid agonist, 40 to 120 mg decreases high risk behaviors associated with heroin use (criminal activity, prostitution, IV drug use); adverse effects include sweating, constipation, nervousness, insomnia, decreased sex drive, difficult ejaculation and low grade opioid withdrawal

        (2)   L-Alpha-Acetylmethadol (LAAM)—longer acting opioid agonist, 80 to 90 mg three times a week

        (3)   Buprenorphine—partial opioid agonist, 4 to 8 mg per day block narcotic effects

4.   Agents to decrease consumption—used with psychosocial therapies

    a.   Alcohol

        (1)   Disulfiram (antabuse)—aversive or alcohol-sensitizing agent, 250 to 500 mg daily interferes with the metabolism of alcohol, producing unpleasant side effects when mixed with alcohol; symptoms include facial flushing, heart palpitations, increased heart rate, dyspnea, nausea, vomiting and decreased blood pressure; clients should be instructed to avoid over-the-counter cough medicines, aftershave lotions, vinegar, mouthwashes, non-alcoholic beer (contains small amount of alcohol) and food cooked with alcohol while taking this drug and for 14 days after drug has been discontinued

    b.   Cocaine/Crack

        (1)   Cocaine vaccine—antibodies that attach to cocaine molecules creating a combined substance that is too large to pass through the blood brain barrier; blunts the effects of cocaine; human trials planned in the near future

    c.   Opioids/Narcotics

        (1)   Naltrexone—50 mg daily or three doses weekly of 100 mg on Monday and Wednesday and 150 mg on Friday will block the euphoric effects

5.   Agents to treat protracted abstinence—continued unpleasant state of low grade withdrawal; includes sleep disruption, anhedonia, anergia, irritability, nervousness, restlessness, conditioned cravings

    a.   5HT reuptake inhibitors—fluoxetine, sertraline, citalopram

      b.   Tricyclic antidepressants—imipramine, desipramine

- Interpersonal Origins

    1.   Psychodynamic Theory

        a.   Substance use is an adaptive attempt to cope with, or compensate for psychological deficits such as dysregulation of affect, poor object relations, internal conflicts and impaired judgement and self care.

        b.   Substance abuse is a response to an underlying internal conflict. This conflict is between an internal need and an external limitation.

        c.   Use of substances to avoid feelings of anxiety, anger, shame, depression, low self esteem

        d.   Use of immature, rigid defense mechanisms such as denial, dependency, regression, displacement and depression accompany substance addiction

        e.   Psychological dysfunctions are often the consequence of substance rather than the cause.

    2.   Social Learning Theory views addiction as the result of maladaptive coping skills.

        a.   Personal experience and past learning

        b.   Situational antecedents

        c.   Biological make-up

        d.   Cognitive processes

        e.   Reinforcement contingencies

- Psychotherapeutic interventions

    1.   Interventions linked to Psychodynamic theory include:

        a.   Promote identification as a "recovering" person

        b.   Foster expression of honest feelings and reinforce efforts to cope in more appropriate ways

        c.   Help client explore, accept and own both positive and negative aspects of self

        d.   Help client identify aspects of self that he/she would like to change

e. Help client regain a feeling of empowerment by pointing out the choices he/she has available

f. Help clients recognize and focus on strengths and accomplishments

g. Confront and explore defense mechanisms such as denial, minimization dependency, regression, projection and displacement

h. Establish parameters such as structure and clear boundaries

2. Interventions linked to Social Learning theory consists of cognitive-behavioral/relapse prevention and behavioral therapies; goals of treatment are to facilitate changes in personal habits and lifestyle so that clients may anticipate and cope with problems and high risk situations; most common high risk situations associated with 75% of relapses include negative emotional states, interpersonal conflict and social pressure

   a. Identify high risk people, places, situations

   b. Identify negative emotions—boredom, loneliness, depression, anxiety, anger, guilt, shame, self-depreciation

   c. Monitor thinking associated with feelings

   d. Plan in advance successful avoidance and coping strategies

   e. Use slips, lapses and relapses as corrective learning experiences not as treatment failures

3. Family Theory

   a. Identifies substance abuse as the presenting symptom of an underlying family system dysfunction (Bowen, 1978). Families are undifferentiated. Members cannot act independently of the whole. Family system is highly stressed and basic nurturing needs are unmet. There is suppression and denial of emotional expression. Communication is indirect, inconsistent and conflictual. Boundaries are weak and constantly changing. Families accommodate to the addiction, thus "enabling" or making it easier for the addicted member to continue using.

   b. Substance abuse is the central theme around which family life is organized. Family rituals and routines, interactional patterns and problem solving revolve around the addict (Steinglass et al. 1987).

     c. Codependency is a condition afflicting the significant other that is characterized by preoccupation, dependency on and obsession with the addicted individual. Codependent individuals are often adult children of alcoholics (ACOA) and/or share similar characteristics.

          (1) Low self esteem and loss of identity

          (2) Seeking external sources of fulfillment

          (3) Need for approval from others

          (4) Fear of abandonment

          (5) Inability to express anger

          (6) Possible behavior that is controlling, rigid, perfectionistic and overresponsible

          (7) Meeting others' needs at the expense of their own needs

4. Strategies in family therapy

    a. Assess the family system—level of denial, level of education and insight—use genogram

    b. Look for strengths to reinforce

    c. Discourage blaming members

    d. Educate family about chemical dependency and refer to AL-ANON / AL-ATEEN for support

    e. Assist with the process of emotional separation and reactiveness to the substance abuse behavior

    f. Model effective communication and attitudes

    g. Support/reinforce healthy change

5. Disease Model

    a. Substance abuse is a medical and spiritual disease

    b. There is a biomedical internal causation for chemical dependency that prevents certain individuals from being able to control and predict their drinking in a consistent manner.

    c. Bio-psycho-social-spiritual maintenance model asserts that excessive alcohol and other drug use leads to profound biological, social, psychological and spiritual, negative consequences. The distress associated with these multidimensional negative consequences leads to further excessive alcohol and drug use. Thus, a vicious addiction cycle develops that maintains the problematic alcohol and drug use.

6. Sociocultural Theories include factors such as ethnic use patterns, religious beliefs and rituals, gender issues and peer pressure as influencing alcohol and drug use.

7. Nursing Light Model developed by Marcia Anderson to assist clients to improve their well being and deliberately change their drug use and associated high risk behavior; uses Martha Rogers Science of Unitary Human Beings in which illness is viewed as a result of an interaction in the human-environmental fields.

    a. Interventions linked to Nursing Light Model

        (1) Nurse develops an understanding of client's perspective throughout the continuum of the nursing process.

        (2) Nurse and client knowingly participate in the continuous process of innovative change.

        (3) See Table 2 for model of interventions

Table 2—Nursing Light Model

Personalized care actions implemented by Nurse	Personalized action implemented by client
Love the client	Love yourself
Intend to help	Identify a concern
Give care gently	Give yourself a goal
Help the client improve well-being	Have confidence and help self
Teach the process	Take positive action

- Group interventions—used more frequently in substance abuse treatment Advantages include:

    1. Peer support and confrontation

    2. Reflection on family of origin issues

    3. Place to practice newly learned interpersonal skills

    4. Specific groups include:

        a. Psychoeducational groups—didactic lectures and discussions on such topics as the disease concept of addiction, the addictive cycle, biopsychosocial consequences of substance abuse, dual diagnosis, relapse prevention, communication skills, assertiveness and relaxation

b. Self help groups

(1) Grounded in the conception that substance abuse is a medical and spiritual disease. The belief is that there is an internal causation for chemical dependency beyond the individual's control.

(2) Groups offer support and mutual sharing. The group is open to all who share the common goal of recovery from a variety of substances and conditions.

(3) The twelve steps provide the roadmap one must follow to reach recovery.

(a) Admitting powerlessness and unmanageability of life

(b) Greater power to restore sanity

(c) Turn life and will over to God

(d) Take a moral inventory

(e) Admitting nature of wrongs

(f) Ready to have God remove character defects

(g) Ask God to remove shortcomings

(h) Make a list of people harmed and willingness to make amends

(i) Make amends

(j) Continue personal inventory

(k) Improve conscious contact with God

(l) Carry message of spiritual awakening to other alcoholics

(4) Critics of the twelve steps believe this approach is not appropriate for everyone and complain about the reference to God. Proponents endorse a broader, more spiritual versus religious definition of God or Higher Power.

- Milieu interventions—based on staff providing a safe, corrective environment that enhances the development of more adaptive coping skills and interpersonal behaviors

  1. Management of withdrawal—detoxification occurs in the early phase of recovery and involves safely tapering off substance of abuse, thereby minimizing the physical discomfort associated with withdrawal

      a. Monitor vital signs and severity of withdrawal (see symptoms associated with specific drugs) and medicate as ordered. Use Clinical Instrument for Withdrawal from Alcohol (CIWA) to measure both objective and subjective symptoms of withdrawal. This enables the nurse to more accurately and safely quantify the amount of detoxification medication that is administered.

      b. Assess and monitor level of consciousness, orientation, thought processes and sensory perceptual alterations

      c. Assess for tremulousness and agitation

      d. Provide a quiet, dimly lit environment with low stimulation

      e. Implement fall precautions

      f. Implement seizure precautions for alcohol, benzodiazepines and sedative/hypnotics

      g. Provide nutritional support—administer vitamin and mineral supplements as ordered; alleviate gastrointestinal distress

      h. Maintain hydration—monitor intake and output, assess water loss from diaphoresis

      i. Implement measures to help client sleep and relax; stress management, breathing retraining, progressive muscle tension relaxation, yoga, meditation, acupuncture, therapeutic touch

      j. Convey acceptance and reassurance

      k. Re-orient when indicated

  2. Psychosocial supportive measures during rehabilitative phase of recovery

      a. Formulate treatment goals and expected outcomes with patient

      b. Role model self-acceptance, assertiveness and responsibility

    c. Maintain consistency in care—requires a high degree of communication among staff

    d. Confront in an empathetic, respectful manner, always focusing on the dysfunctional behavior and not the individual

    e. Identify and work through countertransference issues

    f. Provide structure—use daily activity schedule.

    g. Use of self disclosure only when appropriate and in the context of therapy

    h. Use of behavioral contracts with contingencies

        (1) Reinforce compliance and achievement

        (2) Administer consequences for noncompliance

    i. Provide on the spot conflict management

    j. Assist with task assignments and homework

    k. Use rehearsal and role playing of newly learned skills

3. Clinical nurse specialist interventions

    a. Theory based psychotherapy—individual, group, family

    b. Evaluation, treatment recommendation and appropriate referral

    c. Consultant as an expert in the field of chemical dependency

    d. Staff support and management functions

    e. Interventions for the patient presenting with complex problems

    f. Staff education and supervision

    g. Preventative functions—community awareness and education

    h. Research functions—Participate and/or initiate protocols that may improve future interventions and care of the substance abusing population

    i. Professional development—committee memberships, publications, presentations, learning opportunities

    j. Medication evaluation and monitoring if clinical nurse specialist granted prescriptive authority

4. Community resources

    a. Self-help support group meetings

(1) Alcoholic Anonymous (AA)

(2) Narcotic Anonymous (NA)

(3) Cocaine Anonymous (CA)

(4) Secular Organizations for Sobriety (SOS); geared more toward individuals with agnostic view of spirituality

(5) AL-ANON, NAR-ANON and AL-ATEEN—Family/significant others and teenagers living with or involved with a substance abuser

(6) Adult Children of Alcoholics (ACOA)

b. Prevention groups—special interest groups developed for community awareness and education, public policy making, introducing and changing legislation related to alcohol and substance use

(1) Drug Abuse Readiness Education (DARE)

(2) Mothers Against Drunk Drivers (MADD)

(3) "Just say no" campaign

(4) "Hugs not drugs" campaign

- Impaired nurses—Cahill (1992) and colleagues estimate 7% of registered nurses abuse substances; nurses are at higher risk due to:

1. Accessibility to drugs and addictive substances

2. Mistaken belief that health professionals can "self medicate safely"

3. Role strain and work stress (long working hours, physical and emotional exhaustion)

4. Treatment approaches include:

a. Intervention—structured method of penetrating the delusional system of chemically dependent persons for the purpose of facilitating insight into the addictive problem and entry into treatment.

(1) Use team approach, nonpunitive attitude; 2 -10 professional associates of impaired colleague who share a nonjudgemental attitude (to include one recovering peer and one with experience in chemical dependency if possible)

    (2)   Present documented evidence, always prefacing testimony with positive remarks

    (3)   Give impaired nurse a chance to respond

    (4)   State available options and allow an opportunity for voluntary entry into treatment

        (a)   Diversion programs—facilitate re-entry into practice without licensure sanctions

        (b)   Regulatory legal action—nurse reported to the state board for suspected chemical dependency is dealt with under the Nurse Practice Act and the Administrative Procedure Act

        (c)   Criminal legal action—nurse who diverts a control substance from a facility or obtains a controlled substance by fraud is in violation of the Controlled Substance Act

    (5)   Make arrangements to monitor progress

b.   Specialized inpatient program, AA and/or NA meetings for health care professionals

c.   Employee assistance programs

d.   Peer assistance support from state and district associations

e.   Re-entry back into the workplace

    (1)   Restrictions on handling medications for a certain period of time

    (2)   Urine drug screening

    (3)   Regular documented attendance for outpatient treatment and AA/NA meetings

    (4)   Stable work shifts (minimal shift work)

    (5)   Clear job performance expectations with supervision and regular evaluations.

QUESTIONS

1. Ms. P presents to the community substance abuse center for an evaluation. She states that she does not have a substance abuse problem but agreed to the evaluation at her husband's insistence. The appropriate initial statement would be:

    a. Do you drink often?
    b. Your husband is concerned about your drinking?
    c. What makes you think that you do not have a drinking problem?
    d. How much do you drink?

2. According to Prochaska and DiClemente, at what stage of change would Ms. P be in?

    a. Contemplation
    b. Action
    c. Denial
    d. Precontemplation

3. Mr. C, a 40 year old male with a diagnosis of alcohol dependence, is admitted to the inpatient unit for detoxification. Which of the following measures would NOT be implemented at this time?

    a. Monitor vital signs
    b. Provide quiet, dimly lit atmosphere
    c. Confront denial
    d. Encourage fluids by mouth

4. Mr. C. completes detoxification and rehabilitation and is discharged on Disulfiram (antabuse) 250 mg to be taken every morning. Which of the following substances can Mr. C continue to take?

    a. Mouthwash
    b. Cough elixirs
    c. Non-alcoholic beer
    d. Antidepressant medication

5. When assessing whether or not a patient has a problem with alcohol or drugs, which criteria is the best indicator:

    a. How much a person uses
    b. How often a person uses
    c. The level of interference with physical, emotional and social functioning
    d. Positive laboratory findings

6. Which of the following is NOT a sign of delirium tremens?

   a. Confusion
   b. Tactile hallucinations
   c. Seizures
   d. Stroke

7. Ms. D is admitted to the emergency room with suicidal ideations. Urine drug screen reveals the presence of cocaine in the urine. When questioned with this finding Ms. D denies any use of cocaine. The most appropriate nursing response would be:

   a. "This test is very accurate, Ms. D, you must not be telling the truth."
   b. "You are depressed because you have used cocaine."
   c. "Were you in a room with other people who were smoking crack."
   d. "Have you ever used drugs in the past."

8. Which of the following questions would NOT be important in assessing potential withdrawal from alcohol?

   a. When was your last drink and how much did you consume?
   b. Have you experienced any 'blackouts'?
   c. During the last month, what is the longest period of time that you have gone without alcohol?
   d. Do you experience any physical discomfort when you go without alcohol for a few hours or a few days?

9. Mr. G , a 50 year old chronic alcoholic, ia recently admitted to the inpatient unit. It has been 48 hours since his last drink. Mr. G states that he feels strange and everything around him seems unreal. The nurse notices that Mr. G has scratches on both arms. The nurse should suspect:

   a. Drug seeking behavior
   b. Onset of psychosis
   c. Onset of delirium tremens
   d. Wernicke-Korsakoff syndrome

10. Which laboratory value is NOT necessarily altered by alcoholism?

   a. Aspartate aminotransferase (AST)
   b. Gamma-glutamyltransferase (GGT)
   c. Mean corpuscular value (MCV)
   d. White blood cell count (WBC)

11. Genetic studies in alcoholism support which of the following statements:

    a. Alcoholism is mostly influenced by environmental factors.
    b. Children of alcoholics are four times more likely to have problems with alcohol or drugs.
    c. There is no definitive research that links alcoholism to genetic etiology.
    d. If both parents have alcoholism there is a 75% chance that each child will have an alcohol or drug problem.

12. Mr. F is participating in a six week intensive outpatient substance abuse treatment program for his crack/cocaine addiction. During the third week of treatment he tests positive for cocaine in his urine. The most appropriate intervention would be to:

    a. Refer to inpatient treatment
    b. Dismiss from the Intensive outpatient program
    c. Meet with the patient individually to discuss the slip/relapse
    d. Confront the patient in group

13. Which of the following is NOT necessarily an alcohol-related medical complications?

    a. Arteriosclerosis
    b. Cardiomyopathy
    c. Cirrhosis of the liver
    d. Gastritis

14. There has been an increase in the number of infectious diseases associated with the current drug epidemic. Which of the following infectious diseases is NOT necessarily associated with addictive behavior?

    a. Sexually transmitted diseases
    b. HIV, AIDS
    c. Hepatitis
    d. Encephalitis

15. Nurse K is a nurse counselor working for a university. Ms. G is a 22 year old sophomore that has been referred to nurse K for an evaluation because of her declining grades and poor class attendance. What would be the most appropriate line of questioning for Ms. K to pursue?

    a. Your advisor tells me that you are doing poorly in school?
    b. Have you been spending more time partying than concentrating on your schoolwork?

   c. Can you tell me what has been happening around you that may be affecting your school work?

   d. Are you using any drugs?

16. Ms G continues to smoke marijuana and her school problems are getting worse. Your best intervention would be to:

   a. Call her parents and inform them of her drug use

   b. Tell her she will be expelled if she does not quit using

   c. Refer to substance treatment and monitor compliance and progress

   d. Do not intervene, as patient probably needs to suffer the consequences of her use

17. Which of the following medical complications is NOT necessarily associated with cocaine/crack abuse:

   a. Kidney failure

   b. Seizures

   c. Stroke

   d. Cardiac Arrhythmias

18. Sedative/hypnotics are cross-addicted with:

   a. Alcohol

   b. Opiates

   c. Stimulants

   d. Hallucinogens

19. Mr. L is a 50 year old male with a history of chronic back pain from a car injury that occurred 5 years ago. He has been taking Darvocet-N 100 over the past several years and reports taking up to 15 tablets a day. His medical doctor no longer feels comfortable giving Mr. L prescriptions for pain and refers him to substance abuse treatment. Mr. L is admitted to the inpatient unit for narcotic detoxification. He is very fearful that he will be denied pain medication and left to suffer. The most appropriate nursing intervention would be:

   a. Reassure Mr. L that his pain will be managed while his narcotic is being slowly tapered

   b. Explain to Mr. L that he is addicted to narcotics and must not use them anymore

   c. Explain to Mr. L that his pain threshold has been lowered due to his narcotic abuse and he will not need pain medication

   d. Tell Mr. L that he will have tylenol and aspirin available for pain management

20. Which of the following is NOT a symptom of opiate withdrawal?

    a. Muscle cramps
    b. Tachycardia
    c. Pupillary constriction
    d. Diarrhea

21. Which of the following nursing diagnoses would be the least appropriate for Mr. L 's plan of care?

    a. Injury, potential for
    b. Comfort, alteration in
    c. Self care deficit
    d. Knowledge deficit

22. The benefit of methadone maintenance over heroin use is that it:

    a. Serves as an anticraving agent
    b. Diminishes risky behavior associated with heroin use
    c. Is effective as a detoxification agent
    d. Has no adverse effects

23. Mr. T is a 37 year old male admitted for depression. When the nurse admitting Mr. T asked him about his alcohol use, he stated he had a couple of beers after work every day. He also said that his wife was threatening to leave him..
When Mrs. T came to the hospital to visit her husband, his primary nurse met with them together. Mrs. T stated that she was tired of putting Mr. T to bed every night and calling his job stating he was sick when he was really hungover. Mrs. T states that she also makes herself available at all times to pick up Mr. T if he has been out drinking. She states that she cares about her husband and does not want to see him get hurt. This behavior is typical of:

    a. Caring
    b. Supporting
    c. Controlling
    d. Enabling

24. Ms. K is a 30 year female has finished a cognitive behavioral intensive outpatient treatment program for her crack/cocaine addiction. For follow-up she plans to attend a weekly process group. According to Prochaska and DiClemente, what stage of change would this client be entering?

    a. Action
    b. Maintenance

c. Aftercare
d. Preparation

25. Which of the following is *less* likely to be a limitation of urine drug testing for substances of abuse?

    a. Often produces false positives
    b. ''Short'' window of detection of metabolites
    c. Intermittent abuse patterns of abusers
    d. Issues of civil liberties

26. Which of the following characteristics is NOT necessarily present in fetal alcohol syndrome?

    a. Heart defects
    b. Facial dysmorphology
    c. Growth retardation
    d. Central nervous system dysfunction

27. The CNS leads a multi-family group. Ms.T is a 40 year old housewife who is very angry at her husband because he recently spent the couple's entire savings on cocaine. Ms.T feels very frustrated with her husband's addiction and would like to learn to support him in his recovery. The CNS 's best suggestion would be for Ms. T:

    a. To leave her husband
    b. To take charge of the family finances
    c. To not get involved in her husband's recovery
    d. To attend AL-ANON meetings to explore how significant others cope with their loved one's addiction

28. From a family systems perspective Chemical dependency can be viewed as:

    a. A lack of the family's ability to problem solve
    b. Lack of communication
    c. Lack of family organization and interactional patterns.
    d. A symptom of underlying family dysfunction

29. Ms. R is a 50-year-old women married to an alcoholic. During individual counseling Ms. R states that her husband's drinking interferes with their social activities. His behavior when drinking embarrasses and humiliates her. An appropriate response would be to advise Ms. R to:

    a. Stop going to activities

b. Continue to go to activities without focusing on her husband's drinking, letting him take responsibility for the consequences of his drinking behavior

c. Encourage Ms. R to keep a watchful eye on her husband, frequently reminding him how much he has had to drink

d. Make sure she is available at activities so that she can drive her husband safely home

30. Which of the following goals would NOT be appropriate for the milieu management of a residential substance abuse program?

   a. To maintain a restricted environment
   b. To maintain the safety of the patient
   c. To provide consistent, structured care
   d. To support the patient's recovery effort

31. Ms. G is a 67 year old female with a long history of alcoholism. She currently has cirrhosis of the liver. In order to be put on a list to receive a liver transplant, she must complete an inpatient substance abuse program. Additionally, she must sustain 6 months of abstinence. On admission Ms. G states that the only reason she is here is to receive a new liver. An appropriate initial response would be:

   a. How did you get cirrhosis of the liver?
   b. You sound angry about having to participate in substance abuse treatment?
   c. Treatment requires having insight into your alcoholism.
   d. You are concerned about your liver disease?

32. An evaluation criterion for Ms. G's plan of care would be:

   a. Understand the reasons for her drinking
   b. Verbalize her dependence on alcohol
   c. Recognize situations which put her at high risk for drinking
   d. Discuss her alcoholism openly in group

33. An example of a violation of the Controlled Substance Act would be:

   a. Driving under the influence of alcohol
   b. Drinking or using drugs at work
   c. Possession of an illegal substance outside of work
   d. Diverting a controlled substance from a facility

34. RJ is a 16 year old who presents to the county emergency room one night accompanied by 2 of his peers. His friends state that RJ just started acting very weird while they were attending a concert. The nurse notices that RJ is anxious, agitated, confused, paranoid and his pupils are dilated. RJ is convinced that everything is changing shape and color. Based on this information, the nurse should suspect:

   a. Schizophrenia
   b. A brief psychotic episode
   c. A panic attack
   d. Hallucinogen intoxication

35. The primary nurse is assigned a 24 year old women with a crack cocaine dependence. The nurse meets with the client to discuss a plan of care. The nurse and client decide on an activity that will enhance the client's self esteem and empowerment. Which of the following models is providing the theoretical framework for this intervention?

   a. Disease model
   b. Nursing Light model
   c. Social learning theory
   d. Family systems theory

36. AL-ANON would most probably recommend to the spouse of an alcoholic individual:

   a. Continue the same behavior
   b. You are powerless over the alcoholic individual, so take care of yourself
   c. Learn how you can change the alcoholic individual
   d. Get a divorce

37. A common physical complication of alcohol dependence, which contributes to memory impairment:

   a. Decreased serotonin levels
   b. Elevated liver enzymes
   c. B vitamin deficiency
   d. Gastritis

38. The 12 steps of Alcoholic and Narcotics Anonymous describe:

   a. A spiritual approach to living
   b. How the organizations were developed

c. What goes on in meetings
d. God as a higher power

39. What are the characteristics of therapists who are most successful in treating substance use disorders?

a. They confront and challenge the client's denial
b. They take control, and clearly tell their clients what they need to do to recover
c. They show high levels of empathy
d. They are recovering from addiction themselves

40. Mr. J is a 28 year old male with a diagnosis of polysubstance dependence and panic disorder. Mr. J states that if his anxiety were treated he would have no need to abuse addictive substances. Which statement best supports the nurse's understanding about the treatment of dual diagnosis?

a. The anxiety is probably caused by drugs and will remit with cessation of drug use
b. The substance abuse is an attempt by the patient to self medicate his panic disorder
c. Both the substance abuse and the panic disorder must be treated concurrently to maximize treatment outcome
d. The patient who is adequately treated for panic disorder can return to controlled drug use

ANSWERS TO QUESTIONS

1. b	14. d	27. d
2. d	15. c	28. d
3. c	16. c	29. b
4. d	17. a	30. a
5. c	18. a	31. d
6. d	19. a	32. b
7. d	20. c	33. d
8. b	21. c	34. d
9. c	22. b	35. b
10. d	23. d	36. b
11. b	24. b	37. c
12. c	25. a	38. a
13. a	26. a	39. c
		40. c

BIBLIOGRAPHY

Allen, K. M. (1996). *Nursing care of the addicted client.* Philadelphia: Lippincott.

American Psychiatric Association. (1994). *Diagnostic and statistical manual of mental disorders* (4th ed.). Washington, DC: Author.

Anderson, M. D., & Smereck, A. B. (1992). Consciousness rainbow: An explication of Rogerian field pattern manifestations. *Nursing Science Quarterly, 5(2)*, 72–79.

Bowen, M. (1978). *Family therapy in clinical practice.* New York: Jason Aronson.

Cahill, J., Cassidy, K., Daly, S., Deutisch, D., Hodgson, B., Hodgson, J., Johnson, P. & McMahon, E. (1992). *Nurses Handbook of Law and Ethics.* Springhouse, PA: Springhouse.

Galanter, M. J., & Kleber, H. D. (1994). *Textbook of substance abuse treatment.* Washington, DC: American Psychiatric Press.

Miller, N. S., & Gold, M. S. (1995). *Pharmacological therapies for drug and alcohol additions.* New York: Marcel Dekker, Inc.

Miller, W. R., & C'de Baca, J. (1995). What every mental health professional should know about alcohol. *Journal of Substance Abuse Treatment, 12(5)*, 355–365.

Prochaska, J. O., DiClemente, C. C., & Norcross, J. C. (1992). In search of how people change: Applications to addictive behavior. *American Psychologist, 47*, 1102–1114.

Naegle, M.A. (1992, 1993). *Substance Abuse Education in Nursing* (Vol. I, II, III). New York: National League for Nursing.

Rotgers, F., Keller, D. S., & Morgenstern, J. (1996). *Treating substance abuse: Theory and technique.* New York: Guilford Press.

Steinglass, P., Bennett, L., Wolin, S., & Reiss, D. (1987). *The alcoholic family.* New York: Basic Books.

Sullivan, E. J. (1995). *Nursing care of clients with substance abuse.* St. Louis: Mosby.

Anxiety and Stress-Related Disorders

Karma Castleberry

Anxiety Disorders

Generalized Anxiety Disorder (GAD)

- Definition: Unrealistic or excessive worry accompanied by symptoms of motor tension, autonomic arousal, and vigilance
- Signs and Symptoms
    1. Motor tension—shaky, muscle tension, fatigability
    2. Autonomic arousal—shortness of breath, tachycardia, dry mouth, dizziness, nausea, diarrhea, dysphagia
    3. Vigilance—insomnia, feels "keyed up"
    4. Not limited to discrete periods or discrete stimuli
    5. Often accompanied by depression or another anxiety disorder
    6. Considerable impairment in quality of life
    7. Levels of anxiety
        a. Mild—slight physical arousal, sharp perceptions, ability to learn well
        b. Moderate—physical symptoms apparent, narrowing of perceptual field
        c. Severe—physical symptoms problematic, difficulty concentrating, very apprehensive
        d. Panic—terror, little ability to concentrate, difficulty breathing, palpitations, fear of dying
    8. Anxiety disorders 4–7 times more prevalent than depression in elders; GAD most common (Beck, Stanley, & Zebb, 1996)
- Differential Diagnoses
    1. Physical disorders such as hyperthyroidism and mitral valve prolapse
    2. Caffeine or stimulant abuse
    3. Withdrawal from alcohol or sedatives
    4. Panic or Obsessive Compulsive Disorders
    5. Anxiety disorder due to a general medical condition (APA, 1994)
- Mental Status Variations

1. Appearance—sweating, cold, clammy hands, exaggerated startle response, flushing, or chills

2. Psychomotor Activity—restless, trembling, twitching

3. Mood—irritable, anxious, apprehensive

4. Concentration—difficult to concentrate

5. Insight—impaired; clients often seek treatment for physical symptoms and do not associate physical and emotional responses with anxiety.

- Nursing Diagnoses

    1. Anxiety

    2. Coping, ineffective individual

    3. Family process, altered

    4. Fear

    5. Powerlessness

    6. Parenting, altered, high risk for

    7. Knowledge deficit

    8. Role performance, altered

    9. Sleep pattern disturbance

- Genetic/Biological Origins

    1. Some evidence of genetic link (25% first-degree relatives)

    2. Persons with GAD have increased sympathetic tone, greater response, and slower adaptation to stress.

    3. Gamma aminobutyric acid (GABA), which is a principle inhibitory CNS neurotransmitter, may have diminished activity.

    4. Decreased activity in basal ganglia and paralimbic structures; increased activity in cerebellum and some cortical structures (Johnson & Lydiard, 1995)

    5. Possible genetic link between alcoholism and anxiety disorders

    6. Worry negatively reinforced by decrease in aversive somatic activation (autonomic hyperactivity) (Freeston, Dugas, & Ladouceur, 1996)

- Biochemical Approaches

  1. CNS effects of anti-anxiety agents linked to GABA-chloride channel receptor complex
  2. Benzodiazepines (BZDs) increase the affinity of binding sites for GABA, resulting in a greater influx of chlorine ions into the neuron.
  3. Barbiturates bind to chloride channels, leaving channel open so that chloride flows 4 to 5 times longer.
  4. Both benzodiazepines and barbiturates thus allow neurons to become hyperpolarized and, therefore, more inhibited than by the usual action of GABA alone.

     The following table outlines anti-anxiety medications.

Table 1

Commonly Used Medications for Anxiety Disorders

Generic Name	Trade Name	Dosage (mg/day)
Benzodiazepines		
Alprazolam	Xanax	0.5–6
Chlordiazepoxide	Librium**	5–100
Clonazepam	Klonopin	1.5–10
Clorazepate	Tranxene**	7.5–60
Diazepam	Valium**	2–60
Lorazepam	Ativan *	2–6
Oxazepam	Serax *	30–120
Temazepam	Restoril *	15–30
Triazolam	Halcion *	0.125–0.5
Barbiturates		
Butabarbital	Butisol	45–120
Propanediols		
Meprobromate	Equanil	400–1600
Azaspirodecanediones		
Buspirone	BuSpar	15–25

* short acting
** long acting

5. Special Nursing Concerns
   a. Can cause physical and psychological addiction
      (1) Adhere to prescribed dosage.
      (2) Withdrawal begins 12 to 48 hours after last dose, lasts for 12 to 48 hours, with some symptoms persisting for weeks.
      (3) Reduce drug gradually to prevent seizures.
      (4) Rebound symptoms of intensified anxiety post BZD withdrawal (Blair & Ramones, 1996)
   b. Benzodiazepines with long half lives (1 to 8 days)
      (1) Cumulative effects
      (2) Possible compensatory hyperexcitable state upon withdrawal
   c. Monitor for blood dyscrasias: CBC with differential, sore throat, fever
   d. Monitor for liver dysfunction: nausea, upper abdominal pain, jaundice, fever, rash, liver function studies
   e. May increase depression: monitor, assess for suicide potential
   f. Alcohol potentiates depressant effects
      (1) Behavioral dyscontrol, sedation, and psychomotor effects
      (2) Do not use alcohol
   g. May produce sedation that impairs ability to handle machinery or autos
   h. Teach client to monitor side effects of medication.
   i. Elders and medication (Sheikh & Salzman, 1995)
      (1) Short half-life BZD's (lorazepam, oxazepam, and temazepam) metabolism unimpaired
      (2) Intermediate/long half-life BDZs tend to accumulate in elders

            (3)   BZD toxicity in elderly: decreased cortical arousal, cerebellar toxicity, reduced psychomotor speed/accuracy, and impaired attention and short term recall

- Intrapersonal

1. Origins

   a. Psychodynamic—Anxiety results from unconscious conflict or emergence of unacceptable drives (often related to dependent, sexual, or aggressive content).

      (1) Anxiety serves as a signal that repression of drive or conflict is not working.

      (2) If repression doesn't contain drives, then other defense mechanisms employed (conversion, displacement, regression).

   b. Behavioral—anxiety is a conditioned response to a specific stimulus, or a learned, internal response (perhaps from imitating parental anxiety responses or reinforced by others)

   c. Cognitive—anxiety results from faulty or dysfunctional thoughts about events

      (1) Overestimate danger

      (2) Underestimate ability to cope

2. Psychotherapeutic interventions.

   a. Psychodynamic

      (1) Long-term, insight-oriented therapy

      (2) Focus on resolution of conflicts underlying anxiety

   b. Behavioral

      (1) Relaxation training—Progressive Muscle Relaxation (PMR) or Autogenic Training Techniques

      (2) Breathing techniques

      (3) Biofeedback

      (4) Identification of physical responses that trigger anxiety

      (5) Training components such as problem-solving and social skills (Harvey & Rapee, 1995)

   c. Cognitive

      (1) Identify and challenge dysfunctional thoughts (self-statements) that trigger anxiety

      (2) Replace with positive coping statements

      (3) Evaluate accurately presence of danger

      (4) Encourage use of log (diaries) and homework for subsequent analysis of relationship between thoughts and feeling of anxiety

   d. Solution-focused therapy

   e. Therapeutic touch

- Family Dynamics/Family Therapy

   1. Children of parents with GAD are likely to see the world as dangerous and themselves as vulnerable

      a. May be excessively protected

      b. May be excessively dependent

   2. Family member with GAD may exhibit altered role performance and require other family members to assume greater or inappropriate responsibility (Barloon, 1993)

   3. Family member with GAD may become family's "weak one," or the scapegoat

   4. Family treatment emphasizes the following:

      a. Knowledge of GAD and treatment

      b. Cognitive restructuring for all family members to challenge and correct collective assumptions about danger and coping

      c. Promotion of differentiation, especially in children

      d. Re-establishment of healthy role performance

- Group Approaches

   1. Therapy—group therapy offers opportunities for feedback, realistic self-appraisal, and support when changing behavior patterns

      a. Insight-oriented to resolve unconscious conflicts

      b. Psychoeducational approaches to increase understanding of nature of GAD and learn coping strategies

   c.   Cognitive group therapy to challenge and correct dysfunctional cognitions

   d.   Assertiveness Training

- Milieu Interventions

   1.   Create a safe, supportive environment

   2.   Use goal-oriented contract to focus treatment

   3.   Use diary/logs to record manifestation of anxiety (thoughts, emotions, physiological responses), the situation, course of events, efficacy of intervention

   4.   Teach role of dysfunctional cognitions (danger and inability to cope) in creating/maintaining anxiety

   5.   Teach analysis of negative self-statements and replace with rational, positive statements and receive feedback from other clients

   6.   Teach relaxation techniques, monitor practice of relaxation techniques, and assist to implement when experiencing anxiety

      a.   Breathing techniques

      b.   Progressive muscle relaxation

      c.   Autogenic training

   7.   Assist to develop alternative means of coping such as exercising, taking warm baths, or talking to staff and other clients

   8.   Promote activities that increase self-confidence through progressively more difficult challenges

   9.   Plan leisure activities to deal with ''free time''

   10. Encourage resumption of family, work, and social roles

   11. Refer to partial hospitalization program or outpatient services

- Community Resources

   1.   GAD often treated by primary care providers such as family doctors and nurse practitioners

      a.   CNS may provide consultation, individual, group, and family therapy

      b.   Work collaboratively

2. Provide support groups or parenting classes for persons with anxiety disorders

3. Teach how to access general community resources to enhance support base

Phobias

- Definition: Persistent, excessive, irrational fear of a particular object or situation that actually poses no threat

- Signs and Symptoms

  1. Specific Phobias

     a. Fear of animals (snakes, spiders, dogs)

     b. Claustrophobia

     c. Fear of air travel

     d. Usually little impairment

  2. Social Phobia—fear of being exposed to scrutiny, humiliated, or embarrassed by others

     a. Specific fears—choking on food in restaurant, trembling when writing

     b. General fears—saying foolish things

     c. Usually mild impairment

  3. Agoraphobia—fear of being in a place or situation from which there might be difficult or embarrassing escape, or in which, should symptoms become very embarrassing or incapacitating, there might be no help available—such as:

     a. Fears heart attack, depersonalization, loss of bladder control, etc.

     b. Limits travel, crowds, or being outside the home alone to avoid symptom development

     c. Mild (some avoidance or tolerance of anxiety) to severe (housebound or unable to leave the house unaccompanied) impairment

- Differential Diagnoses

  1. Panic Disorder with Agoraphobia

    2. Avoidant Personality Disorder

    3. Obsessive Compulsive Disorder

    4. Post-traumatic Stress Disorder

    5. Schizophrenia (with delusions)

- Mental Status Variations

    1. Appearance and Behavior—normal unless faced with feared stimulus, then exhibits symptoms of severe anxiety

    2. Mood—commonly depressed, often related to degree of impairment

    3. Thought—persistent, irrational fear of object or situation

- Nursing Diagnoses

    1. Anxiety

    2. Coping, ineffective individual

    3. Family process, altered

    4. Fear

    5. Knowledge deficit

    6. Powerlessness

    7. Role performance, altered

    8. Self-esteem

    9. Social interaction, impaired

- Genetic/Biological Origins

    1. Biological inability to habituate to certain situation

    2. Possible genetic component with higher concordance in first-degree relatives

    3. Serotonergic abnormality

    4. State-dependent abnormalities in caudate and thalamic function

- Biochemical Approaches

    1. Anti-anxiety agents in combination with behavioral approaches

    2. Anti-anxiety agents if behavioral approaches ineffective

    3. Antidepressants for clients with depressive features

    a.   MAOIs in particular for social phobias

    b.   Imipramine for panic disorders with agoraphobia

    c.   Selective serotonin re-uptake inhibitors (Paxil, Zoloft) may be effective

  4. Beta-adrenergic antagonists which block the sympathetic response (e.g., propranolol) are helpful in situational anxiety such as stage fright

- Intrapersonal

  1. Origins

    a.   Psychodynamic—phobia is an outward manifestation of inner, unresolved childhood conflicts

       (1) Anxiety is displaced (when repression fails) upon an object or situation that symbolizes the conflict

       (2) Conflicts are often sexual (oedipal) or related to separation anxiety

       (3) Disturbance of interpersonal attachment & coping

    b.   Behavioral

       (1) Classical conditioned response—phobia develops when anxiety occurs as one is confronted with a naturally frightening stimulus and becomes paired with a neutral stimulus

       (2) Operant theories—person learns to avoid a stimulus for anxiety, and the reduction in anxiety reinforces the behavior

  2. Psychotherapeutic interventions

    a.   Psychodynamic—insight-oriented therapy to resolve childhood conflicts, understand secondary gain, and to find healthy ways to deal with anxiety

    b.   Behavior Therapy (most effective treatment)

       (1) Systematic Desensitization

          (a) Design, with client, list of anxiety-provoking stimuli related to the object/situation from the least to most frightening

        (b) Teach progressive muscle relaxation (PMR) to induce deep relaxation

        (c) Induce/maintain relaxed state, while client imagines each anxiety-provoking stimulus

        (d) When desensitized to one stimulus, move up the scale, until relaxation can be maintained throughout entire list of stimuli

        (e) Apply technique in vivo

    (2) Flooding—intensive exposure to stimulus in vivo or through imagery until fear can no longer be felt

    (3) Neurolinguistic Programming

- Family Dynamics/Family Therapy

    1. When role performance (work, family, social contacts) is impaired, family dynamics are altered, and other members assume additional responsibilities

    2. Children of phobic mothers are encouraged to be overly dependent and solicitous to mother's needs (Barloon, 1993)

    3. Children sense fears of outside world or objects

    4. Family therapy for role restructuring, support of therapy and change, and reduction of secondary gain of all members

- Group Approaches

    1. Therapy

        a. Psychodynamic insight-oriented group therapy

        b. Psychoeducational group—focus on understanding phobic disorders and learning relaxation techniques

        c. Social skills training—modeling, rehearsing, coaching to improve communication

        d. Supportive therapy to provide reality-testing and feedback within a group of others seeking to make similar changes

            (1) May provide "here and now" experience in facing phobic social situations

    2. Self-help groups (affiliated with Phobia Society of America, Rockville, MD) may be present in some communities

- Milieu Interventions (unlikely to be hospitalized unless severely impaired)

    1. Provide safe, supportive environment, free of ridicule for phobia

    2. Goal-oriented contract for treatment

    3. Employ anxiety-reducing techniques (PMR, breathing, etc.) to decrease general arousal

    4. Conduct systematic desensitization (imagined or in vivo)

    5. Engage in activities that increase feelings of power and self-esteem

    6. Reinforce what is learned in individual, group and family sessions

    7. Referral to outpatient support groups

- Community Resources

    1. Outpatient therapy

    2. Support groups

Panic Disorders

- Definition: Recurrent, unexpected, intense periods of extreme apprehension and terror without clear precipitant

- Signs and Symptoms

    1. Begins with rapidly increasing symptoms of fear and doom, palpitations, tachycardia, dyspnea, sweating, hyperventilation

    2. Lasts 30 to 60 minutes; may include symptoms of depersonalization, derealization, paresthesia, fainting, dizziness, choking, nausea, chest pain, flushes or chills

        a. First attacks often in phobogenic situation

        b. Subsequent attacks are spontaneous (uncued, unexpected)

    3. Clients usually try to seek help, focusing on cardiac or respiratory symptoms.

        a. Believe to be dying

        b. Often seen in emergency room

        c. Fear going "crazy"

    4. May be accompanied by agoraphobia, fearing panic attacks will occur in setting without help

5. Between episodes, anticipatory anxiety, vigilant for onset of another attack

6. Ranges from mild (one attack per month or limited number of symptoms), to severe (8 panic attacks per month)

7. Often accompanied by depression

- Differential Diagnoses

  1. Note whether panic disorder is or is not accompanied by agoraphobia.

  2. Physical disorders such as mitral valve prolapse, hyperthyroidism, hypoglycemia, or pheochromocytoma

  3. Withdrawal from psychoactive substances

  4. Caffeine or stimulant abuse

  5. Alcohol abuse

  6. GAD, Post-Traumatic Stress Disorder (PTSD)

  7. Somatization Disorder

- Mental Status Variations

  1. Appearance—anxious, perspiring, choking, difficulty breathing

  2. Behavior—trembling, hyperventilation

  3. Mood—may be depressed (including suicidal)

  4. Speech—stammering, difficulty speaking

  5. Thought—ruminating, preoccupation with fear of death or doom

  6. Memory—impaired

  7. Concentration—decreased, confusion

  8. Orientation—confused

- Nursing Diagnoses

  1. Anxiety

  2. Coping, ineffective individual

  3. Family processes, altered

  4. Fear

  5. Hopelessness

6. Knowledge deficit

7. Parenting, altered

8. Powerlessness

9. Role performance, altered

10. Self-esteem, chronic low

11. Social isolation

12. Violence, high risk for, self-directed

- Genetic/Biological Origins

    1. First-degree relatives of clients with panic disorders affected (20%) and higher concordance rate with monozygotic twins

    2. Mitral valve prolapse present in about half of all persons with panic disorders (cardiac and respiratory symptoms similar in both disorders)

    3. Increased sympathetic responsiveness; sensitivity to CO_2 and lactate; alterations in blood flow and metabolic activity in brain

    4. Enhanced sensitivity to central adrenergic receptors and possible BZD receptor ''set point'' alteration (Johnson & Lydiard, 1995)

    5. Neuro-imaging—possible relationship of CNS lesions with abnormal signal activity or asymmetric right temporal lobe atrophy, abnormal activity in hippocampus and right frontal cortex

    6. Dysfunction of brainstem and parahippocampal areas which usually initiate panic under dangerous physiological or environmental threats

- Biochemical Approaches

    1. Antidepressants, especially imipramine, and some MAOIs

        a. Increase therapeutic dose slowly to decrease adverse effects such as orthostatic hypotension.

        b. Decrease in panic attacks by 2 to 4 weeks

        c. Teach about dietary restriction with MAOIs.

        d. Remain on drug 6 to 12 months after symptom relief, then taper off slowly

      e. Tricyclics (TCAs) problematic with weight gain and toxicity in overdose

2. BZDs, particularly clonazepam, alprazolam, lorazepam, diazepam

3. Plasma levels may identify rapid metabolizers who require higher doses

4. SSRIs (sertraline, fluoxetine, paroxetine) effective with elders and have fewer side effects

5. Panic Disorder responds to pharmacotherapy more readily and rapidly than other anxiety disorders (Pollack & Smoller, 1995)

- Intrapersonal

1. Origins

    a. Psychodynamic—panic occurs when defenses against anxiety (repression, displacement, and avoidance) are ineffective.

      (1) Symbolic nature often related to abandonment and separation anxiety

      (2) Traumatic separations in childhood may increase vulnerability by producing autonomic nervous system stimulation (Shear, 1996)

      (3) Interpersonal problems in assertiveness and sociability (Battaglia, 1995)

    b. Behavioral

      (1) Parental behavior modeling or classical conditioning

      (2) Demonstration of cognitions of exaggerated vulnerability, inability to cope, and general negative views of self; catastrophic interpretations of anxiety symptoms which provide more arousal and symptoms

      (3) Stressful life events—persons with panic disorders report greater frequency of life events that pose danger and threat

2. Psychotherapeutic interventions

    a. Psychodynamic—insight-oriented therapy to focus on origin of anxiety, symbolism, secondary gain, and resolution of early conflicts

    b. Behavioral

       (1) Psychoeducation regarding origin and maintenance of panic attacks

       (2) Desensitization—real or imagined phobic situation

       (3) Cognitive restructuring to decrease self-statements that promote anxiety and to increase positive, coping statements, coupled with exposure to avoided situations or to somatic sensations of anxiety (Otto & Whittal, 1995)

       (4) Reinforcement of mastery

       (5) Relaxation techniques—breathing, PMR, and imagery

       (6) Continued vulnerability and episodic exacerbations after successful symptom removal

- Family Dynamics/Family Therapy

    1. Clients with agoraphobia may always require family members to stay close by resulting in

      a. Marital discord

      b. Dependence upon children

    2. Altered role performance (work, family, social situations) increases responsibility of other family members

    3. Family education about origin, nature, and treatment of disorder

    4. Family therapy to restructure communication and roles to support change

    5. Family work essential due to chronic nature of Panic Disorder (Pollak & Smoller, 1995; Shear, 1995)

- Group

    1. Therapy to improve coping and/or social support

      a. Insight-oriented

      b. Cognitive therapy

      c. Support groups where stable, intimate relationships can buffer anxiety

    2. Self-Help

      a. Community self-help groups encourage acceptance and improved life functioning when residual symptoms persist

- Milieu

1. Provide safe, supportive environment

2. Establish goal-oriented treatment contract

3. Assist client to employ relaxation and cognitive techniques when panic attack first begins

4. Label experience as a "panic attack" and anxiety

5. Promote socialization with peers

6. Engage in activities that promote self-esteem

7. Assist client's use of cognitive strategies to decrease anticipatory anxiety associated with possible future panic attacks

8. Reinforce learning from individual, groups, and family sessions

9. Refer to outpatient therapy

- Community Resources

1. Outpatient therapy

2. Support groups

Obsessive Compulsive Disorder (OCD)

- Definition: Recurrent persistent obsessions and/or compulsions that interfere with functional abilities, occupation, social activities, and interpersonal activities

- Signs and Symptoms

1. Obsession—unwanted, repeated and uncontrollable thoughts, images or impulses

      a. Unable to break thought cycle through distraction in conversation or other tasks

      b. Common themes of losing things, blasphemy, fears of disease, contamination, sexual behavior, or aggression

      c. Increased anxiety if resisted

2. Compulsions—repeated, unwanted patterns of behavior that are often responses to obsessions

   a. Involve excessive cleaning, washing, checking, counting, or repeating

   b. Increased anxiety and dread if compulsions are resisted

3. Intervention usually not sought until basic needs are not met or when physical and/or emotional exhaustion occurs of either client or significant other

   a. Most present with both obsessions and compulsions

   b. Often delay treatment several years

- Differential Diagnoses

   1. Obsessive Compulsive Personality Disorder

   2. Major depression with obsessive thoughts

   3. Hypochondriasis

   4. Tourette's Syndrome

   5. Temporal lobe epilepsy

   6. Schizophrenia

- Mental Status Variations

   1. Appearance—special dress pattern, abraded hands

   2. Behavior—ordering and arranging environment of examiner, touching, licking, spitting, repeating rituals

   3. Mood—depressed, anxious

   4. Thought—intrusive sounds, words, music, sexual images or impulses; thoughts of doom, concerns with germs, dirt, etc.

   5. Insight—understands obsessions and compulsions are irrational

- Nursing Diagnoses

   1. Anxiety

   2. Coping, ineffective individual

   3. Family process, altered

   4. Injury, high risk for

   5. Powerlessness

   6. Role performance, altered

7. Social interaction, impaired

8. Thought process, altered

- Genetic/Biological Origins

  1. Abnormal activity in basal ganglia which may be repository for latent behavior patterns found in both OCD and other neurologically caused movement disorders such as tics, epilepsy, and Sydenham's Chorea

     a. Vigilance and grooming behavior in primitive humans may have been of evolutionary advantage

     b. OCD behavior is remarkably similar regardless of cultures, ethnicity, or age

  2. Serotonin implicated by observations that OCD symptoms decrease with selective serotonin re-uptake inhibitors (SSRIs) and increase with serotonin antagonists.

  3. Some evidence of increased prevalence of disorder in first-degree relatives

- Biochemical Approaches

  1. Clomipramine (antidepressant)

     a. 250 mgm/day ceiling dose because of lowered seizure threshold

     b. Side effects—orthostatic hypertension; anticholinergic effects (dry mouth, constipation, urinary retention, tachycardia) weight gain, ejaculatory failure, impotence, drowsiness

     c. Patient teaching—take at bedtime to minimize side effects; management of side effects; avoidance of alcohol; care in operating machinery or driving; OCD symptom relief in 6 to 12 weeks

     d. Discontinue gradually under supervision

  2. SSRIs effective

- Intrapersonal

  1. Origins

     a. Psychodynamic—unacceptable thoughts and impulses are isolated, but threaten to break through into consciousness so that compulsive acts are performed to undo the possible consequences, should the unacceptable become conscious

- (1) May arise during anal stage since much OCD involves cleanliness or aggressive preoccupation
- (2) Note both ambivalence and magical thinking

b. Behavioral

- (1) Obsessions as conditioned stimulus to anxiety
- (2) Compulsions arise when a behavior reduces the anxiety associated with the obsessions

2. Psychotherapeutic interventions

a. Insight-oriented, psychodynamic therapy to develop acceptable expression of thoughts and impulses

b. Supportive therapy

c. Behavioral therapies have greatest effectiveness

- (1) Combine exposure with response delay (ERD) with pharmacotherapy
- (2) Employ gradual extinction of rituals by exposure to anxiety-producing situations until habituation occurs with strict abstinence from performing rituals (Abramowitz, 1997).
- (3) Reduce obsessive thoughts by thought-stopping (such as snapping a rubber band on the wrist when obsessive thought appears)
- (4) Reduce obsessive thoughts through semantic satiation (write a few words of the obsession and then rewrite or say aloud many times until fear no longer evoked)

d. Therapeutic touch

- Family Dynamics/Family Therapy

1. Family members may constantly reassure the client which reinforces the obsession

2. Family may assist patient to avoid situations which trigger OCD which worsens the fear cycle

3. Family therapy:

      a. Emphasize remaining neutral (not reinforcement through reassurance)

      b. Avoid reasoning with client (increases anxiety)

      c. Avoid ridicule

      d. Assist with response delay

      e. Design with family, ways to use time freed up by successful treatment of symptoms (Shear, 1995)

- Group Approaches

  1. Supportive group therapy

  2. Self-help groups in community are often affiliates of Obsessive Compulsive Foundation Inc. (New Haven, CT)

- Milieu Interventions

  1. Provide safe, supportive environment, free from ridicule

  2. Establish goal-oriented treatment plan and daily structure

     a. Initially, do not interfere with rituals

     b. Plan daily schedule to allow time for rituals

     c. Gradually reduce amount of time spent on rituals in collaboration with treatment team

  3. Assist with self-care if needed

  4. Reinforce what is learned from individual, group, and family session

  5. Assist to implement thought-stopping or response delay as designed by the primary therapist

  6. Promote activities that reduce anxiety such as physical activity, and vary sufficiently in order not to produce a substitute ritual

  7. Promote clear and direct verbal communication of feeling

  8. Engage in developing plan for use of leisure time, involving social interaction and hobbies that are less anxiety producing

  9. Refer to outpatient therapy

- Community Resources—OCD Foundation

Post-traumatic Stress Disorder (PTSD)

- Definition: A response to severe emotional or physical trauma character-ized by (1) intrusive re-experiencing of the trauma, (2) emotional numb-ing, and (3) increased arousal

- Signs and Symptoms

  1. Stressors may include war experiences, assault, rape, serious acci-dents, abuse, and natural catastrophes (van der Kolk, McFarlane, & Weisaeth, 1996)

  2. Common trauma experience—overwhelming fear, loss of control, helplessness, and fear of being annihilated

     a. Person witnesses or experiences events that involve actual or threatened death or severe physical harm

     b. Reacts with fear, helplessness, or horror (APA, 1994)

  3. Recurrent intrusive thoughts of trauma in dreams, thoughts, flash-backs, or events similar to stressor

  4. Numbing or constriction (avoidance)

     a. Avoidance of thoughts/feeling/recollections about trauma

     b. Avoidance of persons/situations which provoke memory of original trauma

     c. Psychogenic amnesia, dissociation

     d. Marked diminished interest in significant activities, persons, or the future

  5. Increased arousal—sleep disturbances, temper outbursts, hypervigi-lance and difficulty concentrating, exaggerated startle response (APA, 1994)

  6. Response may be delayed weeks to many years

  7. Standard definition of PTSD (DSM) tends better to fit survivors of circumscribed events and fails to address symptoms and personality manifestation resulting from prolonged, repeated trauma (Herman, 1992)

  8. Post-traumatic Stress Disorder, dissociation, somatization, and affect dysregulation highly interrelated (van der Kolk, Peclovitz, Roth, Mandel, McFarlane, & Herman, 1997)

- Differential Diagnoses

  1. Factitious Disorder

  2. Borderline Personality Disorder

  3. Schizophrenia

  4. Depression

  5. Panic Disorder

  6. Generalized Anxiety Disorder

  7. Acute Stress Disorder (APA, 1994)

     a. Similar origin and presentation as PTSD, but occurs within 4 weeks of traumatic event

     b. Symptoms last from 2 days to 4 weeks.

  8. Frequently misdiagnosed due to symptoms—hallucinations, depression, addiction, and somatic complaints (Symes, 1995)

  9. High rates of comorbidity (Friedman, 1996)

- Mental Status Variations

  1. Behavior—vigilant, restless

  2. Mood—anxious, depressed, blunted affect, guilty

  3. Perceptual Experiences—flashbacks, derealization, dissociation

  4. Thought—preoccupation with trauma

  5. Memory—impaired

  6. Concentration—impaired

- Nursing Diagnoses

  1. Post trauma response

  2. Grieving, dysfunctional

  3. Self mutilation, high risk for

  4. Spiritual distress

  5. Violence, high risk for, self-directed or directed at others

- Genetic/Biological Origins

1. Increased baseline sympathetic arousal may predispose; after trauma, baseline elevated

2. Trauma response includes the following:

   a. Immediate, excessive arousal, especially cardiovascular and neuromuscular systems

   b. Arousal of sympathetic system that leads to difficulty in distinguishing perceptual cues

   c. Original hyperarousal easily evoked after trauma by variety of cues

   d. Autonomic arousal becomes neurologically entrained (van der Kolk, McFarlane, & Weisaeth, 1996).

3. Regulation of endogenous opioids altered

   a. When stressor subsides, opioids may decrease

   b. Opiod withdrawal symptoms similar to PTSD

   c. May be "addicted" to trauma

- Biochemical Approaches

  1. Antidepressants—tricyclic antidepressants (TCAs) and monoamine oxidase inhibitors (MAOIs)

  2. Propranolol

  3. Carbamazepine

  4. Avoid MAOIs/benzodiazepines if abusing drugs/alcohol

  5. Eye Movement Desensitization and Reprocessing (EMDR)—appears to decrease symptoms of trauma, and continues to be researched (Friedman, 1996; Greenwald, 1996; Shapiro, 1995; Wilson, Becker, & Tinker, 1995)

- Intrapersonal

  1. Origins

     a. Psychodynamic view—trauma reactivates previous, unresolved childhood conflicts.

        (1) Regression, repression, denial and undoing defense mechanisms

        (2) Secondary gain when dependency needs met

b. Cognitive—brain attempts to process through alternate blocking and acknowledging the event until a new mental scheme which incorporates the trauma is devised (Herman, 1992)

c. Personal resilience—persons who construct meaning of the event, connections with others, who actively attempt to cope, and who have strong internal locus of control withstand trauma with fewer symptoms (Herman, 1992)

d. Some evidence that those who dissociate at time of trauma have higher risk for PTSD

e. Epidemiological studies—27% of women and 16% of men experienced sexual abuse as children; 33% of survivors who had physical contact without penetration, and 64% of those with penetration developed PTSD (Rodriguez, Ryan, Vande Kemp, & Foy, 1997)

  2. Psychotherapeutic Interventions (all aimed at empowerment and reconnection with others)

a. Psychoeducation regarding the recovery process (tailor to particular traumas)

b. Expressive therapies (art, dance, music) translate visual and sensorimotor memories, especially those not encoded in cognitive systems, into meaningful symbols and verbal representations to be integrated

c. Purpose of individual therapy to:

  (1) Connect present distress (relationships, work, physical health, mood) to trauma

  (2) Cease minimizing the trauma

  (3) Construct new, caring relationship with self

  (4) Set boundaries on relationships with others

  (5) Confront abusive family-of-origin—mixed results (few admit abuse and usually blame victim)

d. Herman's (1992) three-stage model for recovery

  (1) Safety

    (a) Name the problem

       (b)   Restore control

       (c)   Establish safe environment

       (d)   No harm contract

   (2)   Remembrance and mourning

       (a)   Reconstruct the story, including meaning of the event

       (b)   Transform traumatic memories

       (c)   Mourn traumatic loss

   (3)   Reconnection

       (a)   Learn to fight

       (b)   Reconcile with oneself

       (c)   Reconnect with others

       (d)   Find survivor mission

       (e)   Resolve trauma—van der Kolk's 5 Stage Model (1996)

          (i)   Stabilization

               —Education

               —Identification of feelings through verbalizing somatic states

         (ii)   Deconditioning of traumatic memories/responses

        (iii)   Restructuring of traumatic personal schemes

        (iv)   Reestablishment of secure social relationships and interpersonal efficacy

         (v)   Accumulation of emotional experiences which are restitutive

  e.   Controversy about abuse memories "implanted" by therapist (Loftus, 1993), but empirical support that some survivors forget their abuse experiences (Rodriguez, Ryan, Vande Kemp, & Foy, 1997; Williams, 1994)

  f.   Acute catastrophic stress reactions require immediate support, removal from the trauma scene, antianxiety agents, and crisis intervention (Friedman, 1996)

g. Therapist issues include secondary traumatization, feelings of guilt, needs to rescue or control the client, boundary violations, and numbing strategies. (Crothers, 1995; Friedman, 1996)

h. Additional approaches—hypnosis, systematic desensitization, and cognitive therapy

3. Special Issue—self-injury

a. Self injury helps survivors cope with overwhelming affect, intrusive memories, psychological arousal, and dissociative states (Connors, 1996a)

b. Serves to:

(1) Re-enact original trauma

(2) Express feelings/needs

(3) Reorganize self

(4) Manage dissociation

c. Therapeutic responses (Connors, 1996b)

(1) Present and attentive to disclosure

(2) Help client intervene in own self-injury

(a) Identify patterns

(b) Function of self-injury

(3) Work toward resolution of underlying issues

d. Use no-self-injury contract with caution until resolution of core issues because self-injury recurrence rate is high

(1) Avoid all-or-nothing stances

(2) Clear responsibility of client

4. Special Issue—treatment for male survivors (Draucker & Petrovic, 1997)

a. Treatment often based on models for female survivors, and not geared to men

b. Factors influencing recovery:

(1) Reluctance to seek treatment

(2) Minimizing the experience

(3) Difficulties with male intimacy

(4) Tendency to externalize feelings

c. Common behavioral sequelae include aggression, substance abuse, sexual dysfunction

d. Issues in therapy—disclosure, minimizing victimization, expression of emotions, and identity

- Family Dynamics/Therapy

   1. Family roles altered as PTSD symptoms experienced

   2. Some children develop affective symptoms, become rescuers or disengage from parent who has PTSD

   3. Family may expect quicker recovery than what is possible

   4. Family can help clarify events, listen, and connect distortions

   5. Abusive families-of-origin may deny, punish, and attempt to enforce conspiracy of silence

   6. Family Therapy

      a. Support victim in recovery

      b. Meet needs of all family members

      c. Maintain awareness of how trauma affects views of self, family, and world

      d. Develop shared frame of reference for trauma

      e. Central issues of blame, responsibility, and trust

- Group (group experiences with survivors of similar traumas helpful, length variable)

   1. Adult Survivors of Childhood Sexual Abuse

      a. Long-term group therapy, usually outpatient

      b. Goals

         (1) Reduce isolation, shame, guilt, and sense of deviance

         (2) Restructure family-induced behaviors

         (3) Develop new, more realistic patterns of interaction

  c. Group serves as surrogate family

   (1) Victims often blamed by family for disclosing or over-reacting

   (2) Group serves as training ground for new behaviors

    (a) Analyze effect of family's messages and beliefs on view of self and world

    (b) Learn and practice assertive behaviors

    (c) Do not reinforce helplessness or powerlessness

   (3) Support and validate strengths/worth

   (4) Handle successfully displaced hostility, regression, dissociation, extreme, anxiety or depression, self destructive behaviors

   (5) 12-step groups

   (6) Short-term stress management

   (7) Trauma—focused groups

 2. Combat trauma groups

  a. Often long term

  b. Goals

   (1) Share experiences

   (2) Work through problems in social adaptation

   (3) Manage aggression towards other

   (4) Make sense of trauma in life

- Milieu Interventions

 1. Create a safe environment, including a trusting relationship with staff and no harm contract

 2. Educate client about recovery process

 3. Assist client to employ stress management techniques (relaxation techniques, exercise, cognitive strategies)

  a. Reduce general arousal

  b. Employ techniques when anxiety increases or with intrusive memories

4. Support client's ability to gain control over memories.

   a. To retrieve during therapy

   b. To set aside

5. Teach client to manage physiological symptoms of PTSD, including sleep disorders

6. Listen to client's story, respecting ability to disclose and to stop remembering

7. Engage in activities that promote self-esteem

8. Assist in making plans to use leisure time

9. Encourage social interaction

10. Address spiritual issues

11. Develop system of social support in community

12. Assist to devise realistic plans for future, including therapy, occupation, and relationships

13. Solution focused therapy (Miller, deShazer, Berg, & Hopwood, 1993; Webster, Vaughn, Webb, & Playtor, 1995)

- Community Resources

   1. Twelve-step programs

   2. Community outreach program

   3. Battered Women's Shelter for Domestic (Spouse) Abuse

      a. Includes physical battery, verbal threats, intimidating gestures, forced sexual activity, isolation, and economic deprivation (Campbell, Harris, & Lee, 1995)

      b. Women more commonly hurt than men; 16% of pregnant women abused (McFarlane, Parker, & Soeken, 1995)

      c. Models of explanation

         (1) Perpetrator psychopathology, including substance abuse

         (2) Family violence with generational transmission, and violence within entire system (abused wives use severe violence in conflicts with children)

         (3) Stressful situation arises and perpetrator uses violence instead of appropriate coping

        (4)   Gender relations in which men choose violence when control over women is threatened

    d.   Phases of domestic violence (Weingourt, 1996)

        (1)   Escalation phases—broad spectrum of coercive tactics by perpetrator; isolation of victim

        (2)   Incident phase—intense, dramatic show of force to instill fear of repetition if victim resists control

        (3)   De-escalation phase—perpetrator assuages guilt, expresses remorse, and reassures that this will never happen again; victim wants to believe, desires the relationship, and looks to self for responsibility of the relationship

    e.   Assessment for abuse essential

    f.   Safety planning for family member

    g.   Discussion of options

    h.   Referral to community resources for shelter, legal, and support services, and case management

    i.   Treatment of emotional responses to abuse—anxiety, depression, guilt, substance abuse, isolation

4.   National Organization for Victim Assistance (Washington, D.C.)—a clearinghouse for all victim assistance

Somatoform Disorders

Conversion Disorder

- Definition: Loss or change in physical functioning not explained by any known pathophysiological disorder

- Signs and Symptoms

    1.   Temporally related to psychological factors

    2.   Symptom fulfills a need or deals with a conflict

    3.   Symptom not under voluntary control

    4.   Examples—paralysis, blindness, mutism, paresthesias, pseudocyesis, vomiting

- Differential Diagnosis

  1. Rule out medical disorders, especially neurological diseases

  2. Schizophrenia

  3. Depression

  4. Somatization disorder

  5. Hypochondriasis

- Mental Status Variations

  1. Mood—La belle indifference, inappropriate for physical symptoms

  2. Perceptual disturbances—may be blind, but does not bump into objects; stocking or glove anesthesia

  3. Insight—unaware of relationship between psychological conflict and appearance of symptoms

- Nursing Diagnoses

  1. Anxiety

  2. Communication, impaired verbal

  3. Coping, ineffective individual

  4. Family process, altered

  5. Knowledge deficit

  6. Role performance, altered

  7. Possible—sensory-perceptual alterations, physical mobility, impaired

- Genetic/Biological Origins

  1. CNS arousal disturbance which may diminish awareness of bodily sensations

  2. Subtle impairments in verbal communication, memory, alteration, suggestibility noted in neuropsychological testing

  3. More than half diagnosed with neurological disorder in 3-4 years after Conversion Disorder

- Biochemical Approaches (None indicated)

- Intrapersonal

  1. Origins

     a. Conversion of anxiety into physical symptom

        (1) Conflict usually sexual or aggressive

        (2) Symptom allows both disguising impulse and partially expressing

        (3) Symptoms have symbolic relationship to conflict

        (4) Communicates special needs

     b. Conversion symptoms reinforced by family or society, plus secondary gain

     c. Symptoms replace verbal language

  2. Psychotherapeutic interventions

     a. Psychodynamic insight-oriented psychotherapy to explore conflicts

     b. Focus therapy on stress and coping

     c. Hypnosis to uncover traumatic events

     d. Brief, solution-focused psychotherapy

- Family Dynamics/Family Therapy

  1. Family rules negate direct expression of conflict

  2. Illness may be family-accepted means to avoid taking action

  3. Family may encourage secondary gain

  4. Therapy to improve verbal communication, conflict resolution, and restructuring of family interactional patterns

- Group Approaches

  1. Emphasis on coping with stress

  2. Assertiveness training

- Milieu Interventions

  1. Minimize sick role behavior

  2. Encourage verbal expression of needs and conflicts

3. Assist staff and patients to reinforce verbalization and functional behavior, and ignore impairments to reduce secondary gain

4. Help client understand relationships between conflict, symptoms, and gain

5. Teach new coping skills to decrease anxiety

Hypochondriasis

- Definition: Preoccupation with, and unrealistic interpretation of, physical symptoms and sensations as a serious disease

- Signs and Symptoms

    1. Preoccupation with health state in spite of medical reassurance

    2. Not of delusional quality (can admit possibility of exaggeration)

    3. May be organ-system related or related to a particular bodily function

    4. Experience anguish over physical state

    5. Tend to see multiple practitioners

- Differential Diagnoses

    1. Medical disorders with multiple organ system involvement (AIDS, endocrine disorders, MS, Systemic lupus erythematosus (SLE), some neoplasms)

    2. Generalized Anxiety Disorder

    3. Panic Disorder

    4. Conversion and Somatization Disorders

- Mental Status Variations

    1. Appearance—apprehensive, anguished

    2. Mood—depressed, anxious

    3. Thought—preoccupied with seriousness of physical symptoms

    4. Insight—impaired

- Nursing Diagnoses

    1. Anxiety

    2. Coping, ineffective individual

3. Fear

4. Self esteem disturbance

5. Social interaction, impaired

6. Role performance, altered

- Genetic/Biological Origins

    1. Some evidence of increased prevalence in twins

    2. Physiological lower threshold tolerance for discomfort

- Biochemical Approaches

    1. Medication only for coexistent anxiety or depression

    2. Avoid reinforcing through medication

- Intrapersonal

    1. Origins

        a. Repression of aggressive and hostile impulses with displacement into somatic complaints

            (1) Anger originates in past losses

            (2) Displacement solicits help (which later is rejected)

        b. Cognitive schema focusing on bodily sensations—tendency to amplify and misinterpret symptoms of emotional arousal and to think in concrete rather than emotional terms

        c. Sick role offers respite from responsibilities of life

        d. May begin with physical illnesses in childhood or following a severe medical problem as an adult

        e. Atonement for real or imagined wrong doings (Ford, Katon, & Lipkin, 1993)

    2. Psychotherapeutic interventions

        a. Usually resistant to psychiatric treatment unless occurs in medical setting

        b. Focus on stress reduction and coping

        c. Avoid reinforcements of sick role as a solution to life problems

- Family Dynamics/Therapy

1. Family may reinforce sick role behavior

2. Family conflict over client distress and medical treatment

3. Family roles may be altered

4. Family may have low ability to deal directly with stressful situations or obligations

- Group Psychotherapy

    1. Social support

    2. Social interaction

- Milieu Interventions

    1. Often treated on medical unit

    2. Teach rational interpretation of bodily sensations

    3. Assist to identify relationship between physical symptoms and stress

    4. Teach techniques to cope with anxiety including talking, exercise, and relaxation techniques

    5. Meet physical needs, but avoid reinforcing

    6. Encourage social interaction and constructive use of leisure time

    7. Teach problem-solving techniques for personal difficulties

    8. Refer to outpatient therapy

Somatization Disorder

- Definition: A chronic relapsing syndrome of multiple somatic symptoms for which there is no medical explanation

- Signs and Symptoms

    1. Symptoms include gastrointestinal, pain, cardiopulmonary, conversion, sexual, and female reproductive

    2. History of several years' duration, beginning before age 30

    3. High utilization of health services—physician visits, excessive surgery, psychiatric services, multiple medications

    4. Associated with changes in life style due to illness

    5. Typically, new symptoms arise during times of emotional distress

6. Chaotic social lives

7. Often accompanied by depression and anxiety

8. Existence of primary gain (keep conflicts out of awareness) and secondary gain (benefits of illness)

- Differential Diagnoses

    1. Medical illnesses, especially those with fluctuating presentation such as multiple sclerosis and systemic lupus erythematosus

    2. Anxiety

    3. Depression

    4. Hypochondriasis

- Mental Status Variations

    1. Appearance—may be dressed in exhibitionistic manner

    2. Behavior—seductive, coy

    3. Mood—present as depressed, anxious, with cavalier attitude about symptoms

    4. Thought—medical history disorganized, vague, with dramatic, exaggerated description of symptoms

    5. Insight—none, believes physically ill

- Nursing Diagnoses

    1. Communication, impaired verbal

    2. Coping, ineffective individual

    3. Family processes, altered

    4. Social interaction, impaired

    5. Knowledge deficit

- Genetic/Biological Origins

    1. Inconclusive—dominant hemisphere dysfunction, abnormal cortical function, EEG abnormalities

    2. Possible common genetic background with Antisocial Personality Disorder

    3. Increased risk of Somatization Disorder in first-degree relatives

- Biochemical Approaches

  1. No specific biochemical treatment

  2. If presents with prominent anxiety or depression, may treat with antidepressants or antianxiety agents, but clients tend to misuse

- Intrapersonal

  1. Origins

     a. Substitute somatic symptoms for repressed impulses

     b. Somatization as social communication

        (1) To control or maintain relationships

        (2) Gain disability or divert attention

     c. Somatization as emotional communication

        (1) Symptoms express emotional state

        (2) Coping with environmental stress

     d. Somatic disorders associated with childhood abuse

  2. Psychotherapeutic interventions

     a. Requires close collaboration of medical and mental health practitioners managing chronic condition

        (1) Establish trusting relationship with one medical care provider

        (2) Schedule regular visits at frequent intervals, decrease frequency over time

        (3) Provide physical examination of pertinent organ system, but avoid diagnostic procedures, tests, and surgeries

        (4) Emphasize interest in patient and symptoms and be willing to see patient regularly

        (5) Avoid suggestion that symptoms do not exist or are unsubstantiated

        (6) Treat anxiety or depression if present

        (7) Encourage continued employment or rehabilitation if necessary

     b. Solution-focused, brief therapy approaches

- Family Dynamics/Family Therapy

    1. Children taught to somatize, rather than to deal with issues verbally

    2. Readjust roles to accommodate symptoms and illness behavior

    3. Use somatization as means to mediate relationships

    4. Female clients often choose alcoholics or men with antisocial personality disorders as partners

    5. Family therapy aimed at clear, congruent communication, role restructuring, and increasing self-esteem of family members

- Group Approaches

    1. Time-limited group therapy with emphasis on improving socialization skills and ability to cope

    2. Group therapy with emphasis on how to cope with multiple medical problems

- Milieu Interventions

    1. Monitor and assess client's physical status

    2. Attend to physical needs in supportive, but non-reinforcing way

    3. Reinforce verbal expression of needs and feelings

    4. Assist other staff and patients to understand that physical complaints are experienced as ''real'' (Ford et al., 1993)

    5. Help client realize connection between psychological stress and onset of somatic symptoms

    6. Teach new coping skills including use of social relationships and other techniques to decrease anxiety

    7. Maintain consistent approach by all personnel

    8. Support self-care abilities and appropriate role performance, including occupational

Pain Disorder

- Definition: Severe prolonged pain for which there is no organic basis for the pain and/or the intensity

- Signs and Symptoms
  1. Various manifestations-low back pain, headache, or chronic pelvic pain
  2. Preoccupation with pain
  3. Often follows physical trauma
  4. Analgesics usually do not help
  5. Frequent visits to physicians for relief
  6. Usually refuses to consider psychological origins
  7. Depression usually present
  8. Difficulties in diagnosing because of diverse definitions of pain
- Differential Diagnoses
  1. Organic disorders
  2. Depression
  3. Hypochondriasis
  4. Conversion Disorder
- Mental Status Variations
  1. Appearance—antalgic position, diaphoretic, tense
  2. Behavior—restless
  3. Mood—depressed
  4. Thought—preoccupied with pain
  5. Concentration—impaired
  6. Insight—unaware of psychological factors
- Nursing Diagnoses
  1. Coping, ineffective individual
  2. Family process, altered
  3. Hopelessness
  4. Knowledge deficit
  5. Pain, chronic
  6. Physical mobility, impaired

7. Role performance, altered

8. Self-esteem disturbance

9. Social interaction, impaired

- Genetic/Biological Origins

  1. Greater prevalence in first-degree relatives

  2. Greater incidence of alcoholism and depression in families

  3. Endorphin deficiency

  4. Lower serotonin levels in CNS

- Biochemical Approaches

  1. Analgesics and anxiety agents unhelpful and ineffective; possibility of addiction

  2. Antidepressants, especially amitriptyline, imipramine, and doxepin; anafranil, sertraline

  3. Biofeedback training

  4. Transcutaneous nerve stimulation

  5. Exercise programs/physical therapy

  6. Acupuncture

- Intrapersonal

  1. Origins

     a. Punishment for guilt

     b. Pain behaviors may be reinforced by attentiveness or avoidance of unwanted responsibilities

     c. Control of others

     d. Stabilization of marriage/family relationships

  2. Psychotherapeutic interventions

     a. Rehabilitate client to usual social/occupational roles

     b. Discuss psychological causes and secondary gain common to all pain

     c. Cognitive restructuring

     d. Relaxation techniques

    e.   Supportive psychotherapy

- Family Dynamics/Therapy

  1. Family as a whole may be stabilized by pain experience

  2. Teach family members how to respond to client's pain

  3. Discuss secondary gain and power in sick role behavior

  4. Restructure roles, communication patterns, and responsibilities

  5. Deal with issues of individual and family self-esteem

- Group

  1. Pain support groups

  2. Exercise groups

  3. Psychoeducational (pain management) groups

  4. Assertiveness training

- Milieu Intervention

  1. Help client apply relaxation and cognitive techniques for pain relief and tension reduction

  2. Encourage social interaction and participation in activities

  3. Teach about relationship between stress and pain, and effects of relaxation

  4. Encourage verbal, rather than somatic, communications

  5. Avoid reinforcing pain behaviors

  6. Encourage self-care in ADLs

  7. Help client to find ways of assisting others

  8. Design plan for use of leisure

  9. Refer for rehabilitation, pain management, or vocational training.

- Community Resources—pain management clinics

Factitious Disorder

Factitious Disorder

- Definition: Physical or psychological symptoms intentionally produced or feigned (APA, 1994)

- Signs and Symptoms

    1. Desires role of patient

    2. Compulsive quality

    3. May travel from hospital to hospital, seeking admission for different illnesses under different names

    4. Extremely convincing in presentation of physical or psychological symptoms

        a. With physical presentation of symptoms, may be called "Munchausen" syndrome

        b. Children are presented as the ill one by a parent, but rarely

- Differential Diagnoses

    1. True physical disorder

    2. Somatoform Disorder

    3. Personality Disorders

    4. Schizophrenia

    5. Malingering

- Mental Status Variations

    1. Variance depends upon symptoms produced

    2. Thoughts—conflicts and discrepancies in content

    3. Information not corroborated by significant other

- Nursing Diagnoses

    1. Communication, impaired

    2. Coping, ineffective individual

    3. Role performance, altered

- Genetic/Biological Origins—none identified

- Biochemical Approaches—none
- Intrapersonal
  1. Origins
     a. Found caretakers or hospital as caring with previous illnesses and seek continuance
     b. History of parental deprivation
     c. Those who seek surgery or painful treatment may seek punishment
     d. Identify with relatives with genuine illnesses
     e. Defenses employed—repression, identification, identification with aggressor, and symbolization
  2. Psychotherapeutic intervention
     a. Early recognition and referral for factitious disorder to avoid unnecessary treatment
     b. Avoid setting client up as adversary
     c. Usually avoidance of meaningful therapy
- Family Dynamics/Family Therapy
  1. Psychoeducation about disorder
  2. Assist family not to enable client, but to support therapy
- Group Approaches—none
- Milieu Interventions
  1. Create a safe environment.
  2. Assist caregivers to understand nature of disorder
  3. Avoid reinforcing gain from illness
  4. Assist to find means to meet needs for nurturance

Dissociative Disorders

Dissociative Amnesia

- Definition: Dissociative disorder in which person is suddenly unable to recall memories

- Signs and Symptoms
    1. Not ordinary forgetfulness
    2. Can recall other information, learn, and function coherently
    3. Most common during wars and natural disasters
    4. Amnesia
        a. Localized—short time period
        b. Generalized—for whole lifetime of experiences
        c. Selective—amnesia for some, but not all events
        d. Continuous—forgets successive events as they occur, but alert at the time
    5. Primary and secondary gain
    6. Terminates abruptly
- Differential Diagnoses
    1. Medical conditions—neoplasms, infections, epilepsy, post concussion
    2. Wernicke-Korsakoff syndrome
    3. ECT
    4. Drug-induced (LSD, steroids, benzodiazepines, barbiturates)
    5. Transient global amnesia usually caused by TIAs
- Mental Status Variations
    1. Mood—often depressed
    2. Memory—impaired
    3. Orientation—variable
    4. Insight—impaired
- Nursing Diagnoses
    1. Anxiety
    2. Coping, ineffective individual
    3. Thought processes, altered
    4. Powerlessness

- Genetic/Biological Origins—no definitive explanations

- Biochemical Approaches—thiopental and sodium amytal interviews to recover memories

- Intrapersonal

    1. Origins

        a. Psychoanalytic—expressed or fantasized forbidden wish

            (1) Usually sexual or aggressive

            (2) Cannot deal with, so uses repression and denial

        b. Emotional trauma

            (1) Strong emotional response

            (2) Psychological conflict

    2. Psychotherapeutic intervention

        a. Psychotherapy to deal with emotional responses to trauma

        b. Psychotherapy aimed at resolution of unacceptable impulses or behavior

        c. Hypnosis to uncover memories

        d. Stress management

- Family Dynamics/Family Therapy

    1. If natural disaster affected all family members, reconstruct collective memory

    2. All family members affected by client's distress

        a. Family education to understand condition of individual client

        b. Family therapy to help family members make sense of trauma and/or impulse expression

- Group Approaches

    1. If traumatic event, may benefit from support group of survivors

    2. Group psychotherapy usually not indicated

- Milieu Intervention
    1. Treated primarily on outpatient basis or in general hospital
    2. Create safe environment
    3. Mutually develop contract for care
    4. Provide opportunities to talk about traumatic event and its meaning
    5. Teach coping strategies to deal with anxiety actively (rather than dissociation)
    6. Assist in devising realistic future plans

Dissociative Fugue

- Definition: Dissociative disorder characterized by physically traveling from usual environment, inability to recall important aspects of identity and the assumption of a new identity
- Signs and Symptoms
    1. Old and new identities do not alternate
    2. New identity incomplete
    3. Unaware of having forgotten
    4. Lasts hours to days; rarely months
- Differential Diagnosis
    1. Organic mental disorders such as temporal lobe epilepsy
    2. Psychogenic Amnesia
    3. Malingering
- Mental Status Variations
    1. Memory—amnesia for identity and important aspects of life
    2. Insight—unaware of memory impairment
- Nursing Diagnoses
    1. Anxiety
    2. Coping, ineffective individual
    3. Personal identity disturbance
    4. Thought processes, altered

- Genetic/Biological Origins

  1. Origins—no definitive explanation

  2. Heavy alcohol abuse may predispose, but may be primarily psychological effect

- Biochemical Approaches—amobarbital or Thiopental interviews to uncover identity

- Intrapersonal

  1. Origins

     a. Response of withdrawal (by dissociation) to psychological stressors—war, family, marital, and occupational

  2. Psychotherapeutic interventions

     a. Hypnosis to uncover memories/identity

     b. Psychotherapy

        (a) Uncover identity and memories

        (b) Deal with sources of stress more effectively

     c. Couples therapy if marital situation a source of stress

     d. Stress management

- Family Dynamics/Therapy

  1. Family of origin or current family setting may be source of conflict

     a. Family rules may prohibit overt expression of distress

     b. All family members affected by behavior and loss (for some period of time) of family member

  2. Psychoeducation to understand client's condition

  3. If family dynamics are source of stress, family therapy to improve communication, problem-solve, and deal with crisis

- Group Approaches—if trauma victim (war, natural disaster), support groups

- Milieu Interventions

  1. Treat primarily on outpatient basis

  2. Create safe environment

3. Help to reconstruct memories and identity

4. Assist to create meaning of fugue episode

5. Teach coping skills to deal with anxiety

6. Refer for therapy or other continued assistance in managing stressors

- Community Resources—support groups for managing specific stressors

Depersonalization Disorders

- Definition: Dissociative disorder in which client experiences recurrent alterations in perception of self

- Signs and Symptoms

  1. Described as "detached from reality," "dreamlike," or detached from one's body

  2. Self feels strange, unreal

  3. Able to function during the experience

  4. Client distressed about depersonalization experience

  5. May be episodic or chronic

- Differential Diagnoses

  1. Organic Disorder—neurological, metabolic

  2. Schizophrenias

  3. Anxiety

  4. Obsessive Compulsive Disorder (OCD)

  5. Psychoactive Substance Abuse

- Mental Status Variations

  1. Mood—anxious, depressed

  2. Perception—feelings of detachment from self and/or environment, feeling of physical change in body

  3. Insight—impaired

- Nursing Diagnoses
    1. Anxiety
    2. Coping, ineffective individual
    3. Personal identity disturbance
    4. Sensory—perceptual alterations
- Genetic/Biological Origins
    1. Organic disease—neoplasms, epilepsy, and metabolic disorders
    2. Sensory deprivation
    3. Drug-induced-psychoactive drugs, especially hallucinogens, cannabis
- Biochemical Approaches
    1. Anxiety agents (if anxiety a component)
    2. Treatment of underlying organic disorder
- Intrapersonal
    1. Origin
        a. Internal conflict
        b. Disturbance in ego functioning
        c. Severe emotional distress
    2. Psychotherapeutic Interventions
        a. Insight-oriented psychotherapy
        b. Stress management
        c. Deal with past traumas, if present
- Family Dynamics/Family Therapy
    1. Family may exhibit poor coping mechanisms to deal with internal family conflict or outside stressors
        a. Family myths of strength may prohibit admission of family pain
        b. Family rules may prohibit verbal expression of feelings
    2. Psychoeducation about disorder

      3. Family therapy if family dynamics are stressors or influence coping with anxiety

- Group Approaches

  1. Support groups for specific stressors (parenting, occupational)

  2. Stress management group

- Milieu Interventions (rarely treated inpatient)

  1. Create safe environment

  2. Educate about disorder

  3. Assist client to examine relationship between anxiety and depersonalization

  4. Teach stress management and problem-solving techniques

  5. Plan for use of leisure time

Dissociative Identity Disorder (DID) or Multiple Personality Disorder (MPD)

- Definition: Dissociative disorder in which person has two or more separate, distinct personalities (alters), each with relatively enduring pattern of perceiving, relating to, and thinking about, self and environment

- Signs and Symptoms

  1. At least 2 personalities dominant, recurrent (APA, 1994)

  2. Core personality usually unaware of alters when first seeks treatment

  3. Personalities may represent different ages, genders, races; most have at least one child alter

  4. Personalities with different influence and power over one another

  5. Communicate with one another through executive alter or through inner dialogue

  6. Amnesic symptoms for childhood experiences, or "lose time" when alternate personality present for period of time

  7. Sleep disturbances, self mutilation, substance abuse, headaches

  8. Physiological responses (including allergies) vary in different alters

9. Issue of therapists "creating" memories and alters (North, Ryall, Ricci, & Wetzel, 1993)

    a. Verbal/nonverbal behavior of therapist may create false memories in suggestible client

    b. Public as well as some health care providers doubt validity of the diagnosis

- Differential Diagnoses
  1. Psychogenic fugues
  2. Psychogenic Amnesia
  3. Schizophrenia
  4. Borderline Personality Disorder
- Mental Status Variations
  1. Appearances—dress style, grooming, mannerisms may vary from session to session; marked changes in nonverbal behavior, handedness within sessions; blinking, eye roll, twitches with switching
  2. Speech—marked changes within brief period of time (style, accent, vocabulary)
  3. Mood—depressed, anxious; switches rapidly within sessions
  4. Thought processes—loose association with rapid switches
  5. Perceptual—hallucinations (auditory/visual); voices usually experienced within patient's head
  6. Memory—some long-term memory deficits
  7. Judgment—erratic, depending upon age, personality
  8. Insight—initially not aware of alters
- Nursing Diagnoses
  1. Anxiety
  2. Coping, ineffective individual
  3. Personal identity disturbance
  4. Self-mutilation, high risk for
  5. Violence, high risk for, directed at self and/or others
- Genetic/Biological Origins

1. Higher incidence in first-degree relatives

2. Possible psychobiological ability to dissociate or to be hypnotized

3. Self mutilation possibly biologically entrained

4. Extreme stress has long term effect on memory through release of neuropeptides/neurotransmitters which interfere with laying down of memory (Bremmer, Krystal, Charney, & Southwick, 1996)

- Biochemical Approaches

    1. Generally do not respond to psychotropic medications

    2. Antidepressants, antianxiety agents, or antipsychotics may provide symptomatic relief or help control behavior (Putnam & Lowenstein, 1993)

    3. No specific medication to treat DID

- Intrapersonal

    1. Origins

        a. Prolonged and severe physical, emotional , or sexual abuse as a child

        b. Dissociation helps child cope by creating new personalities to experience and deal with various aspects of time periods of the trauma.

        c. Alters serve various purposes (protection, expression of anger, organizer)

    2. Psychotherapeutic interventions

        a. Individual therapy stages (Putnam, 1989)

            (1) Making diagnosis

            (2) Initial interventions

                (a) Meet personalities

                (b) Take history

                (c) Develop working relationship with system

            (3) Initial stabilization

                (a) Contract with alters

                (b) Contract with entire system

(c) Stabilize uncontrollable behaviors

(4) Acceptance of diagnosis

    (a) Some alters do not accept presence of others

    (b) Issue throughout treatment

(5) Development of communication and cooperation

    (a) Internal communication

    (b) Establish cooperation toward common goals

    (c) Development of internal decision-making process

    (d) Facilitation of switching

(6) Metabolism of the trauma

    (a) Major treatment task

    (b) Uncover trauma

    (c) Abreaction

(7) Resolution and integration

    (a) Some elect integration

    (b) Others remain multiples

(8) Development of postresolution coping skills

    (a) Learn new coping skills

    (b) Take on tasks previously split

    (c) Deal with reactive depression

b. Preparation of patient for therapy re: memory (Kluft, 1996)

(1) Clarification that what emerges in therapy is "food for thought" not grounds for taking action

(2) Recovery as a healing process, not detective work

(3) Recovery can occur even if the truth of the past remains obscure

(4) Memory retrieval techniques may compromise client's credibility in legal proceedings

(5) Determination of what the client will come to believe

about his past must be made by the client, not the therapist

    (6)   Techniques of memory retrieval

        (a)   Clinical interviews

        (b)   Hypnosis

        (c)   Drug-facilitated interviews

        (d)   Dream interpretation

        (e)   Reinstatement of contextual cues

        (f)   Keeping a journal

    (7)   Distortions more likely if client subject to suggestion through leading questions, interviewer bias, reinforcement of subject/material, or focus on material difficult to verify

   c.   Hypnosis uniformly endorsed (Putnam & Lowenstein, 1993)

- Family Dynamics/Family Therapy

   1.   Family of origin characteristics

      a.   United front to community, but internal, severe conflict

      b.   Socially isolated

      c.   One caretaker with severe pathology; one abuses, one labels

      d.   Contradictory messages to child, inconsistent expectations

      e.   Rigid religious/mystical beliefs

      f.   Secrecy and denial

   2.   Family therapy with family of origin; adjunct to primary individual therapy

      b.   Complicated by severe family pathology and secrecy

      c.   Occasionally include selected family members

      d.   Abusers not included in therapy

   3.   Family therapy with partners and children

      a.   Marital therapy helpful adjunct

      b.   Help family members avoid promoting dissociation

    c. Help to deal with hostile personalities

    d. Understand process of therapy and integration

    e. Evaluate children and treat for abuse (if present)

    f. Confirm children's experience with parental behavior and label DID symptoms as illness

- Milieu Interventions

    1. Hospitalize when self-harm or danger toward others

        a. Support during abreaction

        b. Provide structure and safety

        c. Create mutually designed contract so that treatment goals understood by alters

        d. Establish primary nurse for each shift

    2. Maintain consistent, accurate understanding of MPD and client by all staff members to avoid splitting

    3. Provide safe, consistent environment

    4. No-harm contract—homicide, suicide, self-mutilation

    5. Teach techniques to provide:

        a. Anxiety reduction

        b. Personal, emotional safety

        c. Control of switching

        d. Avoidance of self-mutilation, based upon particular meaning of the behavior

    6. Educate about nature of disorder, existence and function of personalities, course of therapy, and integration

    7. Assist staff and clients to treat alters as they present

    8. Help other clients understand MPD client's behavior, attention from the staff, and their own reactions—include inward non-therapy activities, but exclude from general group sessions

Adjustment Disorders

Adjustment Disorders

- Definition: Maladaptive or pathological response to a psychosocial stressor (Strain, Hammer, Huertas, Lam, & Fulop, 1993)

- Signs and Symptoms

    1. Sources of stressors—events, such as job loss, acute or chronic illness, divorce, or specific developmental milestones (beginning school, getting married, etc.)

        a. The more numerous or more disturbing the stressors, the greater effect on adjustment

        b. Previous history of adjustment disorder puts person at more risk

    2. Distress experienced is in excess to what is expected

    3. Significant impairment in social, occupational, or school functioning (APA, 1994)

    4. Occurs within 3 months of stressor's onset

        a. Symptoms may be delayed

        b. Disorder may continue with prolonged stressor or inability to adapt

    5. Commonly diagnosed in medical settings

    6. Manifestations vary:

        a. Depressed mood

            (1) Sadness

            (2) Tearfulness

            (3) Hopelessness

        b. Anxiety

            (1) Palpitations

            (2) Agitation

            (3) Jitteriness

        c. Conduct disturbances

(1)   Violate rights of others

(2)   Violate social norms

d.   Combinations of the above

7.   Physical complaints such as headache or backache are more common in the elderly

- Differential Diagnoses

  1.   Generalized Anxiety Disorder

  2.   Depression

  3.   Somatization Disorder

  4.   Post-traumatic Stress Disorder

  5.   Uncomplicated bereavement

  6.   Conduct Disorder

- Mental Status Variations

  1.   Varies considerably, depending upon manifestation

  2.   Appearance—visibly distressed

  3.   Psychomotor Activity—restless, agitated

  4.   Mood—Anxious, Depressed

  5.   Concentration—Impaired

  6.   Thought—Preoccupation with stressors or physical symptoms

  7.   Insight—May attribute symptoms to onset of stressor

- Nursing Diagnoses

  1.   Coping, ineffective individual

  2.   Family process, altered

  3.   Parenting, altered, high risk for

  4.   Role performance, altered

  5.   Adjustment, impaired

  6.   Grieving, dysfunctional

  7.   Post-trauma response

- Genetic/Biological Origins

1. Psychological insult produces aberration of autonomic regulation and emotional lability

2. Note early responsiveness of REM (rapid eye movement) sleep waves to emotional turmoil

    (1) Decreased delta sleep initially

    (2) Continues if stress unresolved

3. Physical changes associated with aging, particularly sleep deprivation, may contribute to symptoms

4. Possible constitutional predisposition

- Biochemical Approaches

    1. Anti-depressive or anti-anxiety agents on a short-term basis

    2. Limited use of hypnotics to aid sleep

    3. Tendency for overprescription of sedatives and tranquilizers in early phase of coping with stressor

        a. Benzodiazepines which decrease delta sleep may compound problems of insomnia

        b. Beta-blockers decrease anxiety but little effect on depressive component

    4. Teach client to avoid alcohol, caffeine, nicotine, and street drugs

    5. Therapeutic touch

- Intrapersonal

    1. Origins

        a. Psychoanalytic view: early parent-child relationship shapes ability to respond to stressors in later life

        b. Cognitive/Behavioral

            (1) Cognitive coping styles reflect personal attitude and meaning of the event

            (2) Field independent persons use isolation and intellectualization

            (3) Field dependent persons use repression and denial

    2. Psychotherapeutic interventions

    a. Crisis intervention/brief therapies

        (1) Clarify meaning of the event

        (2) Engage social support

        (3) Create active interventions to ameliorate the stressor

    b. Process memories/associations elicited by the stressor

        (1) Dose-by-dose approach to difficult topics

        (2) Teach techniques to keep emotions at tolerable level

    c. Cognitive/Behavioral

        (1) Desensitization

        (2) Flooding

        (3) Stress management techniques

            (a) Autogenic Training/PMR

            (b) Hypnosis

            (c) Meditation

        (4) Assertiveness Training

        (5) Cognitive re-structuring

    d. Interpersonal support and reassurance

- Family Dynamics/Family Therapy

    1. Family members affected by client's response to stressors, or may have experienced the stressors themselves

    2. Family therapy

        a. Clarify meaning of the event

        b. Support effective coping techniques of individuals and entire family system

        c. Decrease secondary gain system-wide

        d. Facilitate decision-making and reality-testing

        e. Educate about the course of adapting to a stressor

- Group Approaches

1. Short-term group psychotherapy with problem-solving, supportive focus

2. Self-help groups developed to deal with particular stressors (e.g., divorce, death, stroke, diabetes)

   a. Common bond

   b. Experience in adjusting

   c. Chance to share coping techniques

   d. Source of continuing support

   e. Pragmatic in nature

- Milieu Interventions (Inpatient or home setting)

  1. Protect from excessive stimulation

  2. Provide structure in activities, environment, and safety

  3. Teach about adjustment process

  4. Support biological functioning (eating, sleeping, etc.)

  5. Emphasize trust in the future, social support, and self-efficacy

  6. Focus on active recollection, re-telling story while differentiating between reality and fantasy (group and/or family helpful)

  7. Reinforce increased communication with others

  8. Reduce external demands to allow for work on stressors

  9. Reinforce conscious control over ruminations or recollections

  10. Deal with recurrent stressors, shame over vulnerability, anger, and sadness

- Community

  1. Refer to community self-help groups

  2. Refer to community resources to deal with specific stressors

  3. Mobilize neighbors, churches, and other naturally occurring groups to lend help

Questions
Select the best answer

1. Ms. Smith, who has panic attacks, comes to where you are sitting and says "it's happening again. I can't breathe. I know I'm going to die." She is breathing with difficulty. She has been attending a group to learn more about panic attacks and how to avert them. Your best response is:

   a. "Let me take your blood pressure."
   b. "You know what to do—start your exercises."
   c. "You're experiencing anxiety; that's what you are feeling."
   d. "Tell me what's been going on."

2. Persons with recurrent panic disorders usually present with:

   a. High level of general anxiety
   b. Cardiac/respiratory symptoms of distress
   c. La belle indifference
   d. Clear precipitants

3. A priority nursing diagnosis for Sandra, an agoraphobic, who will not leave her house without her husband accompanying her is:

   a. Post trauma response
   b. Parenting, altered
   c. Fear
   d. Denial, ineffective

4. Mr. Lee has a generalized anxiety disorder. You will be teaching him some relaxation techniques. When is the best time for him to learn?

   a. When he is only mildly anxious
   b. Immediately after feeling severe distress
   c. In the middle of a time of moderate distress
   d. After taking an anti-anxiety agent

5. Jim, who suffers from severe flashbacks of war experiences, and has just been admitted, sits on the lounge, apart from other clients. Your best response is:

   a. Let him remain apart until he's ready to disclose
   b. Introduce him to two other veterans on the unit with similar problems
   c. Suggest that he work on a crossword puzzle until dinner
   d. Observe him for flashbacks

6. Symptoms of autonomic arousal in the PTSD client include:

    a. Hypersomnia
    b. Tachycardia
    c. Alexithymia
    d. Hypotonic musculature

7. Which mental status variations would you expect for a client diagnosed as having PTSD?

    a. Thought: Delusion of Grandeur
    b. Perceptual: Derealization
    c. Memory: Impaired recent memory
    d. Mood: Inappropriate, silly

8. Physiological monitoring of clients using benzodiazepines includes:

    a. CBC with differential
    b. Kidney function studies
    c. Blood pressure
    d. Serum benzodiazepine levels

9. Jerry, a miner, was injured a year ago and hasn't been able to return to work because of severe low back pain. His neurologist could find no organic reason for his continuing pain. Which of the following psychiatric diagnosis best fits Jerry's clinical picture?

    a. Factitious disorder
    b. Hypochondriasis
    c. Pain disorder
    d. Conversion disorder

10. Nursing diagnoses for Jerry might include all but:

    a. Role performance, altered
    b. Pain, chronic
    c. Post trauma response
    d. Family processes, altered

11. An explanation for Jerry's continued pain in spite of his neurologist's findings is:

    a. Secondary gain
    b. High endorphin levels

   c. High serotonin levels
   d. Repression of unacceptable impulses

12. Treatment of Jerry's chronic pain is likely to include all but which of the following?

   a. Exercise program
   b. Biofeedback-assisted relaxation
   c. Pain support group
   d. Anti-anxiety agents

13. John has been preparing for running a marathon for over a year. "It's my 40th birthday present to myself" he explains. The morning of the race, his wife finds him still in bed, his legs paralyzed. John tells her that he guesses he can't race after all. What mental status variations might you expect?

   a. Mood: Depressed, anxious
   b. Mood: La belle indifference
   c. Mood: Blunted affect
   d. Mood: Relieved

14. The symptoms of a conversion disorder may be related to:

   a. Heightened autonomic arousal
   b. Displacement of aggression
   c. Mid-life crisis
   d. Symbolic relationship with conflict

15. Mae has an intense argument with her 15-year-old daughter who visits her daily in the hospital where Mae is being treated for hypochondriasis. Mae sends her daughter home and asks the nurse for medication for her stomach. "I wonder if she'll regret this when I'm dead of stomach cancer?" she states. Your best reply is:

   a. "Let's talk about what just happened."
   b. "This antacid will help."
   c. "Teenagers just go through those phases."
   d. "Mae, there is *no* sign of stomach cancer. You're not about to die."

16. A client with a conversion disorder hospitalized in a psychiatric facility will require which approach by nursing staff:

   a. Anticipate and meet self-care needs of client
   b. Encourage attendance at expressive therapies

    c. Reinforce verbal expression of needs

    d. Remind the client that his difficulties are not real

17. When an MPD client is hospitalized for serious self-inflicted cuts, the no-harm contract should include:

    a. Ward privileges gained for no self-harm

    b. Clear alternatives to follow when feeling the urge to cut

    c. Provision of antipsychotics for increased agitation

    d. Discharge from the hospital if there is self harm

18. Which is true about the resolution of MPD?

    a. Clients must integrate alters

    b. All traumatic incidents must be remembered

    c. Many clients experience a reactive depression

    d. Some alters always exist, although hidden

19. Given the diagnosis of depersonalization disorder, which nursing diagnosis is most likely to result from assessment?

    a. Powerlessness

    b. Grieving, dysfunctional

    c. Personal identity disturbance

    d. Depersonalization alteration

20. Treatment of dissociative amnesia includes all modalities *except:*

    a. Hypnosis

    b. Stress management

    c. Anti-anxiety agents

    d. Psychotherapy

21. Mrs. Peters who has experienced a traumatic automobile accident in which three persons were burned to death, tells you that she just wants to "put it behind her." She refuses to talk about the accident or attend activities, and says, "I just want my nerve pills." Your best response is:

    a. "Nerve pills are highly addictive. You need to learn to relax."

    b. "I can see why you'd like to put it behind you. It must have been very scary."

    c. "You are right. It's important to carry on and not dwell on the past."

    d. "I hope you'll talk to your doctor about this."

22. Mrs. Peters asks why she has to go to art therapy this morning. "I'm no artist. My hobby is gardening. I'd rather go gardening. I'd rather just stay here and watch a little television." Which is your best response?

    a. "Art therapy is one way to express yourself. You don't have to be an artist—just be willing to try the activity."

    b. "Art therapy may give you an idea about undiscovered talents. You just might be a great artist inside."

    c. "Art therapy is good, but I'll see if we can't schedule you for the green house activity instead."

    d. "I'll stay here and talk with you while you watch TV."

23. Mrs. Peters finally decides to participate in art therapy. She returns to the unit red-eyed and clutching a paper covered with heavy red scrawls. She stops and shows it to you. The best response would be:

    a. "That's really good. That red must be the fire."

    b. "Let's put this up for the other patients to see."

    c. "This is very strong—tell me about it."

    d. "If art therapy was too troubling, I do have some medication for you."

24. Mary has been diagnosed as having a depersonalization disorder. Which experience might she relate during your initial nursing assessment?

    a. "This feeling is so weird—I feel just 'unreal.' "

    b. "I haven't been able to take care of the kids; I just sit around."

    c. "It's no big deal."

    d. "I have dreams that I just can't get out of."

25. Joe, now age 34, was sexually abused by a youth group leader when he was 14. Joe is most likely to present with which of the following statements?

    a. "I have really close friends, both males and females."

    b. "I've told so many people my story that it is getting a little old."

    c. "I don't see how some little thing that happened 20 years ago is influencing my life now."

    d. "I have a great sex life."

26. Mary is thinking about entering a Women's Shelter if her husband starts to abuse her one more time. Her chief concern should be to:

    a. Try to make the relationship work since he has promised to stop abusing her.

    b. Develop a safety plan for her and her children if he begins to escalate.

    c. Let him know she is pregnant because a man is unlikely to hurt a pregnant woman.

    d. Acknowledge her role in causing the abuse.

27. Chris, a successful music major, is preparing for his recital next week. He has experienced severe stage fright in the past and once, refused to perform at all. Which of the following biochemical approaches is most likely to be employed in conjunction with behavioral therapy for his difficulty?

    a. Mono-amine oxidase inhibitor

    b. Tricyclic antidepressant

    c. Beta-adrenergic antagonist

    d. Antiparkinsoniam agent

28. Your client, Fred, attends a men's group for adult survivors of childhood sexual abuse. Some men in the group are currently confronting their families, but Fred is unsure of his course of action. Your best response is:

    a. "Most families welcome the honesty as difficult as it is for everyone."

    b. "You've been learning to be assertive. This is probably the next step."

    c. "If you don't confront your father now, you'll always feel powerless."

    d. "That's a difficult decision. What would you like to have happen with your family?"

29. A Vietnam veteran who served at a field hospital late in the war becomes symptomatic of PTSD after a long period of what seemed excellent adjustment. Her husband and children have joined her in your office to talk about what's happening. They ask if she has PTSD. What is your best response?

    a. Yes, she has PTSD, but we are going to let "bygones" be "bygones" and work on other things in therapy.

    b. "I think there is a different problem. PTSD occurs much sooner."

    c. "She has symptoms of PTSD which are difficult not just for her, but for all of you."

    d. The problem is rooted in the past, family can do nothing now.

30. Family therapy for the PTSD client and her family will meet all but one of the following goals:

    a. Develop a shared frame of reference for the trauma

    b. Support the victim in recovery

    c. Reduce secondary gain by limiting trauma talk to therapy sessions only

    d. Address issues of trust, responsibility, and blame

31. Now, three weeks after the hurricane, Charley cannot remember anything about his 36- hour ordeal, trapped under debris from his house until he was finally rescued. This is best described as:

    a. Dissociative amnesia, localized
    b. Dissociative amnesia, generalized
    c. Dissociative amnesia, continuous
    d. Dissociative amnesia, selective

32. A community support group for flood victims asks you, the CNS, to talk about symptoms of PTSD. The group has been meeting since the disaster six months ago. One woman asks why she continues to have periodic, recurrent dreams and thoughts about the flood. Which is your best reply?

    a. "Your mind is attempting to work through what happened, a little bit at a time."
    b. "You are probably thinking too much. Try to stop these thoughts."
    c. "You could be guilty about surviving."
    d. "At this time, you have a serious problem. Have you seen your doctor?"

33. One hypothesis why PTSD clients may continue to engage in dangerous activities and have recurrent interpersonal difficulties is related to:

    a. Serotonin excesses
    b. Autonomic entrainment
    c. Endogenous opioid withdrawal
    d. Dysregulation of GABA

34. Leonard has recently avoided going out to eat with his family at restaurants. He claims the food is better at home, and that other people may watch him eat and critique his table manners. The most appropriate psychiatric diagnosis is:

    a. Schizophrenia with delusions
    b. Agoraphobia
    c. Avoidant Personality Disorder
    d. Social Phobia

35. The client presenting with a somatization disorder typically:

    a. Exaggerates the seriousness of minor symptoms into major health problems
    b. Refuses medication, preferring to "work it out alone"
    c. Has a chaotic social life
    d. Understands the stress-physical symptoms relationship

36. Joan, who obsessively thinks about her children dying in a house fire, is learning to use thought-stopping techniques. Such techniques include:

    a. Practicing progressive muscle relaxation
    b. Discussing with a staff member the likelihood of a house fire
    c. Snapping a rubber band on her wrist when the thought of fire occurs
    d. Reminding herself of the home fire alarm system

37. Anxiety-reducing techniques such as autogenic\training or progressive muscle relaxation are best employed by a person who fears flying on airplanes:

    a. When anxiety rises to intolerable levels
    b. When the plane takes off and lands
    c. Prior to feeling autonomic arousal
    d. Only in practice settings

38. The psychoanalytic explanation for a phobic disorder involves:

    a. Classical conditioned responses
    b. Reaction formation
    c. Displacement
    d. Avoidance

39. Group therapies for the treatment of agoraphobia include:

    a. Social skills training
    b. Medication education
    c. Art or movement therapies
    d. Gestalt approaches

40. Systematic desensitization includes all but which of the following?

    a. In vivo exposure
    b. Deep muscle relaxation
    c. Understanding why stimuli are anxiety provoking
    d. Cognitive coping self-statements

41. Peggy is hospitalized because of emotional exhaustion. Her husband reports that she has become increasingly preoccupied with cleaning the house over the past year. Always a meticulous housekeeper, she is now afraid that the house is contaminated by environmental toxins. She is up most of the night, trying to clean and decontaminate. When her husband attempts to have her rest, she becomes distraught. The most accurate psychiatric diagnosis is:

    a. Obsessive compulsive disorder
    b. Obsessive compulsive personality disorder
    c. Schizophrenia, paranoid type
    d. Major depression

42. Probable nursing diagnoses include all but:

    a. Coping, ineffective individual
    b. Anxiety
    c. Role performance, altered
    d. Home maintenance management, impaired

43. Clomipramine (Anafranil), 250 mgm every morning, is ordered for Peggy. After taking the medication for a week, she complains of being too sleepy to participate in morning activities. Which of the following actions might the CNS suggest?

    a. Tell her the sleepiness will soon disappear
    b. Recommend the medication be taken at bedtime
    c. Request the medication be discontinued immediately
    d. Reschedule her activities to late afternoon

44. The most effective treatment of panic disorders is:

    a. Reworking previous traumatic separations
    b. Family therapy
    c. Cognitive restructuring
    d. Provision of a stress-free environment

45. Persons prone to high levels of anxiety tend to have which dysfunctional thoughts?

    a. Negative views about the self, world, and future
    b. Overestimation of the support of others
    c. Overestimation of danger
    d. ''Black or white'' thinking

46. Mrs. Stevens has been taking Alprazolam (Xanax) 2.0 mgm/day for six months. She wants to become pregnant and, in preparation, goes off the medication. She currently experiences little anxiety. She has learned a variety of coping techniques in therapy. Your best response to her desire to discontinue the Xanax is:

    a. ''Since you are doing so well, go ahead and stop taking your Xanax.''

b. "You should remain on benzodiazepines for at least one year."

c. "Should you decide to discontinue Xanax, it's important to very slowly reduce the dose."

d. "You might want to try a shorter-acting medication like Oxazepam (Serax) as a substitute."

47. Susan was admitted at 3 a.m. to the emergency department of a medical center, complaining of stomach pain which she believes is cancer. Although she admits to having eaten some "real spicy food" the evening before, she is insistent on having an upper and lower GI series immediately. She is anxious, despite her doctor's reassurance. Which is a likely psychiatric diagnosis?

a. Conversion disorder
b. Hypochondriasis
c. Pain disorder
d. Generalized anxiety disorder

48. A primary focus of treatment for Susan will be:

a. Dietary instructions and antacids
b. Stress management techniques
c. Insight-focused psychotherapy
d. Rehabilitation efforts

49. Upon questioning your client during the intake interview, she relates that she hears voices inside her head, as if in a conversation. Which psychiatric diagnosis best fits these experiences?

a. Schizophrenia
b. PTSD
c. MPD
d. Panic Disorder

50. Family therapy with partners and children of MPD clients is aimed at which of the following?

a. Help children access child alters
b. Help children deal with hostile alters
c. Help children ignore inconsistent parental behavior
d. Help children parent the child alters

51. The most efficacious approach for dealing with a client who has a somatization disorder is to:

    a. Use antidepressants

    b. Closely collaborate with the primary care provider

    c. Confront the unreality of the symptoms

    d. Provide brief, problem-focused therapy

52. Seth, age 72, has almost doubled the amount of Diazepam (Valium) prescribed for him, claiming that his ''nerves are shot'' and the medicine doesn't do enough for him. Which sign of toxicity is the nurse likely to see?

    a. Nausea and vomiting

    b. Rapid speech with flight of ideas

    c Psychomotor excitation

    d. Short-term memory impairment

53. Ellie has a past history of cutting and burning her arms and ankles when anxious or dissociating. She admits to ''little cuts'' last night when thinking about working with a new therapist. Which is the best initial strategy of the advanced practice nurse when beginning therapy with Ellie?

    a. Assist Ellie to identify the patterns and function of self injury

    b. Give her telephone numbers so that the nurse can be reached whenever Ellie begins to feel self-injurious

    c. Define self-injury as unacceptable and as grounds for termination of the therapeutic relationship

    d. Ignore the behavior so as not to reinforce it

Answers

1. c	19. c	37. c
2. b	20. c	38. c
3. c	21. b	39. a
4. a	22. a	40. c
5. b	23. c	41. a
6. b	24. a	42. d
7. b	25. c	43. b
8. a	26. b	44. c
9. c	27. c	45. c
10. c	28. d	46. c
11. a	29. c	47. b
12. d	30. c	48. b
13. b	31. a	49. c
14. d	32. a	50. b
15. a	33. c	51. b
16. c	34. d	52. d
17. b	35. c	53. a
18. c	36. c	

Bibliography

Abramowitz, J. S. (1997). Effectiveness of psychological and pharmacological treatments for obsessive-compulsive disorder: A quantitative review. *Journal of Consulting and Clinical Psychology, 65*(1), 44–52.

American Psychiatric Association. (1994). *Diagnostic and statistical manual of mental disorders* (4th ed.). Washington, DC: Author.

Barloon, D. E. (1993). Effects on children of having lived with a parent who has an anxiety disorder. *Issues in Mental Health Nursing, 14*, 187–199.

Battaglia, M., Bertella, S., Politi, E., Bernadeschi, L., Perna, G., Gabriele, A., & Bellodi, L. (1995). Age of onset of panic disorder: Influence of familial liability to the disease and of childhood separation disorder. *American Journal of Psychiatry, 152*(9), 1362–1364.

Beck, A. T., Sokol, L., Clark, D. A., Berchick, R., & Wright, F. (1992). A crossover study of focused cognitive group therapy for panic disorder. *American Journal of Psychiatry, 149*(6), 778–783.

Beck, J. C., Stanley, M. A., & Zebb, B. J. (1996). Characteristics of generalized anxiety disorder in older adults: A descriptive study. *Behaviour Research and Therapy, 34*(3), 225–234.

Blair, D. T., & Ramones, V. A. (1996). The undertreatment of anxiety: Overcoming the confusion and stigma. *Journal of Psychosocial Nursing, 34*(6), 9–18.

Bremmer, J. D., Krystal, J. H., Charney, D. S., & Southwick, S. M. (1996). Neural mechanisms in dissociative amnesia for childhood sexual abuse: Relevance to the current controversy surrounding the "false memory syndrome." *American Journal of Psychiatry, 153*(7), 71–82.

Campbell, J. C., Harris, M. J., & Lee, R. K. (1995). Violence research: An overview. *Scholarly Inquiry for Nursing Practice, 9*(2), 106–126.

Connors, R. (1996a). Self-injury in trauma survivors: 1. Functions and meanings. *American Journal of Orthopsychiatry, 66*(2), 197–206.

Connors, R. (1996b). Self-injury in trauma survivors: 2. Levels of clinical response. *American Journal of Orthopsychiatry, 66*(2), 207–216.

Crothers, D. (1995). Vicarious traumatization in the work with survivors of childhood trauma. *Journal of Psychosocial Nursing and Mental Health Services, 33*(4), 9–13.

Davis, M., Eshelman, E. R., & McKay, M. (1988). *The relaxation and stress reduction workbook* (3rd ed.). Oakland, CA: New Harbinger.

Draucker, C. B. (1992). The healing process of female adult incest survivors: Constructing a personal residence. *Image, 24*(1), 4–8.

Draucker, C. B., & Petrovic, K. (1997). Therapy with male survivors of sexual abuse: The client perspective. *Issues in Mental Health Nursing, 18,* 139–155.

Ford, C. V., Katon, W. J., & Lipkin, M. (1993). Managing somatization and hypochondriasis. *Patient Care, 27*(2), 31–34.

Freeston, M. H., Dugas, M. J., & Ladouceur, R. (1996). Thoughts, images, worry, and anxiety. *Cognitive Therapy and Research, 20*(3), 265–273.

Friedman, M. J. (1996). PTSD diagnosis and treatment for mental health clinicians. *Community Mental Health Journal, 32*(2), 173–189.

Greenwald, R. (1996). The information gap in the EMDR controversy. *Professional psychology: Research and practice, 27*(1), 67–72.

Harvey, A. L., & Rapee, R. M. (1995). Cognitive behavioral therapy for generalized anxiety disorder. *Psychiatric Clinics of North America 18*(4), 859–870.

Herman, J. (1992). *Trauma and recovery.* NY: Basic Books.

Johnson, M. R., & Lydiard, R. B. (1995). The neurobiology of anxiety disorders. *The Psychiatric Clinics of North America, 18*(4), 681–725.

Katon, W. J., Lin, E., VonKorff, M., Russo, J., Lipscomb, P., & Bush, T. (1991). Somatization: A spectrum of severity. *American Journal of Psychiatry, 148*(1), 34–40.

Kline, M., Sydnor-Greenberg, N., Davis, W. W., Pincus, H. A., & Frances, A. J. (1993). Using field trips to evaluate proposal changes in DSM diagnosis criteria. *Hospital and Community Psychiatry, 44*(7), 621–623.

Kluft, R. P. (1991). Clinical manifestations of multiple personality disorder. *Psychiatric Clinics of North America, 14,* 605–629.

Kluft, R. P. (1996). Treating the traumatic memories of patients with dissociative identity disorder. *American Journal of Psychiatry, 153*(7), 103–110.

Lydiard, R. B., Brawman-Mintzer, O., & Ballenger, J. C. (1996). Recent developments in the psychopharmacology of anxiety disorders. *Journal of Consulting and Clinical Psychology, 64*(4), 660–668.

Loftus, E. F. (1993). The reality of repressed memories. *American Psychologist, 48,* 518–537.

Lowenstein, R. J. (1991). An office mental status examination for complex chronic dissociative symptoms and multiple personality disorder. *Psychiatric Clinics of North America, 14,* 567–604.

McFarlane, J., Parker, B., and Soeken, K. (1995). Abuse during pregnancy: Frequency, severity, perpetrator, and risk factors of homicide. *Public Health Nursing, 12*(5), 284–289.

McKay, M., Davis, M., & Fanning, P. (1981). *Thoughts and feelings: The art of cognitive stress intervention.* Oakland, CA: New Harbinger.

Miller, S. D., de Shazer, S., Berg, I. K., & Hopwood. (1993). *From problem to solution: The solution focused brief therapy approach.* New York: Norton.

North, C. S., Ryall, J. M., Ricci, D. A., & Wetzel, R. D. (1993). *Multiple personalities, multiple disorders.* NY: Oxford University Press.

Otto, M. W., & Whittal, M. L. (1995). Cognitive-behavior therapy and the longitudinal course of panic disorder. *The Psychiatric Clinics of North America, 18*(4), 803–821.

Pollack, M. H., & Smoller, J. W. (1995). The longitudinal course and outcome of panic disorders. *The Psychiatric Clinics of North America, 18*(4), 785–801.

Pollock, D. (1992). Structured ambiguity and definition of psychiatric illness: Adjustment disorder among medical inpatients. *Social Science and Medicine, 35*(1), 25–35.

Putnam, F. W. (1989). *Diagnosis & treatment of multiple personality disorder.* New York: Guilford.

Putnam, F. W., & Lowenstein, R. J. (1993). Treatment of multiple personality disorder: A survey of current practices. *American Journal of Psychiatry, 150*(7), 1048–1052.

Rodriguez, N., Ryan, S. W., Vande Kemp, H., & Foy, D. W. (1997). Post-traumatic stress disorder in adult female survivors of childhood sexual abuse: A comparison study. *Journal of Consulting and Clinical Psychology, 65*(1), 53–59.

Shapiro, F. (1995). *Eye movement desensitization and reprocessing: Basic principles, protocols, and procedures.* New York: Guilford.

Shear, K. M. (1996). Factors in the etiology and pathogenesis of panic disorder: Revisiting the attachment-separation paradigm. *American Journal of Psychiatry, 153*(7), 125–136.

Shear, M. K. (1995). Psychotherapeutic issues in long-term treatment of anxiety disorder patients. *The Psychiatric Clinics of North America, 18*(4), 885–893.

Sheikh, J. I., & Salzman, C. (1995). Anxiety in the elderly. *The Psychiatric Clinics of North America, 18*(4), 871–883.

Spratto, G. R., & Woods, A. L. (1993). *RN's nurses drug reference.* Albany, NY: Delmar.

Strain, J., Hammer, J., Huertas, D., Lam, H. T., & Fulop, G. (1993). The problem of coping as a reason for psychiatric consultation. *General Hospital Psychiatry, 15*(1), 1–8.

Symes, L. (1995). Post traumatic stress disorder: An evolving concept. *Archives of Psychiatric Nursing, 9*(4), 195–202.

van der Kolk, B. A., McFarlane, A. C., & Weisaeth, L. (Eds.). (1996). *Traumatic Stress.* New York: Guilford.

van der Kolk, B. A., Pelcovitz, D, Roth, S., Mandel, F., McFarlane, A., & Herman, J. L. (1997). Dissociation, somatization, and affect dysregulation: The complexity of adaptation to trauma. *American Journal of Psychiatry, 153*(7), 83–93.

Webster, D. C., Vaughn, K., Webb, M., & Playtor, A. (1995). Modeling the client's world through brief solution-focused therapy. *Issues in Mental Health Nursing, 16,* 505-518.

Weingourt, R. (1996). Connection and disconnection in abusive relationships. *Perspectives in Psychiatric Care, 32*(2), 15–19.

Williams, L. M. (1994). Recall of childhood trauma: A prospective study of women's memories of child sexual abuse. *Journal of Consulting and Clinical Psychology, 62,* 1167-1176.

Wilson, S. A., Becker, L. A., & Tinker, R. H. (1995). Eye movement desensitization and reprocessing (EMDR) treatment for psychologically traumatized individuals. *Journal of Consulting and Clinical Psychology, 63*(6), 928–937.

Schizophrenia and Other Psychotic Disorders

Mary Fultz Spencer
Mary Ann Camaan

Schizophrenia

- Definition: Disorder of the brain producing disturbances in reality, thought process and social development (Johnson, 1993); seen as persistent, long-term illness with alternating periods of exacerbation and remission

- Epidemiology

  1. 1.5% of U.S. population has been diagnosed with disorder

  2. New diagnoses occur in 0.3 to 0.6 per 100 persons per year in the U.S.

  3. Age of onset later in females than males

- Signs and Symptoms (APA, 1994)

  1. Presence of two (or more) of the following for a significant portion of time during a one month period (or less if successfully treated)

     a. Delusions

     b. Hallucinations

     c. Disorganized speech—derailment or incoherence

     d. Grossly disorganized or catatonic behavior

     e. Negative symptoms—affective flattening, alogia or avolition

  2. Only one of the above symptoms is necessary in the presence of:

     a. Bizarre delusions (involving a phenomenon that the person's culture would regard as totally implausible, e.g., thought broadcasting, being controlled by a dead person)

     b. Hallucinations of a voice with content having no apparent relation to depression or elation, or a voice keeping up a running commentary on person's behavior or thoughts

     c. Two or more voices conversing with each other

  3. Social/ocupational dysfunction for a significant portion of time since onset

     a. In adults—work, interpersonal relations or self-care below level achieved before onset

     b. In children or adolescents—failure to achieve expected level of interpersonal, academic or occupational achievement

4. Continuous signs of the disturbance for at least six months including:

   a. At least one month of active symptoms (or less if successfully treated) and

   b. Prodromal and residual phases including the following negative symptoms

      (1) Withdrawal or social isolation

      (2) Impairment in role functioning

      (3) Odd behavior (e.g., talking to self in public)

      (4) Little attention to personal hygiene, bathing, manner of dress, overall self-care and activities of daily living

      (5) Odd speech characterized by circumstantiality, tangentiality, poverty of speech, or poverty of content of speech

      (6) Magical thinking including ideas of reference

      (7) Recurrent illusions or other perceptual experiences

      (8) Decrease in motivation, energy, or initiative

   c. Prodromal and residual phase may also consist of two or more active phase symptoms in an attenuated form (e.g. odd beliefs, unusual perceptual experiences) or only negative symptoms

- Subtypes of Schizophrenia

  1. Paranoid Schizophrenia—characterized by preoccupation with one or more delusions which may be persecutory, or by frequent auditory hallucinations

  2. Disorganized Schizophrenia—characterized by a flat or incongruous affect; exhibits bizarre mannerisms and social isolation occur; onset occurs early in life and often has persistent symptoms

  3. Catatonic Schizophrenia—identified by intense psychomotor disturbance; disturbance may take the form of stupor or excitement and is manifested by such psychomotor disturbances as posturing, immobility, catalepsy, mutism and negativism

4. Undifferentiated Schizophrenia—meets active phase criteria but does not fit the criteria of other subtypes; manifested by fragmented delusions, visual hallucinations, bizarre and disorganized behaviors, disorientation and incoherence (Fortinash & Holoday-Worret, 1995)

5. Residual Schizophrenia—absence of hallucinations and delusions; two or more residual symptoms are continued

- Differential Diagnosis/Related Disorders: Important that the presence of psychotic symptoms be assessed in relationship to other related, concomitant, or neurological disorders

  1. Mood disorder with psychotic features

  2. Organic illnesses—medical work-up important to rule this out

  3. Substance abuse/use/toxic psychosis—acute intoxication with legal and illegal substances and/or drug reactions to medicinal drugs may induce psychotic behaviors and thought disorders, e.g., alcohol withdrawal, amphetamines, bromides, corticosteroids, ephedrine, levadopa, LSD, phencylidine, propranolol, tricyclic antidepressants (Vallone, 1997)

  4. Other Psychotic Disorders

     a. Delusional disorders

     b. Schizophreniform disorder

     c. Schizoaffective disorder

     d. Brief Psychotic Disorder

  5. Brain disorders—e.g., emboli, ischemia, trauma, tumor, epilepsy, narcolepsy, encephalitis, Huntington's disease (Vallone, 1997)

  6. Systemic Disorders—vitamin B_{12} deficiency, AIDS, Syphilis, tuberculous meningitis, pellagra, hypoglycemia, hepatic encephalopathy, hyperthyroidism, lead, mercury poisoning, multiple sclerosis (Burgess, 1997)

  7. Dementias and Delirium—especially in the elderly; may be manifested by irritability, anxiety, isolation and agitation

Schizophreniform Disorder

- Definition/Signs and Symptoms

  1. Episode of symptoms of schizophrenia which last at least one month but less than six months

  2. Good prognosis indicated by:

     a. Psychotic symptoms within 4 weeks of onset

     b. Confusion during psychosis

     c. Good social and occupational functioning before onset

     d. Blunted or flat affect absent (APA, 1994)

- Differential Diagnosis

  1. Schizophrenia, schizoaffective and mood disorders

  2. Medical illness or medication response

Delusional Disorder

- Definition/Signs and Symptoms: Active Phase

  1. Nonbizarre delusions

  2. None of the folowing for more than a few hours

     a. Hallucinations

     b. Disorganized Speech

     c. Grossly disorganized or catatonic behavior

     d. Negative symptoms

  3. Functioning not markedly impaired except for the impact of the delusions

  4. In the elderly, mood may be manifested by anger, paranoia and anxiety; behaviors may include suspiciousness, aggression and isolation

- Types of delusions (Townsend, 1993)

  1. Persecutory—belief that others are after them or "out to get them"; may feel they are being followed by the CIA or that others are poisoning their food

  2. Jealous—belief that one's sexual partner is unfaithful

3. Erotomania—belief that someone in a higher status or position is in love with them

4. Grandiose—belief that they have special knowledge or powers; may believe they are Jesus Christ or the President of the United States

5. Somatic—belief that one's appearance is abnormal or some physical illness is present

- Differential Diagnosis: Schizophrenia

Schizoaffective Disorder

- Definition: Major depressive episode, or manic episode which occurs concurrently with active phase schizophrenia symptoms; during same period of illness, there have been delusions or hallucinations for at least 2 weeks in the absence of prominent mood symptoms, but mood symptoms are present during a substantial part of the illness (APA, 1994)

Brief Psychotic Disorder

- Definition/Signs and Symptoms

  1. One of the following is present and not culturally sanctioned

     a. Delusions

     b. Hallucinations

     c. Disorganized speech

     d. Grossly disorganized or catatonic behavior

  2. Onset is generally sudden with duration of symptoms of one month or less, but at least one day

  3. Individual recovers to a normal level of functioning

  4. Presence or absence of marked stressors should be noted, as should onset within four weeks of postpartum

- Differential Diagnosis

  1. Schizophrenia—symptoms are similar due to hallucinations and delusions, but thought disorder is not as evident (Torrey, 1988)

  2. Drug-induced psychosis

3. No mood disorder is present.

4. Schizoaffective disorder—no mood disorder

Shared Psychotic Disorder (Folie à deux)

- Signs and Symptoms (APA, 1994)

    1. Delusional system develops in the context of a close relationship with a person who already has a psychotic disorder with delusions

    2. Delusion is similar in content to that of the person who already has the established delusion

- Differential Diagnosis

    1. Schizophrenia or another psychotic disorder

    2. Substance abuse or a general medical illness

Psychotic Disorder Due to a General Medical Condition

- Signs and Symptoms (APA, 1994): Delusions or hallucinations which:

    1. Do not occur during course of delirium or dementia

    2. Are not better accounted for by another mental disorder

    3. Are related to a medical condition as determined by

        a. History

        b. Physical examination

        c. Laboratory findings

Substance Induced Psychotic Disorder

- Definition: (APA, 1994) Delusions or hallucinations (these are not included if the client has insight that they are substance induced) which:

    1. Develop during or within a month of significant substance intoxication

    2. Are in excess of what would be expected for the amount and type of substance abused

    3. Do not occur during the course of delirium or dementia

- Differential diagnosis: Other psychotic disorders

Psychotic Disorder not Otherwise Specified

- Signs and Symptoms (APA, 1994)

    1. Postpartum psychosis which does not meet other DSM criteria

    2. Persistent auditory hallucinations with no other symptoms

    3. "Persistent nonbizarre delusions with periods of overlapping mood episodes that have been present for a substantial portion of the delusional disturbance"

    4. Psychosis where a more specific diagnosis is impossible

    5. Psychotic symptoms which have lasted for less than 1 month but have not yet remitted, so that the criteria for Brief Psychotic Disorder are not met

THE FOLLOWING INFORMATION APPLIES TO SCHIZOPHRENIA AND OTHER PSYCHOTIC DISORDERS

- Mental Status Variation/Related Nursing Diagnosis

    1. Alteration in sensory Input—internal senses, emotions; external senses, sight, sound, touch, taste, smell; problems in pain recognition

    2. Alteration in cognitive function—difficulty with memory, impaired short term/long term memory; difficulty maintaining attention, distractibility

    3. Alteration in thought process—loose associations, tangentiality, incoherence, illogical, pressured, distractible speech, circumstantiality; illogical thinking, lack of planning skill, difficulty in making decisions, concrete thinking

    4. Alteration in thought content—delusions (paranoid, grandiose, religious, somatic, thought broadcasting, thought insertion, thought control; hallucinations (auditory, visual)

    5. Social isolation—related to difficulties in thought process as well as stigma and difficulty communicating

    6. Self care deficits—related to difficulty with attention, may include personal hygiene, grooming, lack of volition, and lack of perception of self and others

    7. Impaired verbal communication—related to alteration in thought process and content

8. Altered sleep patterns—decreased rapid eye movement (REM) sleep

9. Potential for violence (self or others)—related to command hallucinations or persecutory delusions

10. Past trauma response—possible for Brief Psychotic Disorder

11. Alteration in Nutrition—related to delusions about food

- Genetic/Biological Theories of Schizophrenia and Other Psychotic Disorders:

  1. Genetic (Torrey, Bowler, Taylor & Gottesman, 1994)

     a. The lifetime risk of developing schizophrenia when one has a parent, identical twin or sibling with schizophrenia is much higher than in the population at large

     b. Torrey et al. (1994) studied 66 pairs of identical twins and noted that 27 pairs were discordant for schizophrenia and 13 pairs were concordant for schizophrenia.

  2. Immunologic/Risk Factor Models

     a. Exposure to viruses, especially influenza prenatally—theorized that such exposure may create maternal antibodies which become autoantibodies in the fetus and create source of development changes which present risk factor for schizophrenia (Cannon & Marco, 1994)

     b. Risk factors associated with schizophrenia

        (1) Studies of childhood encephalitis, head trauma under age 10, hemorrhage into the ventricles, ischemic damage to cortex associated with schizophrenia

        (2) Twin studies established indicators of liability, but do not predict the disease (Torrey, Bowler, Taylor & Gottesman, 1994)

  3. Neuroanatomic Models—structural functional abnormalities according to magnetic resonance imaging (MRI) and computerized tomography (CT) scans

     a. Ventricular enlargement

     b. Prominence of cortical sulci

     c. Defects in limbic brain structure

    d.   Cortical atrophy/ decrease in number of cortical neurons (usually more pronounced in the left hemisphere) possibly linked with negative symptoms (Walker, 1997)

    e.   Subtle neuroanatomical differences in part of the thalamus, septum, hypothalamus, hippocampus, amygdala and cingulate gyrus (Bendik, 1996)

    f.   5% reduction in brain weight and slight decrease in brain length (Keltner & Folks, 1997)

    g.   Decrease in volume of temporal lobe structures and decrease in substantia nigra and putamen (Walker, 1997)

    h.   Thickening of corpus callosum on MRI

    i.   Abnormalities in brain density and symmetry

    j.   Atrophy of portion of cerebellum

4.   Neurofetal Development Factors (Fox & Kane, 1996)—enlarged lateral and third ventricles, decrease in cranial, cerebral and frontal brain tissue, delivery complications (may affect fetal neural development)

5.   Neurophysiological Models

    a.   Decreased cerebral blood flow (as measured by Single Photon Emission Computed Tomography (SPECT)) (Keltner & Folks, 1997) and decreased glucose metabolism in the frontal lobes (as measured by Positron Emission Tomography (PET))

    b.   Hypofrontality may be related to changes in abstract thinking and social judgement

6.   Neurotransmitter Models

    a.   Theories about schizophrenia include specific and interconnected roles of various neurotransmitters

    b.   Serotonin ($5HT_2$) deficiency may be responsible for some forms of schizophrenia

    c.   Norepinephrine (NE) may be insufficient in clients with schizophrenia that display prominent negative symptoms

    d.   Dopamine (DA) is likely to be excessive at certain receptor sites or persons with schizophrenia may have more dopamine receptors.

D_2 receptors are present in limbic and motor neuron center; over activity of D_2 receptors may be related to positive symptoms of schizophrenia (Harris & McMahon, 1997)

e. More recently the **interaction** of various neurotransmitters have been studied relative to schizophrenia

f. Recent studies have examined effect of interactions between hormones and neurotransmitters in schizophrenia; patterns of dopamine-thyroid interactions and dopamine pituitary hormone secretions were found to be related to symptoms of schizophrenia

7. Theory of Two Types of Schizophrenia

    a. Type I—characterized by *positive* symptoms of schizophrenia e.g., delusions, hallucinations, disorganized thinking; responds well to typical antipsychotic medications

    b. Type II—characterized by *negative* symptoms including withdrawal, flattening of affect, decreased motivation; respond better to newer antipsychotics (clozapine and risperidone); negative symptoms may be more related to structural defect and not dopamine function (Keltner & Folks, 1997)

- Biochemical Interventions for Schizophrenia and Other Psychotic Disorders

1. Typical Antipsychotics

    a. Used to decrease psychotic symptoms including hallucinations, delusions, and paranoia (Sherr, 1996)

    b. Used short term in Schizophreniform Disorder

    c. Mode of action—block dopamine receptors in post-synaptic neuron

        (1) Potency related to D_2 receptor affinity in primarily four major pathways in the brain

        (2) Blockade of dopamine receptors in the cortex potentially makes negative symptoms worse

        (3) D_2 receptor blockade responsible for many side effects of typical antipsychotics (Sherr, 1996)

    d. Medications (See Table 1)

    (1)   Fluphenazine (Prolixin) 12.5 to 50 mg every 6 hours and haloperidol (Haldol) 6 to 20 mg daily are available in intramuscular, injectable forms that are long-acting and released over two to three weeks

        (a)   Reduces need to take daily oral medications

        (b)   Helps reduce ambivalence

    (2)   Dosages vary widely among patients

  e. Potential side effects of typical antipsychotics

    (1)   Anticholinergic effects occur due to interference of nerve impulses by acetycholine and epinephrine; include constipation, dry mouth, blurred vision, urinary retention and hesitancy; bethanecol is sometimes given for urinary retention

Table 1

Typical Antipsychotics

Classification	Generic (Trade name)	Dosage Range
Phenothiazines	Chlorpromazine (Thorazine)	100–1400mg
	Thioridazine (Mellaril)	200–800mg
	Mesoridazine (Serentil)	100–500mg
	Perphenazine (Trilafon)	8–64mg
	Trifluoperazine (Stelazine)	2–80mg
	Fluphenazine (Prolixin)	5–40mg
Thioxanthenes	Thiothixene (Navane)	6–60mg
Butyrophenones	Haloperidol (Haldol)	4–40mg
Dibenzoxazepines	Loxapine (Loxitane)	50–250mg
Dihydroindolones	Molindone (Moban)	20–225mg

(2) Extrapyramidal symptoms due to medication's effects on the extrapyramidal tracts of central nervous system

    (a) Acute Dystonia—muscle spasms may occur early in treatment sometimes after first dose; occurs in up to 10% of clients

        (i) Blepharospasm (eye closing)

        (ii) Torticollis (neck muscle contraction, pulling head to side)

        (iii) Oculogyric crisis (severe upward deviation of the eyeballs)

        (iv) Opisthotonos (severe dorsal arching of neck and back)

        (v) Severe spasms of tongue and larynx can result in dysphagia (difficulty swallowing) and compromise airway

        (vi) Treatment—Anticholinergic drugs; severe painful symptoms benefit from IM dose cogentin 2 mg or benedryl 50 mg which may be repeated in 30 minutes if no resolution of symptoms

    (b) Neuroleptic-Induced-Pseudoparkinsonism— dopamine blockade in nigrostriatal pathways results in clinical symptoms such as:

        (i) Tremors

        (ii) Bradykinesia/akinesia (slowness, absence of movement)

        (iii) Cogwheel rigidity (slow, regular, muscular movements)

        (iv) Postural instability, shuffling gait, loss of mobility in the facial muscles (mask like facies), hypersalivation and drooling

        (v) Pillrolling of fingers

        (vi) Affects up to 15% of clients

    (c) Akathisia—may occur weeks or months after treatment; occurs in approximately 25% of persons treated with neuroleptics

        (i)   Objective symptoms—restlessness, pacing, rocking (shifting from one foot to another) and foot tapping

        (ii) Subjective symptoms—descriptions of inner restlessness, tension, irritability and inability to sit still or lie down

        (iii) Differentiation between akathisia and anxiety and psychomotor agitation of worsening psychosis is important

        (iv) May respond to reduction of antipsychotic medication

        (v) Anticholinergic treatment generally has limited effect except in high doses which are often not well tolerated

        (vi) Beta-blockers may be most effective adjunctive treatment—propanolol (Inderal) 160 mg/day; nadolol (Corgard) 80 mg/day

    (d) Tardive Dyskinesia (TD)—abnormal repetitive movement which is irreversible in 50% of cases even after withdrawal of drug

        (i)   Oral (lip smacking, puckering), buccal, lingual (tongue protrusion) masticatory and eyelid (blinking) movement; choreiform movements which may at first occur anywhere in the body, including arms, legs, fingers, feet and trunk

        (ii) Less commonly involves muscles in swallowing reflex or diaphragm—can lead to choking or respiratory compromise

        (iii) Clients are often less aware of the movements than those around them who generally report them

(iv) Careful assessment of symptoms of TD using standard instruments, such as Abnormal Involuntary Movement Scale (AIMS) is a nursing responsibility

(v) Pathophysiology of TD is only partially understood, but includes an understanding of posssible increase in dopamine receptors after long term blockade with neuroleptics and/or development of supersensitivity of dopamine receptors

(vi) Discontinuing drug may result initially in withdrawal dyskinesia

(vii) Benzodiazepines may bring temporary relief

(viii) Approximately 50% will not return to normal movement even after withdrawl of drug

(ix) Some clients seem to respond to treatment with clozapine (Clozaril)

(3) Treatment of EPS and Pseudoparkinsonism

(a) Anticholinergic drugs

(i) Contraindication—narrow angle glaucoma

(ii) Relative contraindications—dehydration, cardiac arrythmias, and benign prostatic hypertrophy

(iii) Caution—older clients and those on additional medications with anticholinergic effects must be monitored

(iv) Excess anticholinergic medication may result in urinary retention, paralytic ileus and memory problems, sometimes called anticholinergic delirium (includes disorientation)

(v) Other side effects may include blurred vision, dry mouth and tachycardia

(b) Dopamine agonists (See Table 2 for medications to treat extrapyramidal symptoms)

Table 2

Medications Used to Treat Extrapyramidal Symptoms (EPS) and Pseudoparkinsonism

	Generic name	Trade name	Dose & Route
Anticholinergics	Benztropine	Cogentin	1-8 mg PO or Injectable
	Trihexyphenidyl	Artane	2-15 mg capsule, extended release, elixir
Antihistamine	Diphenhydramine	Benadryl	50-200 mg capsules, liquid, injectable
Dopamine Agonist	Amantadine	Symmetrel	100mg-300mg capsules and liquid

(4) Neuroleptic Malignant Syndrome (NMS)—potentially fatal idiosyncratic reaction to antipsychotics

    (a) Characterized by muscular rigidity, hyperthermia, autonomic instability

    (b) Laboratory findings can include leukocytosis (15,000 to 300,000), elevated creatinine phosphokinase (CPK) (may be > 3000 IU/mL); myoglobinuria

    (c) May occur any time during treatment but is more frequent shortly after initiation of antipsychotics or dose increases; rapid administration of a high potency antipsychotic and an increased number of IM injections may increase risk

    (d) Treatment of NMS requires discontinuation of antipsychotic drugs and maintenance of nutrition, cooling and hydration

    (e) Ventilation may be required for respiratory failure; renal dialysis for renal failure

    (f) Muscle relaxant IV to reduce rigidity

    (g) Dopaminergic drugs such as bromocriptine (Parlodel), amantadine (Symmetrel) and anticoholinergics

(5) Other side effects of typical antipsychotics

    (a) Reduction of seizure threshold, especially with the use of low-potency agents

    (b) ECG changes (conduction delays); and rarely sudden death; more common with low-potency drugs

      (c)   Photosensitivity—may continue up to a month after drug discontinued

      (d)   High doses of thioridazine (Mellaril) can lead to pigmentary retinopathy and permanent blindness

      (e)   Sexual dysfunction, including retrograde ejaculation, impaired erection, inhibition of orgasm and amenorrhea

      (f)   Orthostatic hypotension, sedation, weight gain

      (g)   Cholestatic jaundice—in chlorpromazine, usually self-limiting

      (h)   Agranulocytosis—signs of an infection such as sore throat, flu like symptoms and fever may indicate medical emergency and require immediate evaluation

   (6)   Treatment of side effects—dose reduction, changing to another drug and adding an adjunctive agent are considered in light of efficacy of antipsychotic drug and side effect profile of individual client

2. Atypical Antipsychotics

   a.   Clozapine (Clozaril)

      (1)   Indicated for treatment of refractory schizophrenia (Littrell, 1994)

         (a)   Found to improve response in clients who have failed to respond to two antipsychotics of different chemical classes given at doses of 800 chlorpromazine equivalents a day for at least 6 weeks

         (b)   Restricted indication due to 1% risk of agranulocytosis (Littrell, 1994)

      (2)   Mode of Action—blocks Dopamine receptors; considerable $5HT_2$ blockade

      (3)   Side effects

         (a)   Agranulocytosis

            (i)   Complete blood count prior to therapy and

white blood cell count (WBC) weekly for duration of treatment

    (ii)   Greatest risk period is first 6 months of treatment and risk peaks at approximately 3 months; cases have occurred after 2 years of treatment

    (iii)   Recovery from agranulocytosis usually complete if drug stopped before clinical symptoms of infection appear

    (iv)   If agranulocytosis occurs, drug not restarted

(b)   Because there is less penetration into the striatum where EPS occur, there is minimal EPS or tardive dyskinesia compared to typical antipsychotics

(c)   Seizures—dose related side effect

    (i)   Maximum daily dose is 900 mg

    (ii)   Overall seizure incidence is approximately 3%

    (iii)   Valproate (Depakote), most common antiseizure medication may be added; carbamazepine (tegretol) is avoided because of possibility of decreased white blood cells

    (iv)   Myoclonic jerking may precede seizures and may indicate need to hold or reduce total daily dose

(d)   Anticholinergic effects—generally moderate, however, there is a 30% incidence of hypersalivation; dose reduction or addition of anticholinergics may help night time hypersalivation

(e)   Rapid changes in clozapine dose or sudden discontinuation can result in serious rebound psychosis and anticholinergic rebound; nausea, vomiting and diarrhea

(f)   Non-compliance for several days and reintroduction at previous dose could result in syncopal episodes, orthostatic hypotension or seizures

      (g) Other side effects

          (i) Sedation, tachycardia, hypotension, GI upset, benign hyperthermia, constipation, headaches (most diminish substantially with time)

          (ii) Tachycardia (increases of 25 beats /minute) may persist—can be treated with beta blockers

          (iii) Benign hyperthermia usually develops in first 3 weeks of treatment; usually remits on its own

          (iv) Some clients complain of vague burning in stomach; may be relieved by food with resultant weight gain

  (4) Dosage and efficacy

      (a) Start at 12.5 mg with increases of 25 mg each day for 5 to 7 days; low dose initiation reduces risk of orthostatic hypotension

      (b) Most clients respond to 300 to 600 mg/day, usually given in divided dose two times per day or at bedtime

      (c) Medication is distributed to outpatients for 7 days if WBC > 3000

      (d) Effective with both "positive" and "negative" symptoms of schizophrenia

      (e) Gradual improvement over several months with possibility of continued improvement throughout first year

      (f) Some clients have remarkable response in psychotic symptoms, daily function and social organization; report "thinking more clearly" leading to medication and treatment compliance

      (g) Nurse is pivotal in setting up atmosphere that improves compliance

  b. Risperidone (Risperdal)

(1) Mode of Action

    (a) Blocks serotonin and dopamine (D_2) receptors in limbic tract which improves positive symptoms

    (b) Also blocks $5HT_2$ receptors in cortical regions of brain; frees dopamine in area and improves negative symptoms (Keltner & Folks, 1997)

(2) Side Effects

    (a) Unlikely to cause tardive dyskinesia; however clients should be monitored over time

    (b) EPS—dose related side effects

    (c) Does not cause agranulocytosis

    (d) Has mild alpha blockade and histamine blockage, resulting in some risk of orthostatic hypotension and sedation

    (e) Other side effects—anxiety, dizziness, constipation nausea, tachycardia (Keltner and Folks, 1997); insomnia, agitation, headache, rhinitis, weight gain

(3) Dosage and Efficacy

    (a) Starting dose in adults is 1 mg b.i.d. increased by 1 mg b.i.d. daily to initial daily dose of 4 to 6 mg/day

    (b) In geriatric clients, dosing should be reduced by half, starting at 0.5 mg b.i.d. titrating to 1.5 mg

    (c) In doses beyond 8 mg/day potential loss of improvement in negative symptom response

    (d) May take up to 6 to 8 weeks to become maximally effective

    (e) Absorbed well orally, IM form not available

c. Olanzapine (Zyprexa)

(1) Mode of Action

(a) Like risperidone is a serotonin/dopamine antagonist (Littrell, 1997) and is known as a Multi-Acting Receptor Targeted Antipsychotic (MARTA)

(b) Binds to both serotonin $5HT_2$ and dopamine D_2 receptors with a greater affinity for serotonin, decreasing positive and negative symptoms

(2) Side Effects

(a) Decreased risk for causing EPS

(b) Minimal risk of prolactin elevation

(c) Neurological side effects—limited to akathisia (5%), tremor (47%), and hypertonia (4%)

(d) Other side effects include somnolence (26%), agitation (23%), and insomnia (20%)

(e) Nervousness and dizziness also reported

(f) To date, no reported cases of tardive dyskinesia

(3) Dosage and Efficacy

(a) Recommended initial dose is 5 to 10 mg with a target dose of 10 mg within a few days

(b) Because of the relatively short time to steady state, recommended that patient remain on a dose for 5 to 7 days before increasing

(c) Mean 30 hour half-life of olanzapine allows for once a day dosing, usually at bedtime

(d) Effective in treating positive and negative symptoms

3. Medications used for Schizoaffective Disorder—antidepressants, lithium or tegretol or depakote may be utilized, in addition to a variety of neuroleptics, depending on presenting problems

- Intrapersonal Origins/Psychotherapeutic Interventions for clients with Schizophrenia and other Psychotic Disorders

1. Interactional model for schizophrenia delineates that biologic vulnerability along with environmental factors, social skills, and support of individual are factors in development of the illness

2. Psychotherapeutic Intervention

    a. Establishment of trust on inpatient unit

        (1) Nurse should set a tone of quiet confidence in treatment process that conveys a sense of caring rather than judgement

        (2) Delivery of simple and short instructions about the facility, daily schedule and treatment process are important to building a relationship that conveys respect and concern for individual as well as their illness

        (3) Expected outcome of patient care for persons experiencing schizophrenia is patient will live, learn, and work at a maximum possible level of success as defined by individual (Moller & Murphy, 1995)

        (4) Initial treatment efforts are directed at correcting instability related to major symptoms experienced and resulting disruption in activities of daily living

        (5) Medication management is joint effort, and must include careful attention to observed behaviors, client description, and client response to medication therapies

        (6) Careful record keeping of descriptive information and use of Brief Symptom Rating Inventory (BSRI) assists in initial assessment phase of treatment and determines client outcome profile related to treatment and medication

        (7) Treatment milieu organized to reduce sensory stimulation, while providing opportunities for simple and brief social and professional interactions

        (8) Schedule should provide time for rest, structured activity and set times to speak with providers

        (9) Use of soft lighting, uncluttered space, and sound control can create an environment for recovery

    b. Moller and Murphy (1995), describe early acute stage as unstable neurobiological responses that require constant observation and monitoring; nursing interventions should focus on restoration of adaptive neurobiological responses while providing for safety and well being

    (1)   Assess and monitor health status and medications

    (2)   Identify symptoms of relapse and/or factors that increase symptoms

    (3)   Assist in management of delusions and hallucinations

    (4)   Allow for sufficient rest for brain responses to stabilize

    (5)   Provide a safe, protective, quiet environment

    (6)   Reduce pressure to perform

    (7)   Allow to verbalize fears, concerns

    (8)   Use clear, concise, concrete communication

    (9)   Facilitate communication with significant others

    (10)   Assist with activities of daily living as needed

    (11)   Assist with anger, anxiety management, and problem solving

    (12)   Simplify decision making

    (13)   Assess risk to self and others

c. Communication—patient may communicate in symbols; listen actively for theme

d. Hallucinations

    (1)   Observe patient attending to internal stimuli

    (2)   Note if patient talks or smiles to himself/herself

    (3)   Encourage involvement in real conversations and/or structured activities

    (4)   Administer medication as ordered and observe response

    (5)   Assess for content of hallucination; if patient is having command hallucinations to harm self or others, provide for safety

    (6)   Utilize judgment when providing for increased levels of observation as patient with command hallucinations may not be able to contract for safety

e. Delusions—delusional individual may have delusions of grandeur, paranoia, or poverty; may think he is a public figure or may believe he is being followed by CIA

(1) Do not argue with client or deny belief; does not eliminate delusion nor is trust gained by this approach

(2) Focus on reality and talk about reality-oriented issues in order to redirect the client from delusional topics

(3) Accept client's need for belief without actually reinforcing the belief

(4) For paranoid client, helpful to assign same staff member consistently to build trust

(5) Note stressors or any escalation in anxiety that may precipitate delusional thinking; assist individual in anxiety reduction

(6) If client feels food is poisoned, serve food in sealed containers

(7) Paranoid thinking may cause elderly to need assistance with nutrition and hydration

f. Withdrawn behavior

(1) Assist with food and fluid intake as well as hygiene.

(2) An accepting attitude and unconditional positive regard may decrease sense of isolation

(3) Gradually introduce patient into activities

(4) Give positive reinforcement for participating

(5) Allow time for being alone as well as structure

g. Potential for harm to self

(1) Inquire about suicidal thoughts

(2) Create safe environment by removing sharp and other harmful objects

(3) Encourage patient to contract for safety; if command hallucinations are present, contracting may not be feasible

h. Social Isolation

(1) Spend time with patient

(2) Make brief, frequent contacts

(3) Gradually encourage participation in activities

       (4)   Encourage structure in the day

  i. Alteration in nutrition

       (1)   Encourage balanced diet with high fiber

       (2)   Intake, output, and caloric count when needed

       (3)   Limit caffeine intake

       (4)   Small, frequent meals

  j. Potential for injury

       (1)   Decrease stimulation in environment.

       (2)   Encourage quiet time in room

       (3)   Promote safe environment

  k. Management of violent behavior

       (1)   Violence against self may be in the form of suicide or self-mutilation, particularly if there are command hallucinations present

       (2)   Violence towards others is also possibility

       (3)   Assess characteristics such as increased pacing, clenched fists, tense expression, irritability, agitation, threatening verbalizations

       (4)   Early intervention is important, keeping in mind use of least restrictive measures

          (a)   Decrease stimulation in the environment

          (b)   Administer prn medications and observe response

          (c)   Provide for safe environment by removing dangerous objects

          (d)   Encourage patient to spend quiet time in room or in quiet room

          (e)   When approaching patient, do so from the side and not in a direct manner.

          (f)   A show of force may be necessary and is sometimes sufficient in redirecting the client and de-escalating a situation

        (g) If redirection and medication as well as decrease in stimulation are not effective, and client is at risk of harming self or others, seclusion and restraint may be needed as a last resort; may not be used as punishment

        (h) Protocol for restraints varies from hospital to hospital and may include:

            (i) Positioning client to prevent aspiration

            (ii) Glasses, jewelry, shoes, or belts are removed to prevent injury

            (iii) Constant observation is recommended due to possibility of laryngeal spasms from neuroleptic medications

            (iv) Range-of-motion to extremities should be performed every two hours and pulses, color, and temperature assessed and documented; at risk for thromboembolic events

            (v) Nursing care includes hydration, nutrition, and attention to elimination

            (vi) Need for seclusion and/or restraint should be documented; flowsheet should be available to record care given and patient response

            (vii) Assessment is ongoing and patient may gradually be moved from 5-point restraints to 3-point and 2-point restraints; patient should *never* be left in only one restraint

            (viii) Client is released from seclusion when behavior is under control and he/she is not in danger of hurting self or others

- Family Dynamics/Family Therapy

  1. No proof that schizophrenia or other psychotic disorders are caused by family interaction patterns therefore family therapy is not used; important family is involved in care of individual; family is an integral part of treatment plan and has best knowledge of individual's illness and ability to function

2. Illness affects entire family system including careers, finances, schedules, and social life; problems which recur most frequently are:

   a. Failure to care for personal needs/hygiene

   b. Difficulty handling finances

   c. Withdrawal

   d. Odd personal habits

   e. Suicide threats

   f. Concern for safety of client and family

3. Eliminating blame is important if family members blame each other; acceptance of illness is first step toward management of illness; expectations of patient should be realistic

4. Anger may have to be addressed

5. Other questions to consider include:

   a. Devotion of time to other family members

   b. Respite for caregiver

   c. Home care versus boarding home or halfway house

5. Family members require education and instruction; discharged client may require reintegration within family and role shifting may occur; nurse should assess family attitudes toward client overall atmosphere in family, and available emotional/social supports

6. Some aspects of family life have been linked to relapse in schizophrenia; concept of expressed emotion is implicated; three main components of expressed emotion are criticism, hostility, and overinvolvement; for individuals with schizophrenia with high expressed emotion, there is a higher probability of relapse. (Haber, 1997)

7. Family needs to be educated on the role of stress in the exacerbation of symptoms

8. Environment for medication compliance is also important; 70% relapse rate if medications are not taken regularly and 30% relapse rate if medication regimen is followed

9. Family members can be taught to recognize symptoms that may require medication adjustment or hospitalization

10. Family can provide responsibilities for client such as simple chores to introduce a sense of routine and accomplishment

11. Family should encourage participation in vocational rehabilitation and other therapeutic activities

12. Role of the Psychiatric/Mental Health Clinical Nurse Specialist

   a. Help client and family learn more about illness, treatment options, and ways to live with disease in a productive fashion

   b. Plan psychoeducational approaches that maximize times when client symptoms are relatively stable

   c. Simplify instruction, reduce distracting stimuli, provide both visual and verbal information, and provide instruction in small segments with frequent reinforcement (Moller & Murphy, 1995)

   d. Initiate family education that accentuates the family's belief in their own expertise, and focuses on symptom management and self-care skills for client

   e. Discuss with client and family, rationale for selection of medication regimen, options available, expected benefits, side effects and time lag in response

   f. Establish a partnership with client, family members and other health care professionals to develop treatment and rehabilitative goals

   g. Provide Case Management

      (1) Identify and coordinate services

      (2) Understand appropriate use of day treatment programs, clubhouse programs, and companion programs etc., so they may be used as part of comprehensive treatment program

      (3) Make appointments and accompany client if needed

      (4) Asssist during crises

- Group Approaches/Therapy and Self-help

   1. Traditional group therapy, insight-oriented groups or groups that are

primarily interactional in nature are generally not helpful, as the individual has difficulty filtering stimuli

2. Self-help groups may be more beneficial—focus on educational issues, support, and destigmatization of mental illness

3. Social skills training can occur in groups and would include introducing oneself, starting a conversation, and listening skills; staff act as role models for implementation of these skills

- Milieu Interventions

  1. Regular daily activities can provide a sense of predictability as well as sense of accomplishment and reward

  2. Treatment environment should emphasize involvement, organization and standards of safety; should be established norms and rules

  3. Client may feel safer if periods of time are scheduled to be spent in his/her room.

  4. If client feels threatened by milieu activities, encourage involvement with only one other client

- Community Resources

  1. The National Alliance for the Mentally Ill (NAMI) and Friends and Family of the Mentally Ill provide advocacy, support groups and educational programs

  2. Local chapters of Companion Peer (COMPEER) develop community connections by providing companion matching services

  3. Local community services boards plan, implement and evaluate a variety of programs including outpatient, day treatment, case management, crisis services, club houses, employment and job coaching

  4. Local community mental health center is also valuable resource; patient is followed on an outpatient basis through mental health center and receives medication through this setting

  5. Day treatment programs

  6. Possibilities for residential placement include halfway houses or boarding homes depending on patient's abilities and skills

  7. Supplementary security income can provide small, fixed income and may pay residential costs in boarding home

  8. Transportation services are key resources to promote access

9. Psychiatric Home Care

   a. Allows for careful identification and monitoring of target symptoms and relapse prevention

   b. Promotes involvement of client in self-assessment

   c. Focuses on attainment of specific goals related to rehabilitation and maximization of functional ability

   d. Nurse in psychiatric home care is essentially a "guest" in client's home, which is an empowering position for the client and family and supports process of continuing outpatient care for persistent but treatable mental illness.

   e. Nurse in psychiatric home care uses a rehabilitative model that supports client self-care and develops appropriate goals for successful, feasible outcomes that are compatible with the limitations of illness and abilities of client

Questions
Select the best answer

1. Mr. Jones is a patient diagnosed with schizophrenia who is hospitalized on a psychiatric unit. You notice him standing motionless on one leg in the day area. This would most likely be an example of:

    a. Attention-seeking behavior
    b. Catatonic posturing
    c. A side-effect of neuroleptic medication
    d. Catatonic stupor

2. During the initial assessment, the nurse inquires of Mr. Jones, "What brought you to the hospital?" Mr. Jones replies, "An ambulance." This is an example of:

    a. Deductive reasoning
    b. Abstract thinking
    c. Concrete thinking
    d. Poverty of content of speech

3. Mr. Jones is informed during his hospital stay that his brother has been diagnosed with cancer and will be undergoing surgery. Mr. Jones laughs upon hearing the news. Your understanding of this is:

    a. Mr. Jones is obviously not close to his brother.
    b. Mr. Jones possibly has a mood disorder.
    c. Mr. Jones is obviously anxious and upset by this news.
    d. Mr. Jones is displaying incongruence between content of communication and his emotions

4. Mr. Jones comments that he hears voices of men telling him "bad things about myself. They say I should hurt myself." Your most appropriate initial response would be to:

    a. Reassure Mr. Jones of his safety and security by telling him the voices aren't real
    b. Provide for Mr. Jones' comfort and security by reminding him that he has never hurt himself in the past
    c. Assess the command hallucinations for potential destructiveness by asking specifically for the content
    d. Tell him to ignore the voices and administer prn medications

5. When John, a 25 year old graduate student, diagnosed with paranoid schizophrenia is ready for discharge which of the following is important for the client and his family?

    a. To understand all of the causal explanations of the illness so they can be discussed at home
    b. To set up a plan to improve the outlook of the client that includes daily rules for acceptable behaviors
    c. To understand the treatment plan, including prescribed medication, expectations concerning effects and plans for continuity of care and professional resources
    d. To understand that all activity is to be avoided, so that John will not get upset

6. The patient remarks repeatedly that he believes he is Jesus Christ and has come to save the world. This can best be described as:

    a. Defense of identification
    b. A delusion of grandeur
    c. An illusion
    d. An idea of reference

7. Mr. Brown continues to remark that the CIA is following him and that they are waiting outside the door to the emergency room. Your best response would be:

    a. "Mr. Brown, the CIA is not following you."
    b. "We've told the CIA to leave you alone."
    c. "I understand you feel that they are outside, but the CIA is not there and you're safe here."
    d. "Why do you think the CIA is out there?"

8. You notice during the assessment period that Mr. Brown is rocking back and forth on his feet and appears to be restless. This could be an indication of:

    a. Extreme anxiety
    b. Neuroleptic Malignant Syndrome
    c. Catatonic rigidity
    d. Acute dystonia

9. Ms. Smith was recently admitted to an inpatient psychiatric facility. During the assessment she seems to be mimicking your body movements. This is an example of:

    a. Echopraxia

    b. Echolalia

    c. Mirroring the therapist

    d. Akathisia

10. Several hours after being admitted, Ms. Smith complained of feeling bugs crawling on her skin. This could be indicative of:

    a. Alcohol withdrawal

    b. A hallucination common among patients with schizophrenia

    c. A side-effect of neuroleptic medications

    d. A seizure disorder

11. Ms. Smith displays paranoid behavior on the unit and becomes particularly suspicious. She comments that she suspects the food is being poisoned. A possible intervention would be to:

    a. Serve the food in sealed containers

    b. Serve small, frequent meals

    c. Have Ms. Smith eat away from the other patients

    d. Have Ms. Smith prepare her own meals

12. Mr. Brown has been treated for the past several years with Prolixin. You notice that he is drooling, has a tremor, and there is slight pillrolling of the fingers. These are the extrapyramidal symptoms known as:

    a. Anticholinergic side effects

    b. Pseudoparkinsonism

    c. Tardive dyskinesia

    d. Dystonic reaction

13. Several days into the hospitalization, Mr. Brown complains of urinary retention, an anticholinergic side effect. Which of the following medications would be best to ease the urinary retention?

    a. Cogentin

    b. Artane

    c. Lasix

    d. Bethanecol

14. Mr. Brown has been on cogentin along with haldol. You notice that in addition to the urinary retention, his face is flushed, and he has become disoriented. This is an example of:

    a. An exacerbation of the psychosis

   b. Anticholinergic delirium
   c. Early-onset dementia
   d. Brief reactive psychosis

15. Mr. Johnson is being treated with haldol. He develops a fever of 102°F, muscular rigidity, altered mental status, and diaphoresis. It is determined that he is suffering from neuroleptic malignant syndrome. Which laboratory findings are *most* likely to occur?

   a. An elevated haldol level
   b. A decrease in the CPK and an elevated white blood cell count
   c. An increase in the CPK level and an elevated white cell count
   d. A decrease in the white cell count

16. Possible complications from Neuroleptic malignant syndrome include the following:

   a. Muscle rigidity, hyperthermal, autonomic instability
   b. Liver failure
   c. Increased intracranial pressure
   d. Agranulocytosis

17. Nursing care for the patient with Neuroleptic Malignant Syndrome will include:

   a. The discontinuation of the neuroleptic, maintenance of skin integrity and hydration, and administration of bromocriptine
   b. The gradual tapering of the neuroleptic, the administration of cogentin, and maintenance of skin integrity and hydration
   c. The gradual tapering of the neuroleptic, administration of bromocriptine, and maintenance of skin integrity and hydration
   d. The discontinuation of the neuroleptic, maintenance of skin integrity and hydration, and the administration of cogentin

18. Which of the following statements best describes characteristics about the onset and development of Neuroleptic Malignant Syndrome?

   a. It is noted most commonly in female patients taking haldol, so they are most at risk
   b. The initial onset is insidious and is therefore difficult to detect
   c. It develops only after months to years of treatment with neuroleptic medications
   d. The onset may be sudden and can occur after the first dose of the medication

19. Mr. Jones has not been eating and has difficulty bringing food to his mouth. The most appropriate intervention would be:

    a. Place the spoon in the patient's hand, scoop food into it and say, "Eat a bite of this apple sauce."
    b. Place the patient on a liquid supplement as this may be more easily tolerated
    c. Spoon feed the patient
    d. Allow patient to eat in his room as he will be more comfortable away from the other patients

20. Which best describes the action of antipsychotic medications?

    a. They block dopamine receptors
    b. They decrease available amounts of serotonin and norepinephrine
    c. They enhance the availability of dopamine
    d. They block re-uptake of dopamine to increase availability at receptor sites

21. As a nurse employed at the community mental health center, you are a case manager for several patients taking clozapine. The advantages of taking clozapine include:

    a. Follow-up is less frequent since tardive dyskinesia does not occur
    b. It is less likely to cause orthostasis
    c. Restlessness and tremors are less likely to occur
    d. It is more potent than phenothiazines

22. Medication teaching about clozapine *should include* which of the following:

    a. Cautioning the patient to report any signs of infection including sore throat, flu-like symptoms and fever
    b. The importance of being compliant with having a complete blood count drawn at least monthly
    c. Notifying the physician *immediately* about lip-smacking or vermiform movements of the tongue
    d. Notifying the physician immediately at the onset of diarrhea and hand tremors

23. You are caring for a patient who suffers from epilepsy and has been diagnosed recently as having schizophrenia. Teaching should include which of the following:

a. Antipsychotic medications should be used cautiously as they increase seizure threshold

b. Antipsychotic medications should be used cautiously as they decrease seizure threshold

c. Antipsychotic medications do not affect seizure threshold

d. Antipsychotic medications are contraindicated

24. The following is indicative of a dystonic reaction:

a. Oculogyric crisis and spasms of the back muscles
b. Cogwheel rigidity and lip-smacking movements
c. Shuffling gait and mask-like facies.
d. Urinary retention and leg stiffness.

25. Nursing actions during a dystonic reaction may include:

a. Turning patient on side
b. Notifying physician, administration of cogentin and making certain respiratory support equipment is available
c. Administration of IM physostigmine and bethanecol
d. Decreasing stimulation in environment as dystonia and agitation may appear similar

26. Which of the following statements about tardive dyskinesia is *most* accurate?

a. Symptoms are generally reversible, particularly in younger patient population
b. Symptoms may appear 1-10 days following administration of neuroleptic medication
c. Occurs most often in dehydrated patients
d. All patients on long-term neuroleptic therapy are at risk

27. Your patient on neuroleptic medication complains of dizziness. Your *initial* intervention would be:

a. Taking the patient's blood pressure sitting and standing
b. Forcing fluids
c. Prompt discontinuation of the medication and notifying the physician
d. Instructing patient to place their head between knees

28. You are working with Mr. Green who has recently been prescribed thorazine. He comes to the nurses' stations and complains of blurred vision and constipation. Your most appropriate response would be:

a. "I'll notify the physician right away as your dose is probably too high."
b. "Those are possible side effects to the medication and tolerance usually develops in several weeks. We can order a bulk diet for you."
c. "I'll notify the physician right away and see if we can try a different medication."
d. Administer an anticholinergic medication

29. A common hypothesis regarding the biological origin of schizophrenia is:

a. Dopamine hypothesis which postulates that some cases may be due to excess of dopamine in the brain and/or an excessive number of dopamine receptors
b. Disease is caused by enlarged lateral ventricles in the brain
c. Norepinephrine hypothesis which states that schizophrenia is due to an excess of this neurotransmitter which causes hallucinations
d. All cases of schizophrenia are caused by viruses contracted in utero

30. The most current family theory states:

a. Research has indicated schizophrenia is a direct result of dysfunctional family interaction
b. The individual with schizophrenia withdraws and hallucinates as a defense against a hostile family environment
c. There is no proof that schizophrenia is caused by family interaction patterns
d. An individual with schizophrenia is most likely to be product of a cold, aloof mother and absent, distant father

31. According to genetic studies of schizophrenia:

a. Genetic factors are not important to one's risk of developing schizophrenia
b. A twin of a monozygotic (identical) twin with schizophrenia has a greater chance of having schizophrenia than the general population
c. A twin of a monozygotic (identical) twin with schizophrenia has a lesser chance of having schizophrenia than the general population
d. Genetic inheritance is most likely the only cause of schizophrenia since family interactional patterns cannot be empirically studied

32. Mr. Jones reports that he is hearing voices telling him to cut his wrists and he is highly agitated with complaints of fear and anxiety. The *most appropriate* intervention would be to:

   a. Administer medication and encourage Mr. Jones to contract for safety and to notify nursing staff should voices increase

   b. Administer prn medication and encourage Mr. Jones to spend time in his room, after checking for sharp objects and ensuring the environment is safe

   c. Administer prn medication, remove dangerous objects from patient's environment, and place him on constant observation

   d. Administer prn medication and place him in closed door seclusion with safety checks every 15 minutes

33. Ms. Williams who was admitted to the unit yesterday is withdrawn and keeps to herself on the unit. An appropriate intervention would be:

   a. Encouraging Ms. Williams to attend all activities as prescribed in order to integrate into the milieu and feel a part of the group

   b. Encouraging Ms. Williams to spend all day and early evening on the unit and locking the door to her room

   c. Encouraging Ms. Williams to attend activities gradually with a supportive staff member

   d. Electing Ms. Williams as the patient representative to increase her sense of confidence

34. Ms. Williams has difficulty trusting the staff members on the unit. Which of the following interventions is *most* likely to promote trust?

   a. Using therapeutic touch in order to convey caring and concern for Ms. Williams

   b. Encouraging patient to engage in a one-to-one session for an hour on both morning and evening shifts to convey acceptance of her

   c. Assigning the same staff to work with Ms. Williams as often as possible

   d. Encouraging Ms. Williams to play a game of cards with the other patients

35. David has responded well to clozapine with a maintenance dose of 400 mg per day. The psychiatric home health nurse draws blood for a weekly WBC and distributes a week's supply of medication if the WBC > 3,000. She explains the importance of compliance to the daily dose as prescribed and instructs David to call his doctor if he misses more than two doses of medication because:

   a. He will need to begin the titration process from the beginning

   b. Non-compliance for several days and reinstatement at the previous dose could result in syncopal episode, orthostatic hypotension or seizure

   c. His doctor will discontinue the medication

   d. He is at risk for immediate acute exacerbation of psychosis

36. The CNS assesses the relationship between David and his family and together they work out a plan for David to attend a social club house program 3 afternoons a week, and a referral to COMPEER. His family is told about the meeting times for the local chapter of the Alliance for the Mentally Ill. The purpose of the Alliance for the Mentally Ill is to:

    a. Provide a companion matching service to develop community connections for those with mental illness
    b. Provide advocacy and support programs for clients and their families
    c. Provide housing and supervision on a continuum from professional caregivers to managed properties
    d. Provide transportation 24 hr a day

37. Mr. Parker has been diagnosed with Paranoid Shizophrenia and has stated that he believes that other patients are out to get him. Mr. Parker has escalated to the point where he is threatening others and he is having difficulty staying in his room. The decision is made to assist Mr. Parker by having him spend some time in the quiet room. Which of the following interventions will *most likely* promote safety?

    a. Approach Mr. Parker with several other staff members in a quiet manner and escort him to the quiet room
    b. Approach Mr. Parker alone as he may feel more threatened with more than one staff member
    c. Place Mr. Parker in 4-point restraints and check on him every 15 minutes
    d. Force medicate him according to hospital policy

38. Mr. Parker begins banging his head against the wall. It becomes necessary to place Mr. Parker in mechanical restraints in order that he not hurt himself. Nursing care should include the following:

    a. Checking on Mr. Parker at least once an hour
    b. Performing range-of-motion exercises every 2 hours and assessing circulation to the extremities
    c. Removing all restraints if Mr. Parker becomes less agitated within 10 minutes
    d. Gradually removing restraints until Mr. Parker has only one restraint remaining

39. The individual with schizophrenia may benefit from a group-oriented approach. Which of the following groups would be *most* appropriate?

    a. A didactic as well as supportive group that provides social skills training

    b. Insight-oriented

    c. Cognitive-behavioral in order to assist with difficulties with self-care

    d. Any of the above, depending on the individual patient

40. Mr. Williams who has been hospitalized for over a month due to exacerbation of schizophrenia will soon be discharged to his home where he will live with his parents and one younger brother. Which of the following recommendations will be most helpful to the family?

    a. Provide Mr. Williams with a structured routine, including chores and other responsibilities

    b. Do not encourage spending time alone as this will increase a sense of isolation from the family

    c. Encourage Mr. Williams to take complete responsibility for medications and follow-up appointments

    d. Set goals for Mr. Williams as he may have difficulty doing this for himself

41. After a short period on a typical antipsychotic, a client complains that she can't sit still and taps her foot continuously. The nurse should:

    a. Administer a prn dose of medication because she is still agitated

    b. Understand that these symptoms are akathisia, and obtain an order for diphenhydramine and/or reduce the dosage of medication

    c. Help client relax in bed and obtain an order for an antianxiety medication

    d. Provide for vigorous activities until she settles down

Answers

1. b	15. c	29. a
2. c	16. a	30. c
3. d	17. a	31. b
4. c	18. d	32. c
5. c	19. a	33. c
6. b	20. a	34. c
7. c	21. c	35. b
8. a	22. a	36. b
9. a	23. b	37. a
10. a	24. a	38. b
11. a	25. b	39. a
12. b	26. d	40. a
13. d	27. a	41. b
14. b	28. b	

BIBLIOGRAPHY

American Nurses Association (1994). *A statement on psychiatric mental health clinical nursing practice and standards of psychiatric mental health clinical nursing practice.* Washington: DC: Author.

American Psychiatric Association. (1994). *Diagnostic and statistical manual of mental disorders* (4th ed.). Washington, DC: Author.

Bendik, M. (1996). The Schizophrenias. In K. Fortinash & P. Holoday-Worret (Eds.). *Psychiatric mental health nursing* (pp. 285-316). St. Louis: Mosby.

Burgess, A. W. (Ed.). (1997). *Psychiatric nursing: Promoting mental health.* Stanford: Appleton & Lange.

Cannon, J., & Marco, E. (1994). Structural brain abnormalities as indicators of vulnerability to schizophrenia. *Schizophrenia Bulletin, 20(1),* 89-102.

Chesla, C. (1992). Applying the nursing process for clients with schizophrenia and other psychotic disorders. In H. S. Wilson & C. R. Kneisl (Eds.). *Psychiatric nursing* (pp. 258-284). Redwood City: Addison-Wesley Nursing.

Farnsworth, B., & Biglow, A. (1997). Psychiatric case management. In J. Haber, B. Krainovich-Miller, A. McMahon, & P. Price-Hoskins (Eds.). *Comprehensive psychiatric nursing* (5th ed., pp. 318-331) St. Louis: Mosby.

Fortinash, K., & Holoday-Worret, P. (Eds.). (1996). *Psychiatric mental health nursing.* St. Louis: Mosby.

Fox, J. C., & Kane, C. F. (1996). Information processing deficits in schizophrenia. In A. B. McBride & J. K. Austin (Eds.). *Psychiatric mental nursing: Integrating behavioral and biological sciences* (pp. 321-347). Philadelphia: W. B. Saunders.

Haber, J. (1997). Psychiatric homecare. In J. Haber, B. Krainovich-Miller, A. McMahon & P. Price-Hoskins (Eds.). *Comprehensive psychiatric nursing* (5th ed., pp. 366-381). St. Louis: Mosby.

Harris B., & McHahon, A. (1997). Psychobiology. In J. Haber, B. Krainovich-Miller, A. McManon, & P. Price-Hoskins (Eds.). *Comprehensive psychiatric nursing* (5th ed., pp. 219-238). St. Louis: Mosby.

Johnson, B. (1993). Thought disorder: The schizophrenic disorders. In B. Johnson (Ed.), *Adaptation and growth: Psychiatric mental health nursing* (3rd ed., pp. 463-494). Philadelphia: J. B. Lippincott Co.

Kanter, J. (1989). Clinical case management: Definition, principles, components. *Hospital and Community Psychiatry, 40,* 361-367.

Keltner, N. L., & Folkes, D. G. (1997). *Psychotherapeutic drugs.* St. Louis: Mosby.

Laraia, M., & Stuart, G. (1995). *Quick Psychopharmacology Reference* (2nd ed). St. Louis: Mosby.

Littrel, K. (1994). *Clozaril: Guide to clozaril therapy.* East Hanover: Sandoz Pharmaceuticals Corp.

Littrell, K. (1997). *Clanzapine: A new atypical antipsychotic.* Indianapolis: Eli Lilly & Company.

Moller, M., & Murphy, M. (1995). Neurobiological responses and schizophrenia and psychotic disorders. In G. W. Stuart & S. J. Sundeen (Eds), *Principles & practice of psychiatric nursing.* (5th ed., pp. 475-507 St. Louis: Mosby.

Sherr, J. (1996). Psychopharmacology and other biologic therapies. In K. P. Fortinash & Holoday-Worret (Eds.), *Psychiatric mental health nursing* (pp. 532-563). St. Louis: Mosby.

Torrey, E. F., Bowler, A., Taylor, E., & Gottesman, I. (1994). *Schizophrenia and manic-depressive disorder: The biological roots of mental illness as revealed by the landmark study of identical twins.* New York: Basic Books.

Townsend, M. C. (1993). *Nursing diagnosis in psychiatric nursing: A pocket guide for care plan construction.* Philadelphia: F. A. Davis.

Vallone, D. (1997). Schizophrenia. In A. W. Burgess (Ed). *Psychiatric nursing: Promoting mental health* (pp. 503-517). Stamford: Appleton & Lange.

Walker, M. (1997). Schizophrenia and other psychotic disorders. In J. Haber, B. Krainovich-Miller, A. McMahon, P. Price-Hoskins (Eds.) *Comprehensive psychiatric nursing* (5th ed., pp. 567-604). St. Louis: Mosby.

Mood Disorders

Mary D. Moller

- Definition

  1. Mood disorders are characterized by a disturbance of mood (a prolonged emotion that colors the whole psychic life)

     a. Generally involves single or recurring depressive (unipolar) and/or manic (bipolar) episodes

     b. Also occurs as part of other non-mood conditions (eating, panic, obsessive-compulsive disorders)

     c. Occurs in drug or alcohol intoxication or withdrawal

     d. Occurs as consequences of non psychiatric medical conditions (cerebrovascular accident (CVA), dementia, diabetes, cancer, acquired immunodeficiency syndrome (AIDS), chronic fatigue syndrome (CFS), fibromyalgia, multiple sclerosis (MS) or as consequences of the use of selected prescription medications (See Table 1)

- Prevalence (U.S.)

  1. Mood disorders 8–9% in general population; 24% in 1st degree relatives; 10–15 million American people experience mood disorders at any given time.

  2. Major depressive episode—17.1% lifetime, 10.3% one year

  3. Manic episode—1.6% lifetime, 1.3% one year

  4. Dysthymia—6.4% lifetime, 2.5% one year

  5. First-degree relatives of persons with mood disorders have a higher rate of depression and mania than occurs in the general population.

  6. Bipolar disorder (manic-depressive illness) lifetime prevalence is 1–2%; 8% in first-degree relatives; represents 25–35% of mood disorders; mean age of onset is early 20s.

  7. Recurrence rate—over 50% for unipolar and bipolar illness.

  8. Suicide rate—1% in general population; people with a history of affective disorder—18%

  9. Fifty percent of the annual suicides are associated with depression.

  10. Fifteen percent of people with Bipolar I Disorder (BPI) untreated commit suicide.

  11. Suicide occurs more frequently > 60; at risk are white single males.

12. Suicide rate is increasing in < 24 age cohort.

- Sex distribution

    1. Unipolar Disorder females to males 2:1

    2. Bipolar Disorder—equal male-female distribution; females have a higher depression to mania ratio

Depressive Disorders

Major Depression (Unipolar, Endogenous)

- Definition: Depressed mood or loss of interest or pleasure in all or almost all activities, and associated symptoms for a period of at least 2 weeks, persisting and representing a change from previous functioning; can be mild, moderate or severe, with or without psychotic features.

- Signs and Symptoms: Presence of at least 5 of the following (1–10) including presence of (1) or (2) (APA, 1994):

    1. Depressed mood most of day, nearly every day

    2. Markedly diminished interest or pleasure in all, or almost all, activities

    3. Significant weight loss or gain when not dieting (>5% of body weight in a month)

    4. Insomnia or hypersomnia

        a. Initial insomnia/difficulty falling asleep (DFA)

        b. Middle insomnia (waking up during sleep and difficulty falling back to sleep)

        c. Terminal insomnia/early morning awakening (EMA)

    5. Psychomotor retardation or agitation (observable by others)

        a. Slowed speech/pressured speech/muteness/poverty of thought

        b. Slowed body movements/pacing, handwriting, inability to sit still, rubbing of hair, skin, clothing

    6. Fatigue or loss of energy

    7. Feelings of worthlessness or excessive or inappropriate guilt

    8. Diminished ability to think or concentrate or indecisiveness

9. Recurrent thoughts of death (not just fear of death); recurrent thoughts of suicide without a plan, a suicide attempt or a specific suicide plan

*   Differential Diagnosis

    1. Substance abuse

    2. Medications that may cause depressive symptomatology (See Table 1).

    3. Physical health problems that may cause or be associated with depressive symptoms.

    4. Non-mood psychiatric disorders

    5. Prior episodes of unipolar depression or bipolar disorder and/or suicide attempts

    6. Nodal events/stressful life events (postpartum, death of a spouse, job loss, geographic move, illness)

    7. Bereavement (symptoms persist longer than 2 months after loss of a loved one or include psychotic symptoms)

    8. Mixed state episode

Table 1
Medications Associated with Depression

Cardiovascular Drugs	*Hormones*
Alpha-Methyldopa	Oral Contraceptives
Reserpine	ACTH (corticotropin and glucocorticoids)
Propanolol	Anabolic steroids
Guanethidine	
Clonidine	*Psychotropics*
Thiazide diuretics	Anxiolytics
Digitalis	Anticonvulsants
Antihypertensives	Antiparkinsonian Drugs
	Neuroleptics
Anticancer Agents	Sedatives
Cycloserine	
Interferon	*Others*
	Opioids
Anti-Inflammatory/Anti-Infective Agents	Cocaine (withdrawal)
Steroids	PCP
Non-steroidal anti-inflammatory agents	Amphetamines (withdrawal)
Ethambutol	Anti-ulcer
Sulfonamides	L-dopa
Baclofen	Cimetidine
Metoclopramide	Rantidine
Analgesics	Hallucinogens
	Muscle relaxants
	Anesthetic agents
	Inhalants

Depression With Melancholic Features

- Definition: A severe form of major depressive episode occurring more commonly in older persons; believed to be particularly responsive to somatic therapy; applied to the current episode only if it is the most recent episode

- Signs and Symptoms: The presence of 1 or 2 below and 3 of the remainder (3–8) (APA, 1994):

  1. Loss of interest or pleasure in all, or almost all, activities

  2. Lack of reactivity to usually pleasurable stimuli

  3. Depression regularly worse in morning

  4. Early morning awakening (EMA)—at least 2 hours before usual time

  5. Psychomotor retardation or agitation

  6. Significant anorexia or weight loss

  7. Distinct quality of depressed mood

  8. Excessive or inappropriate guilt

Depression With Seasonal Pattern (Seasonal Affective Disorder)

- Definition: Regular temporal relationship between the onset of an episode of major depression or bipolar disorder, recurrent and a particular period of the year; in the absence of obvious seasonal stressor such as regular winter unemployment; full remissions or a change from depression to hypomania or mania also occur at a characteristic time of the year (APA, 1994)

- Differential Diagnosis

  1. At least 2 episodes of major depression that demonstrate the temporal, seasonal relationships in 2 consecutive years

  2. Seasonal major depressive episodes substantially outnumber the non-seasonal episodes that may have occurred over the individual's lifetime.

  3. No non-seasonal major depressive episodes have occurred during the same 2 years

Dysthymic Disorder

- Definition: Chronic depressed mood for most of the day, for more days than not, as indicated by subjective account or observations made by others, for at least 2 years (APA, 1994)

- Signs and Symptoms: The presence while depressed of at least 3 of the following that cause clinically significant distress or impairment in school, occupation or other important areas of functioning:

    1. Low self-esteem

    2. Feelings of hopelessness

    3. Poor concentration or difficulty making decisions

    4. Low energy or fatigue

    5. Insomnia or hypersomnia

    6. Poor appetite or over-eating

- Differential Diagnosis

    1. During the two year period of the disturbance, the person has not been without symptoms for more than two months at a time

    2. No major depressive episode during the first two years of the disturbance

    3. Has never had a manic, hypomanic, or mixed episode

    4. Does not occur exclusively during the course of a chronic psychotic disorder such as schizophrenia

    5. Not due to the direct effects of a substance (i.e. drug of abuse or other medication) or a general medical condition (i.e. hypothyroidism)

Major Depression With Postpartum Onset

- Definition: Depressive episode, ranging from moderate to severe, following childbirth with or without psychotic features and/or manic episodes

- Signs and Symptoms

    1. Onset within 4 weeks following delivery

    2. Evidence of increased risk with family history of bipolar disorder

- Prevalence

  1. Recurrence rate for psychotic postpartum depression at future deliveries is 30 to 50 percent

  2. Occurs in 1:500–1000 deliveries and may be more common in primiperous women

Bipolar Disorders

A disorder of mood in which there is at least one or more manic or hypomanic episodes, usually with a history of one or more major depressive episodes (APA, 1994).

Bipolar I Disorder (BPD I)

- Definition: Frank manic or hypomanic episdodes with or without major depressive episodes that occur in an alternating pattern separated by hours, weeks, months or years, interspersed with periods of euthymia (normal mood)

  1. Manic episode

     a. A distinct period during which the predominant mood is elevated, expansive, or irritable, causing marked impairment in occupational functioning, social activities, and relationships for at least one week.

     b. Presence of at least 3 of the following during the same period:

        (1) Inflated self-esteem or grandiosity

        (2) Loquaciousness/pressure of speech

        (3) Flight of ideas/thoughts racing/looseness of associations

        (4) Distractibility

        (5) Increase in goal-directed activity ranging to frantic, disorganized activity

        (6) Excessive involvement in pleasurable activities with harmful consequences (i.e., spending sprees, promiscuity, reckless business decisions and investments)

        (7) Decreased need for sleep

    c.   Differential Diagnosis

        (1)   Mixed-state Episode

        (2)   Schizoaffective Disorder

        (3)   Substance abuse

        (4)   Response to somatic antidepressant treatment, e.g., ECT, light therapy, antidepressant medication

2.   Hypomanic Episode

    a.   A distinct period of sustained, elevated, expansive, or irritable mood, lasting throughout four days, that is clearly different from the nondepressed mood.

    b.   At least 3 of the following symptoms (1–7) have been present to a significant degree:

        (1)   Inflated self-esteem or grandiosity

        (2)   Decreased need for sleep

        (3)   More talkative or pressure to keep talking

        (4)   Flight of ideas/thoughts racing

        (5)   Distractibility

        (6)   Increase in goal directed activity

        (7)   Excessive involvement in pleasurable activities

    c.   Associated with:

        (1)   Unequivocal change in functioning

        (2)   Disturbance in mood and change in functioning are observable by others

        (3)   Episode not severe enough to cause marked impairment in social or occupational functioning, or to necessitate hospitalization

        (4)   No psychotic features

    d.   Differential Diagnosis—medication, substance abuse or general medical condition, (e.g., hyperthyroidism)

3. Depressive Episode

    a. Definition: Previously has had at least one manic episode, but currently in a major depressive episode

    b. Signs and Symptoms—see Major Depression

Bipolar II Disorder (BP II)

- Definition: One or more major depressive episodes with at least one episode of hypomania that cause clinically significant distress or impairment in social occupational or other imporant areas of functioning (APA, 1994)

- Differential Diagnosis

1. Has never had a mixed episode

2. Has never had a manic episode

3. Mood symptoms not accounted for by Schizoaffective Disorder; not superimposed on Schizophrenia, Schizophreniform Disorder, Delusional Disorder, or Psychotic Disorder Not Otherwise Specified (N.O.S.)

4. Not precipitated by somatic antidepressant treatment

Bipolar Disorder not Otherwise Specified (APA, 1994)

- Definition: Mood Disorders with bipolar features that do not meet full criteria for a specific bipolar disorder

- Signs and Symptoms

1. Very rapid alternation between manic and depressive symptoms

2. Recurrent hypomanic episodes without intercurrent depressive symptoms

3. Manic or mixed episode superimposed on Delusional Disorder or Psychosis N.O.S., or Residual Schizophrenia

4. Episode in which the clinician has determined that a Bipolar Disorder is present but is unable to determine whether it is primary, substance induced, or due to a general medical condition.

Cyclothymic Disorder

- Definition: A chronic mood disturbance of at least 2 years duration involving numerous hypomanic episodes and periods of depressed mood or loss of interest or pleasure

- Differential Diagnosis

  1. Person not without hypomanic or depressive symptoms for more than 2 months during a 2 year period

  2. Has not met criteria for a Major Depressive, Mixed or Manic Episode

- Signs and Symptoms

  1. For symptoms of depression, see Depressive Disorders

  2. For symptoms relating to hypomania, see Bipolar Disorders

Mood Disorder Due to...(Indicate General Medical Condition) (APA, 1994)

- Definition: Prominent and persistent disturbance in mood judged to be due to direct physiological effects of a general medical condition; e.g., stroke, endocrine or autoimmune conditions, viral or other infections that causes *clinically significant* distress or impairment in social, occupational or other important areas of functioning

- Signs and Symptoms:

  1. Depressed mood or markedly diminished interest or pleasure in all or almost all activities

  2. Elevated, expansive or irritable mood

  3. Evidence from history, physical exam or laboratory findings that the mood disturbance is the direct physiological consequence of a general medical condition

- Differential Diagnosis:

  1. Not better accounted for by another mental/psychiatric disorder

  2. Does not occur exclusively during the course of delirium

Depressive Disorder Not Otherwise Specified (APA, 1994)

- Definition: Disorders with depressive features that do not meet criteria for Major Depressive, Dysthymic Disorder, Adjustment Disorders

- Signs and Symptoms

  1. Symptoms associated with premenstrual dysphoric disorder severe enough to markedly interfere with work, school or usual activities, that are absent for at least one week post menses

  2. Minor depression—episodes of at least 2 weeks of depression, but with fewer than the 5 items required for Major Depressive Disorder

  3. Recurrent brief depression—episodes lasting 2 days to 2 weeks that occur at least once a month for 12 months (not associated with the menstrual cycle)

  4. Post-psychotic depression of schizrenia

  5. Can be superimposed on Delusional Disorder, active phase of Schizophrenia or Psychotic Disorder N.O.S.

  6. The clinician has determined a depresssive disorder is present but is unable to determine whether it is primary, due to general medical condition or substance induced.

Major Depression with Catatonic Features (APA, 1994)

- Definition: Severe state characterized by marked psychosomatic disturbance that can occur in Major Depression, Mania, Mixed Episode, Bipolar I or Bipolar II Disorder

- Signs and Symptoms:

  1. Motor immobility manifested by catalepsy, waxy flexibility, or stupor

  2. Excessive motor activity that is generally purposeless, and not influenced by external stimuli

  3. Extreme negativism as shown by an apparently motiveless resistance to all instructions; mutism or maintenance of a rigid posture that resists movement by an outside force

  4. Peculiarities of voluntary movements as shown by assumption of inappropriate or bizarre postures; stereotyped movements, prominent mannerisms or prominent grimacing

  5. Echolalia or echopraxia

Mood Disorder with Rapid Cycling (APA, 1994)

- Definition: At least 4 episodes of a mood disturbance in the previous 12 months that meet criteria for a manic depressive, manic, mixed or hypo-manic episode

- Signs and Symptoms

  1. May be applied to Bipolar I and Bipolar II Disorder (occurs in 5-15% of Bipolar I)

  2. Episodes are demarcated either by partial or full remission for at least 2 months or a switch to an episode of opposite polarity (i.e. Major Depression to manic episode)

  3. Women comprise 70 - 90% of individuals

  4. May be associated with hypothyroidism, certain neurological conditions, i.e., multiple sclerosis, mental retardation, head injury, antidepressant therapy

  5. Can appear at anytime and may appear and disappear, particularly when associated with antidepressant therapy

  6. Associated with a poorer long-term prognosis

Mood Disorder, Most Recent Episode: Atypical (APA, 1994)

- Definition: Mood reactivity—defined as the capacity to be cheered up when presented with positive events; mood may become euthymic (not sad) for extended periods if circumstances remain favorable; not associated with melancholic or catatonic features

- Signs and Symptoms: Must include 1 below and 2 or more of 2-5

  1. Mood reactivity—the mood brightens in response to actual or potential positive events

  2. Significant weight gain or increase in appetite

  3. Hypersomnia

  4. Leaden paralysis, i.e., heavy feeling in arms and/or legs

  5. Long-standing pattern of interpersonal rejection sensitivity, not limited to episodes of mood disturbance, that results in significant social or occupational impairment; may include using substances

  6. Two to three times more common in women

  7. Patients report an earlier age at onset of depressive episodes

Substance Induced Mood Disorder (APA, 1994)

- Definition: Permanent and persistent disturbance in mood that is judged to be due to the direct physiological effects of substance; e.g., drug abuse, medications, somatic treatments for depression, toxin exposure that arises *only in association* with intoxication or withdrawal states causing clinically significant distress or impairment to social, occupational, or other important areas of functioning

- Signs and Symptoms

    1. Prominent and persistent mood disturbance that predominates the majority of time characterized by either depressed mood, a markedly diminished interest in most activities and/or elevated, expansive or irritable mood

    2. Evidence from history, physical exam and/or laboratory results that either occurrence within a month of intoxication or withdrawal of medications is etiologically related to the disturbance

- Differential Diagnosis

    1. Mood disorder that is not substance induced

    2. Does not occur exclusively during a delirium

Suicide

- Definition: A self-directed act to end one's life that may be associated with:

    1. Major Depression

    2. Bipolar Disorder

    3. Schizophrenia (command hallucinations)

    4. Alcohol and Drug Use or Withdrawal

    5. Impulse Control Disorders

- Involves:

    a. Behavior Changes

    b. Anxiety

    c. Insomnia

    d. Anorexia

    e. Expression of anger, helplessness, or hopelessness

      f. Giving away personal possessions, closing bank accounts

      g. Sudden calmness or improvement in a depressed client

      h. Questions about guns, poisons or other lethal instruments

      i. Social withdrawal/isolation (physical or social)

      j. Stress (i.e. loss of health, significant other, job)

      k. Feelings of worthlessness (e.g. everyone would be better off without me)

- Risk Factors Related to Suicide, (See Table 2)

Table 2

Risk Factors Related to Suicide

- History of Suicidal Ideation and/or Attempts
- Hopelessness
- Physical Illness
- Family History of Substance Abuse
- Family History of Depression or Suicide
- Caucasian Race
- Male Gender
- Advanced Age
- Depression
- Living Alone/Isolation
- Presence of Psychotic Symptoms
- Lethality of Suicide Plan

Etiology of Mood Disorders

- Genetic/Biologic Theories

    1. Neurotransmitter Hypotheses

        a. Imbalances in nerve cells whose neurotransmitters are biogenic amines (e.g.) serotonin (5 HT), norepinephrine (NE) and other related modulating neurohormones, acetylcholine and gamma acetyl buteric acid (GABA); the feedback between messenger hormones and target organs suggest many types of defective neuro-endocrine secretion.

        b. Overactivity of the limbic hypothalamic-pituitary-adrenal axis (LHPA) leading to hypercortisolism

    2. Circadian Rhythm Hypothesis

a. A disturbance in regulation of biological rhythms that synchronize body functions is congruent with rhythmical cyclical nature of mood disorders.

b. Depressed persons may be in a chronic state of sleep satiety (arousal) leading to REM sleep abnormalities. Acetylcholine may be involved in shortened REM latency in depression (phase advance of circadian rhythms) leading to advances in cortisol secretion (which normally surges in early morning to prepare for wakefulness).

c. Depressed persons may dispense earlier with central nervous system (CNS) programs that promote vegetative functions or overcome the restraints of arousal systems sooner than non-depressed persons.

d. The phase delay hypothesis posits that for individuals with seasonal affective disorder (SAD) circadian rhythms occur at a later time relative to sleep onset and temperature, and predicts an antidepressant response to morning photo-therapy. This shifts the onset of melatonin production and secretion to an earlier time in the evening, which results in a correction of the disrupted relationship between sleep, temperature and circadian rhythms.

e. Bipolar patients in the manic phase may have phase shifting, loss of patterning, and disorders of amplitude

3. Kindling and Behavioral Sensitization Hypothesis

a. Kindling refers to electrical stimulation (shock) leading to nerve depolarization and seizure activity, which can later occur spontaneously when animals are placed in the environment in which original electrical stimulation occurred; animals also exhibit dysphoria

b. Stress, like shock, is hypothesized to lower the threshold for stimulant induced sensitization, especially inescapable stress, resulting in behavioral and neurochemical abnormalities associated with depression

c. Bipolar patients in the manic phase may have repeated daily subthreshold electrical stimulation producing seizure-like activity. Features of this seizure are irritability, rapid mood swings, and epileptic auras.

4. Genetic Hypothesis

   a. Data consistently demonstrate higher rates of depression among lst degree relatives of people with unipolar depression and bipolar disorder and among monozygotic versus dizygotic twins

   b. Prevalence

      (1) Unipolar

         (a) General population—7%

         (b) First-degree relatives—18%

      (2) Bipolar

         (a) General population—1–2%

         (b) First-degree relatives—8%

      (3) Any major affective disorder

         (a) General population—8–9%

         (b) First-degree relatives—24%

   c. No genetic factor consistently identified

- Psychoanalytic Theory

   1. Object Loss Hypothesis—infants experiencing loss of the maternal love object in infancy experience separation anxiety and grief related to loss of the primary love object; early loss is thought to predispose the adult to respond dysfunctionally to losses that occur later in life, becoming depressed significantly more often than those not experiencing such early losses

   2. Aggression-Turned-Inward Hypothesis—depression is proposed to be a turning inward of the aggressive instinct that is not directed at the appropriate object, with accompanying feelings of guilt

      a. This process is initiated by loss of an object toward whom a person feels love and hate (ambivalence).

      b. The person is unable to express the angry feelings because they are thought to be irrational or inappropriate and are unacceptable to the superego.

    c. The person may develop a pattern of containing angry/aggressive feelings and directing them inward against the self leading to self-hatred.

    d. Suicide viewed as a strike against the hated and loved object as well as the self; manic episode is viewed as a defense against depression

- Cognitive Theory

  1. Depression is a cognitive problem originating from disturbed thinking in which the depression-prone person explains an adverse event as a personal shortcoming.

  2. Developmental experiences sensitize certain people and make them vulnerable to depression. The constellation of negative thoughts that characterize depression remains dormant until a person becomes depressed. When depression occurs after a life stressor, the dormant cognitive set appears; negative cognitive processes replace objective thinking.

  3. Cognitive Elements of Depression

    a. Cognitive triad—the person's negative view of self, the world and the future, which is a distortion of reality

    b. Silent assumptions—irrational beliefs or rules that significantly affect the depressed person's cognitive, affective, and behavior patterns

    c. Logical errors—faulty information processing and errors in thinking that maintain the person's belief in the validity of his/her negative concept despite contradictory evidence

- Hopelessness Theory of Depression (Learned Helplessness)

  1. Based on attribution theory—a chain of perceived negative life events are hypothesized to be the ''occasion setter'' for people to become hopeless and depressed.

  2. Depression consists of four classes of deficits: motivational, cognitive, self-esteem, and affective.

  3. Three types of influences determine whether a person will become hopeless, and, in turn depressed, when negative life events are experienced.

    a. When highly desired outcomes are believed improbable or

when highly aversive outcomes are perceived probable, and the person anticipates that no response in his or her repertoire will positively affect the outcome (helplessness), depression occurs.

b. When negative life events are attributed to stable versus unstable and global versus specific causes, and are viewed as important, helplessness, low self-esteem and depression ensue.

c. Inferred negative consequences are most likely to lead to depression. The consequence is viewed as important, not remediable, likely to change, and affecting many areas of life. When inferred characteristics about the self (self-worth, abilities, desirability, etc.) are negative and will interfere with attainment of important outcomes, hopelessness and depression may ensue.

- Family Theory

1. Developmental experiences within the family system (abuse, conflict, divorce, death) can be antecedents of depression.

   a. Nodal events (significant exits and entries of people, places, objects, activities, and roles in a family system), especially those perceived as undesirable, can precipitate depression, especially when an event generates stress or anxiety not openly dealt with in the family system.

   b. Multiple nodal events occurring within a brief period may escalate the likelihood of stress (cluster stress) and depression.

   c. Anniversary reactions (affective responses around anniversary of nodal event), which reactivate feelings associated with original nodal event, can take form of depression, suicidal thoughts, gestures attempts, and other stress-related symptoms.

2. Family precursors of mood disorders include early developmental family experiences related to strong nurturing in early childhood followed by cutting off of nurturing supplies in early childhood, coupled with unrealistic expectations, unquestioning acceptance of parental values, and frustrated efforts to obtain family approval and love. Underlying resentment toward parents may erupt briefly, followed by quiet and fear of rejection. Manic episode masks guilt, loss, and rejection. Depressive episode represents internalization of disappointment, loss, and perceived failure.

Screening Instruments

- Patient Self-Report Questionnaires
    1. General Health Questionnaire (GHQ)
    2. Center for Epidemiological Studies—Depression Scale (CES-D)
    3. Beck Depression Inventory (BDI)
    4. Zung Self-Rating Depression Scale (ZSRDS)
- Clinician-Completed Rating Scales
    1. Hamilton Rating Scale for Depression (HRS-D)
    2. Montgomery-Asberg Depression Rating Scale (MADRS)
    3. Schedule for Affective Disorders and Schizophrenia (SADS)
    4. Inventory for Depressive-Symptomatology-Clinician Rated (IDS-C)
    5. Minnesota Multiphasic Personality Inventory (MMPI)
    6. Symptom 90 Checklist

Laboratory tests—experimental

- Thyrotropin releasing hormone (TRH) stimulation test and corticotropin-releasing hormone (CRH)—differentiate unipolar from bipolar disorders and mania from schizophrenia

- Dexamethasone suppression test (DMST)—dexamethasone is an exogenous steroid that suppresses blood levels of cortisol. Based on the premise that many depressed patients exhibit hypersecretion of cortisol, a single (11 p.m.) dose of cortisol does not depress late afternoon cortisol levels. If the post dexamethasone cortisol level is ≥ 5 mg/mL, then it has escaped suppression, and support is added for a diagnosis of biological depression.

- Urinary MHPG—a major metabolite of norepinephrine (NE) is 3-methoxy 4-hyroxy-phenylglycol (MHPG); because this metabolite crosses the blood-brain barrier, its CNS activity can be estimated by measuring MHPG elimination in urine (peripheral MHPG is also secreted in urine); proposed that patients with low MHPG have less norepinephrine to metabolize and would respond to antidepressants that block norepinephrine reuptake; patients with normal or high NE levels may have a serotonin deficient depression and may respond to drugs that block serotonin reuptake

- Sleep EEG (REM Latency Measurement)—Sleep EEGs indicate that depressed patients spend less time in the more refreshing slow-wave phases of sleep and have a shorter pre-REM phase (decreased REM latency) of 2–30 minutes versus 90 minutes.

Nursing Diagnoses (See Table 3)

Table 3

Comparison of DSMIV Criteria and Nursing Diagnosis Related to Mood Disorders

DSMIV Criteria	Nursing Diagnoses
Depression	
1. Psychomotor retardation or agitation	Mobility, alteration in
2. Loss of interest in usual pleasures	Coping, ineffective individual/impaired social interaction
DSMIV Criteria	**Nursing Diagnoses**
3. Decreased ability to concentrate	Thought processes, alteration in
4. Feelings of worthlessness, guilt	Self-concept, disturbance in
5. Insomnia or hypersomnia	Sleep pattern disturbance
6. Fatigue or loss of energy	Fatigue/self-care deficit
7. Recurrent thoughts of death or suicide	Potential for self-harm
	Dysfunctional grieving
8. Appetite disturbance	Nutrition, alteration in less than body requirements more than body requirements
9. Depressed mood with psychotic features (hallucinations, delusions)	Alteration in perception or cognition
Mania	
1. A distinct period of abnormally elevated, expansive, or irritable mood	Emotional lability
2. Grandiosity	Self-concept, disturbance in
3. Hyperverbal, pressured speech	Communication, impaired verbal
4. Distractibility	Thought process, alteration in
5. Poor Judgement	Sensory perceptual alteration; potential for self-harm
6. Decreased need for sleep	Sleep pattern disturbance
7. Racing thoughts, flight of ideas	Thought processes, alteration in
8. Increased activity	Impaired social interaction/self-care deficit
9. Excessive involvement in pleasurable activities	Altered impulse control/manipulation
10. Mania with psychotic features (delusions, hallucinations)	Alteration in perception/cognition

Nursing Interventions

- Pharmacological Interventions

    1. Objectives

        a. Symptom reduction (initial objective)

        b. Improved function

        c. Recurrence prevention

    2. Role of the nurse

        a. Collection of pretreatment assessment data

    b.   Coordination of treatment modalities

    c.   Client education

        (1)   Provide information about medication and its side effects (See Tables 4, 5, 6 and 7)

        (2)   Clarify misinformation

        (3)   Explore perceptions and feelings about medication

        (4)   Medication management strategies

    d.   Monitoring drug effects/minimize side effects

    e.   Prescribing and/or administering medications

3.   Antidepressant drugs

    a.   First-line treatment modality for depressive disorder when:

        (1)   Client requests medication

        (2)   Medication and psychotherapy are planned treatment strategy

        (3)   Psychotherapy not available

        (4)   Prior positive response to medication

        (5)   Maintenance/treatment is planned

    b.   Mode of action

        (1)   Exact mechanism of action unknown

        (2)   Equilibrate effects of biogenic amines through various mechanisms

            (a)   Blocks reuptake of neurotransmitters (norepinephrine, serotonin) at presynaptic neuron

            (b)   Blocks reception of neurotransmitters at post-synaptic neuron forcing up or down regulation of neurotransmitters

            (c)   Inhibits metabolism of neurotransmitters (norepinephrine, serotonin)

            (d)   Regulates the locus ceruleus, the part of the brain where most norepinephrine is made

        (3)   MAOIs—inhibit the action of monoamine oxidase, an enzyme that metabolizes neurohormones responsible for

Table 4

Pharmacology of Antidepressant Medications

Drug	Therapeutic Dosage Range (mg/day)	Increase in Neuro-transmitter Function		Sedative Effect	Therapeutic Blood Levels ng/ML	Elimination Halflife (h)
		5–HT	NE			
Tricyclics						
Amitriptyline (Elavil, Endep)	75–300	3	2	4	150–250	10–46
Clomiprimine (Anafranil)	75–300	3	1	2	100–250	17–28
Desipramine (Norpramin, Pertoframe)	75–300	0	4	1	125–300	12–76
Doxepin (Sinequan, Adapin)	75–300	2	2	4	150–250	8–36
Imipramine (Tofranil, Janimine)	75–300	2	3	3	150–250	4–34
Nortriptyline (Aventyl, Pamelor)	40–200	2	3	2	50–150	13–88
Protriptyline (Vivactil)	20–60	2	4	1	70–250	54–124
Trimipramine (Surmontil)	75–300	2	3	4	150–250	7–30
Heterocyclics						
Amoxapine (Ascendin)	100–600	1	4	3	200–600	8
Bupropion (Wellbutrin)	225–450	1	1	1	25–100	10–14
Maprotiline (Ludiomil)	100–225	0	4	3	200–600	27–58
Trazodone (Desyrel)	150–600	4	0	4	800–1600	4–9
Selective Serotonin Reuptake Inhibitors (SSRIs)						
Fluvoxamine (Luvox)	50–300	3	1	2		15
Fluoxetine (Prozac)	10–40	3	1	1	200–700	24–96
Paroxetine (Paxil)	20–50	3	1	2	100–400	24
Sertraline (Zoloft)	50–200	3	1	2	20–500	24
Selective Serotonin Norepinephrine Reuptake Inhibitors						
Venlafaxine (Effexor)*	25–400	3	3	1		5–11
Nefazodone (Serzone)*	50–600	2	2	4		1.5–18

* These new agents are very unique in action and require further study.

Drug	Therapeutic Dosage Range (mg/day)	Increase in Neuro-transmitter Function		Sedative Effect	Therapeutic Blood Levels ng/ML	Elimination Halflife (h)
MAOIs						
Phenelzine (Nardil)	45–90	u	u	3	u	
Tranylcypromine (Parnate)	10–60	u	u	2	u	
Selective Norepinephrine Reuptake Inhibitors						
Mirtazapine (Remeron)	15–60	2ndary	4	1–4 dose dependent		28–34

High = 4   5HT = Serotonin
Moderate = 3   NE = Norepinephrine
Low = 2
Slight = 1
None = 0
Potency Unknown = u

Table 5

Selected ANTI-DEPRESSANT Drug Side Effects

Pharmaceutical Company	Generic Name	Anticholinergic	Sedation	Orthostatic Hypotension	1/2 Life (Hours)	Active Metabolites	1/2 Life of Metabolites
Geigy	Imipramine	**	**	***	4-34		
Marion Merrill Dow	Desipramine	*	*	*	12-76		
Stuart	Amitriptyline	***	***	***	10-46		
Sandoz	Nortriptyline	**	**	*	13-88		
Merck	Protriptyline	**	*	?*	54-124		
Roerig/Lotus	Doxepin	**	***	**	8-36		
Wyeth-Ayerst	Trimipramine	**	**	?**	7-30		
Lederle	Amoxapine*	*	**	?*	8		
Ciba	Maprotiline*	*	**	?*	27-58		
Wallace	Trazodone	0	***	**	4-9		
Burroughs	Bupropion*	*	0	*	10-14		
Dista/Lilly	Fluoxetine	0	0	*	24-72	Norfluoxetine	168-360
Roerig	Sertraline	*	0	*	24-30	Desmethyl-sertraline	66
SmithKline	Paroxetine	*	0	*	3-65		
Wyeth-Ayerst	Venlafaxine	0	0	*	5	O-desmethyl-venlafaxine	11
Bristol Myers	Nefazodone	0	**	*	2-4	Hydroxyne-fazodone	1.5-18
Upjohn	Fluvoxamine *neurotoxic*	0	0	*	15		
Organon	Mirtazapine	*	0-****	*	20-40		

Table 6

Adverse/Side Effects of Antidepressants and Nursing Interventions

Side Effect	Nursing Intervention
Neurological Sedation, psychomotor slowing, difficulty concentrating and planning	Inform the client, especially if he operates machinery or must perform mental tasks; tolerance can develop and thus side effects do decrease or dose can be lowered
Muscle weakness, fatigue, nervousness, headaches, vertigo neuropathies, tremors, ataxia, paresthesias, twitching	Not common; tolerance can develop and thus side effects do decrease or dose can be lowered
Lowered seizure threshold	Start drugs at lower dose and increase more gradually with seizure disorder clients
Extrapyramidal side effects (EPS): acute dystonic reactions, akathisia, Parkinson's syndrome, tardive dyskinesia	Rare, since they do not block dopamine; amoxapine, the exception, can cause all the common EPS reactions, possibly tardive dyskinesia with long-term use
Psychiatric symptoms: increased anxiety, depression, insomnia, nightmares, psychotic reactions, or confusional states with delusions, hallucinations, and disorientation; mania	Uncommon, may have to discontinue drug; mania may be precipitated if client has prior history of mania in self or family (avoid tricyclics if possible in patients predisposed to mania)

Table 6 - Continued

Side Effect	Nursing Intervention
Gastrointestinal	
Heartburn, nausea, vomiting	Take with meals; switch medication if discomfort becomes severe or vomiting occurs
Decrease in intestinal motility, paralytic ileus	Monitor elimination patterns
Dry mouth	Increase fluids
Hematological	
Leukopenia and thrombocytopenia	Monitor; rarely clinically significant
Agranulocytosis: Allergic response of sudden onset; appears 40 to 70 days after initiation of drug (low WBC, normal RBC, infection of the pharynx, fatigue, malaise)	Very rare; discontinue drug and place patient in reverse isolation immediately; never administer drug again; try antidepressant with a different chemical structure and follow client closely
Cardiovascular	
Postural hypotension: light-headedness or dizziness on rising due to decrease in blood pressure	Occurs frequently; take vital signs sitting and then standing $\frac{1}{2}$ hour after dose; rise slowly, dangle feet, tolerance can develop in first few weeks; not dose related, can continue to raise dose
Tachycardia: rapid heart beat EKG changes	Occurs frequently; tolerance usually develops; can increase symptoms of angina in clients with coronary artery disease; very frightening to panic disorder clients; worsening of intraventricular conduction problems; take a careful cardiac history and do a pretreatment EKG, especially with clients over 40 years of age
Sudden death	Rare; clients at risk for cardiac heart block; over 50 years of age, family history of heart disease, preexisting cardiac disease or recent myocardial infarction, or bundle-branch block
Opthalmological	
Blurred vision caused by ciliary muscle relaxation	Tolerance can develop over the first few weeks of treatment; distant vision is usually intact; do not use with clients with narrow-angle glaucoma
Hepatic	
Liver toxicity within first 8 weeks of treatment: abdominal pain, anorexia, fever, mild transient jaundice, abnormal liver function tests	Rare hypersensitivity response; discontinue drug; switch to another type of antidepressant
Endocrine	
Amenorrhea, galactorrhea	Due to increased prolactin caused by amoxapine; rare with other tricyclics
Menstrual irregularities	Rare and reversible; decrease dose; change to a different tricyclic
Cutaneous	
Maculopapular rashes, petechiae, photosensitivity	Rare; can give an antihistamine; anti-depressant

Table 6 - Continued

Side Effect	Nursing Intervention
Genitourinary Increased or decreased sexual desire, delayed ejaculation	Decrease dose, change to a less anticholinergic drug; take daily dose after sexual intercourse, not immediately before, for delayed ejaculation
Urinary retention	Lower dose, change to a less anticholinergic drug, try bethanechol; rare: acute renal failure following an atonic bladder
Miscellaneous Tinnitus, weight loss, increased appetite and weight gain, psychomotor stimulation, parotid swelling, alopecia, allergic response: edema, generalized on face, tongue, and orbits	Very rare; weight control; decrease dose; may have to discontinue drug and try an antidepressant that is structurally different
Pathological sweating	Occurs in 25% of patients; head, neck, and upper extremities; episodic, or occurs only at night
Withdrawal syndrome Mild withdrawal after sudden discontinuation: malaise, muscle aches, coryza, chills, nausea, dizziness, anxiety	Taper client off drug gradually (one to several weeks)
Intoxication syndromes Poisoning, usually seen in overdose; CNS depression and/or cardiotoxicity; hallucinations, delirium, agitation, sensitivity to sounds, dilated pupils, hypothermia, hyperpyrexia, seizures, coma, arrhythmias, respiratory arrest	Treat aggressively; recovery can be slow; induce emesis, gastric lavage, cardiac monitoring, respiratory support, blood chemistry, arterial blood gases, monitor tricyclic plasma levels, carefully administer physostigmine, valium, mannitol, lidocaine, and other symptomatic treatments
Anticholinergic syndromes Confusion, delirium, disorientation, agitation, hallucinations, anxiety, motor restlessness, seizures, delusions, constipation, urinary retention, decreased sweating, increased pupillary size, dry mouth, increased temperature, motor incoordination, flushing, tachycardia	Usually occurs with high doses of psychoactive drugs with anticholinergic effects; physostigmine, cardiac monitoring, respiratory support; in sensitive or aged clients, may occur at normal, therapeutic levels

stimulating physical and mental activity (serotonin, norepinephrine, and epinephrine); usually used when client is unresponsive to non-MAOI anti-depressants

    (4)   Pharmacology outlined in Table 4

  c. Administration

    (1)   Oral route

    (2)   Begin with low dosage administered at bed time to minimize side effects (e.g., 25 to 50 mg/day of desipramine)

    (3)   Increase dosage in increments over 1 to 3 weeks (except fluoxetine because of long half life)

    (4)   Fluoxetine and paroxetine administered in morning, others at night or bid

    (5)   Note time lag in onset of therapeutic effect, 7–28 days

    (6)   Monitor blood levels and side effects weekly/biweekly and adjust dosage after 3 days

    (7)   Evaluate side effects weekly/biweekly

    (8)   Assess outcomes at 6 weeks and 12 weeks

    (9)   Continue medication for 4–9 months

    (10) Continuation of medication may be indicated if depression is recurring

  d. Side/adverse/toxic effects of non-MAOIs

    (1)   Incidence of side/adverse effects most common at beginning of treatment subside over time and/or clients adapt to many side effects over time (See Tables 5 & 6) and/or develop tolerance

    (2)   Toxic effects same as side effects but intensified

       (a)   Anticholinergic, CNS stimulation followed by CNS depression

       (b)   Cardiac irregularities (except fluoxetine and fluroxamine); extends duration of QRS complex ≤ 0.125)

  e. Side/Adverse Effects of MAOIs

    (1)   Most common effects are: constipation, anorexia, nausea, vomiting, dry mouth, urinary retention, skin rash, transient impotence, drowsiness, headache, dizziness, orthostatic hypotension

    (2)   Occasional stimulant effect (insomnia, restlessness, anxiety)

    (3)   Hypomania in patients with bipolar disorders (35%)

    (4)   Parasthesias (tingling at periphery, electric-shock-like sensations)

(5)   Hypertensive crisis (See Tables 7 & 8)

4.   Mood Stabilizers

a.   Lithium

(1)   First-line treatment modality for bipolar disorders

(a)   In manic and depressive episodes

(b)   As prophylaxis against further episodes

(c)   In other disorders with an affective component

- Recurrent unipolar depression
- Schizo affective disorder
- Catatonia
- Alcoholism

(d)   In non-affective disorders

- Aggressive conduct disorder
- Eating disorders
- Borderline personality disorder

(2)   Mode of Action

(a)   Exact mode of action not fully understood—affects calcium gate mechanism

(b)   Corrects anion exchange abnormality

(c)   Alters sodium transport in nerves and muscle cells

(d)   Normalizes synaptic transmission of norepinephrine, serotonin, and dopamine

(e)   Increases reuptake and metabolism of norepinephrine

(f)   Changes receptor sensitivity for serotonin

(3)   Administration

(a)   10–14 days before complete effect is observed

(b)   Acute mania often initially treated with neuroleptics to manage psychotic symptoms and/or behavioral excitement until lithium is effective

Table 7

Signs and Symptoms of Hypertensive Crisis and Nursing Interventions

Signs and Symptoms	Nursing Intervention
Warning Signs	
Increased blood pressure	Hold next MAOI dose
Palpitations	Do not lie client in supine or prone position (elevated BP
Frequent Headaches	in head)
Symptoms of Hypertensive Crisis	
Sudden elevation of blood pressure	Monitor vital signs
Explosive headache (occiptal radiating frontally)	Chlorpromazine 100 mg IM (blocks Norepinephrine, repeat
Palpitations; chest pain	if necessary)
Sweating	Phentolamine slowly administered in 5 mg IV doses (binds
Fever	with norepinephrine receptor sites, blocking
Nausea; vomiting	norepinephrine)
Dilated pupils	Manage fever with external cooling techniques
Photophobia	Assess intake of tyramine containing foods
Neck stiffness	
Nosebleed	
Intracranial bleeding	

Table 8

Dietary Restrictions for Patients Taking MAOIs

Food and Beverages to Avoid	Safe Food, Beverages and Medication
Cheese, especially aged or matured (Cheddar, Mozzarella, Parmesan, Gruyre, Stilton, Brie, Swiss, blue, Camembert)	Cottage Cheese
	Farmer's Cheese
Fermented or aged protein (salami, mortadella, sausage, bologna, pepperoni)	Cheese Whiz
	Ricotta
Pickled or smoked fish	Havarti
Beer, red wine, Sherry, Cognac, liqueurs	Boursin
Yeast or protein extracts (Marmite, Oxo, Bovril)	Fresh fruits
Broad bean pods	Bread products raised with yeast (bread)
Beef or chicken liver	
Yogurt	
Sauerkraut	
Over ripe fruit	

Foods and Beverages to be Consumed in Moderation
Chocolate
Sour cream
Avocado
Clear spirits and white wine
Soy sauce
Caffeine drinks

Medications to Avoid	Safe Medications
Cold Medications	Aspirin, Tylenol
Nasal and sinus decongestants	Pure steroid asthma inhalants
Allergy and hay fever remedies	Codeine
Narcotics, especially meperidine	Plain Robitusin or Terpin-hydrate with codeine
Inhalants for asthma	All laxatives
Local anesthetics with epinephrine	All antibiotics
Weight reducing pills	Antihistamines

  (c) Dose guided by plasma level; increase slowly to minimize side effects until symptoms are reduced, side effects are too great as upper limit of therapeutic blood level is reached.

  (d) Acute treatment: 900–2400 mg daily (.08–1.2 mEq/L) (300 mg tid)

  (e) Maintenance: 400–1200 mg daily (0.6–1.0 mEq/L) (tid, or bid if sustained release form is used)

  (f) Blood levels drawn

- 7 days after tx begins (12 hours after last dose)
- 2× weekly × 2 weeks
- 1× weekly × 2 weeks
- q 3 months × 6 months
- q 6 months thereafter

  (g) Therapeutic Range 0.6–1.4 mEq/L for adults; 0.6–0.8 mEq/L in geriatric clients or those with medical illness

 (4) Side/adverse/toxic effects of Lithium

  (a) Incidence of side effects most common at beginning of treatment disappear after a few weeks (See Table 9)

  (b) Symptoms coincide with peaks of lithium concentration due to rapid absorption of lithium ion

  (c) Lithium toxicity—usually dose related (see table 10)

 b. Anticonvulsants

 (1) Depakote approved for first-line treatment for mood stabilization in Bipolar Disorder;

  (a) When lithium is contraindicated or ineffective

  (b) For rapid cyclers (> 4 episodes/year)

  (c) Prevention of recurrence

 (2) Other anticonvulsants; (see Table 11)

Table 9

Lithium Side Effects and Nursing Interventions

Side Effect Symptom	Nursing Intervention
Polyuria, with possible progression to diabetes insipidus. Urine output is large in volume and so dilute that it may be colorless	Reassure client that increased urination is common and benign.
Client may complain of urinating so frequently that it interferes with activities of daily living, including sleep.	Urine volume may diminish if the physician reduces the lithium dose or changes to a slow release form or a single daily dosage. When severe, the physician usually orders 24-hour urine volume. If volume is greater than 3 L, a further renal workup is usually requested. When severe, polyuria is often treated by the physician with a thiazide or potassium-sparing diuretic (taking care to reduce the lithium dose). Lithium is contra-indicated for clients with renal dysfunction.
Increased thirst	Recommend that clients quench their thirst and maintain a fairly stable intake of liquids from day to day. The best thirst quencher is water or a low-calorie beverage that will not cause weight gain when taken in large amounts. Gum or hard candies may help moisten the mouth.
Tremor: A fine tremor that worsens with intentional movements. It can make writing, drinking hot beverages, and many other motor tasks difficult.	Reassure that this is benign and may be temporary. In some clients it is persistent. The physician may order a reduction in dose, more frequent doses, or a change to a slow-release form. When the tremor is severe or incapacitating, the physician may treat it with a beta blocker, usually propranolol (Inderal). Recommend that the client reduce or eliminate caffeine-containing beverages.
Nausea, abdominal discomfort, diarrhea, or soft stools	Reassure that this is benign and usually temporary. Recommend that the client take lithium with meals, a glass of milk, or a snack. If symptoms persists, the physician may change to another lithium preparation.
Muscle weakness or fatigue	Reassure that this is benign and usually temporary. Since this is not a very common side effect of lithium, ascertain whether it is being caused by another medication being taken by the client. Encourage the client to remain active and get regular physical exercise. If symptom persists, the physician may reduce the dose, order more frequent divided doses, change to slow-release, or reduce the dose and more gradually increase to the present dose level.
Edema of the feet or other body parts	Reassure that this is benign and may be temporary. A moderate salt restriction may reduce the edema. If moderate salt restriction is undertaken, the serum lithium level usually rises somewhat. It then becomes necessary to monitor for signs of toxicity and keep the physician informed in case it becomes necessary to reduce the lithium dose.
Hypothyroidism (5%)	Explain that this is reversible and treatable. The physician usually orders thyroid hormone replacement, such as levothyroxine (Synthroid) or desiccated thyroid.

Table 9 - Continued

Side Effect Symptom	Nursing Intervention
Weight gain (60%)	Explain that this is fairly common and benign. Moderate calorie restriction and increased exercise usually help. Advise against fluid restriction or sodium restriction unless undertaken with knowledge of the physician and nurse, since either intervention can cause the serum lithium level to rise.
Hair thinning or loss	Explain that this may be temporary. Since hair loss can be a symptom of hypothyroidism, inform the physician so that thyroid function can be checked. If hair does not return, lithium is usually stopped so that hair can regrow.
	During periods of hair loss, encourage the client to consider wearing a wig.
Benign, reversible granulocytosis	Explain that this is benign. This side effect is the basis for its use as a treatment in some granulocytopenic conditions.
Decreased Libido	Suggest timing sexual activity to not coincide with peak action time of medication.
	Explore strategies for continuing relationship intimacy.

Table 10

Lithium Toxicity and Related Treatment

Mild
- At lithium levels of 1.5–2 mEq/L; occasionally occurs at normal levels
- Develops gradually over several days
- Symptoms: ataxia, coarse tremor, confusion, diarrhea, drowsiness, fasciculation, slurred speech
- Treatment: Hold all lithium doses
  - Obtain lithium blood level
  - Check vital signs
  - Patient education

Moderate to Severe
- At lithium levels > 2 mEq/L
- Gradual or sudden onset
- Symptoms: muscle tremor, hyperreflexia, pulse irregularities, hyper or hypotension, EKG changes, visual or tactile hallucinations, oliguria or anuria, seizures, coma, death
- Treatment: Rapid assessment of clinical signs and symptoms of lithium toxicity
  - Hold all lithium doses
  - Monitor vital signs and LOC
  - Protect airway and provide standby oxygen
  - Obtain lithium level stat; BUN, creatinine, urinalysis; CBC; monitor electrolytes EKG; monitor cardiac states
  - Limit lithium absorption; provide an emetic; N–G suctioning may be appropriate
  - Vigorously hydrate 5 to 6 L/day IV; indwelling catheter; monitor intake and output; ROM; deep breathing
  - Maintain bed rest

Table 11

Anticonvulsant Used in Treatment of Bipolar Disorder

Drug	Dose	Effects Side/Adverse/Toxic
Carbamezapine (Tegretol)	Begin at 200 mg/day in divided doses and increase progressively by 100 mg 2×/wk to as much as 1600 mg/day until attaining serum levels of 6–12 mg/l. First serum level drawn > 5 days after starting therapy Usual dose 300–1200 mg daily (less in Orientals and elderly) Slow-release tablets available; may decrease side effects due to peak levels of drug	skin rash sore throat mucosal ulceration low-grade fever drowsiness vertigo ataxia diplopia blurred vision nausea vomiting hepatotoxicity benign ↓ in WBC agranulocytosis
Valproate/Valproic Acid (Depakene, Depakote)	Begin at 500–1000 mg/day until serum level of 50–125 μg/ml is achieved Response occurs in 1–2 weeks	anorexia nausea vomiting diarrhea tremor sedation ataxia increased appetite pancreatitis
Clonazepam (Klonopin)	4–24 mg/day (indication not approved by FDA)	ataxia drowsiness cognitive impairment increased salivation behavioral dyscontrol (disinhibition) blurred vision paradoxical agitation

(3) Mode of Action

    (a) Structurally related to tricyclic antidepressants

    (b) Anticonvulsant activity mediated through a ''peripheral'' type benzodiazepine receptor

    (c) Effective in inhibiting seizures kindled from repeated stimulation of limbic structures

    (d) GABA antagonist activity

(4) Administration

(a) Fourteen days before peak effect

(b) Dose guided by plasma levels (See Table 11)

(c) Complete laboratory tests prior to beginning therapy

- CBC

- Liver function tests

- Serum electrolytes

- EKG

(d) Blood tests q 2 weeks × 3 months; q 3 months thereafter to monitor hematopoetic suppression and hyponatremia

(5) Reinforce teaching after each treatment.

- Electroconvulsive Therapy

  1. Mode of action

     a. Largely unknown

     b. Therapeutic effect may be due to seizure activity in brain producing changes in post-synaptic response to neurotransmitters similar to antidepressants.

  2. Indications

     a. Emergency therapy for suicidal or hyperactive clients who are in physical danger

     b. Clients unresponsive to or cannot tolerate medications

     c. During time lag between initiation of pharmacotherapy and establishment of therapeutic medication level

  3. Treatment

     a. 6–12 treatments on alternate days

     b. Atropine sulfate administered for vagolytic effect 30 minutes prior to treatment

     c. Short-acting barbiturate (Brevital Sodium) administered IV to induce anesthesia

      d.   Succinyl choline (Anectine) administered IV as muscle relaxant after anesthetic

      e.   100% O_2 administered 1–2 min. to prepare for apneic period from muscle relaxant and convulsion

      f.   Client positioned in supine position; mouth gag inserted; jaw supported; suctioning, prn

      g.   Electrodes applied unilaterally (less amnesia) at non-dominant side temple or bilaterally (more amnesia) at temples

      h.   Fingers and toes observed for twitching

      i. O_2 administered by bag breathing when twitching stops until spontaneous respiration resumes.

      j.   Patent airway maintained; client positioned on side

      k.   Vital signs monitored until stable

      l.   Patient begins to respond in 10–15 minutes.

4.   Side Effects

      a.   Anoxia during seizure

      b.   Memory loss—temporary

      c.   Cardiac arrhythmias

      d.   Mortality 1:10,000 patients

5.   Nursing intervention

      a.   Complete physical assessment including EKG, EEG, X-rays of spine and chest

      b.   Provide opportunity to express feelings about ECT

      c.   Assess client's response

      d.   Client education

          (1)   Assess patient and family anxiety level and ability to understand.

          (2)   Individualize amount of information shared (i.e., treatment, post ECT confusion, memory loss, etc.).

          (3)   Provide time to discuss concerns and answer questions

      (4)   Instruct accompanying adult in dealing with post ECT effects.

          (a)   Orienting to time, place, and person

          (b)   Headache

          (c)   Nausea

   e.   Treatment responsibilities

      (1)   Check emergency equipment

      (2)   Maintain NPO status

      (3)   Remove harmful objects (dentures, jewelry, etc.)

      (4)   Monitor vital signs

      (5)   Position on side until reactive

      (6)   Maintain airway

      (7)   Assist to ambulate

      (8)   Orient to environment

      (9)   Offer antiemetic or analgesea as needed

   f.   Ethical considerations

      (1)   Provide patient/family education

      (2)   Obtain informed consent

      (3)   Act as patient/family advocate

- Monitoring Physical Needs

   1.   Alteration in nutrition

      a.   Record intake and output

      b.   Weigh clients daily

      c.   Monitor electrolytes

      d.   Assist clients in identifying food preferences

      e.   Offer small, frequent high calorie meals and fluids

      f.   Provide nutritional meals that can be "eaten on the run" by manic clients

      g.   Assist as needed with feeding

    h. Promote weight management strategies for clients who overeat

2. Alteration in Sleep Patterns

    a. Discourage daytime sleeping

    b. Administer antidepressants hs (except Prozac, which may increase insomnia)

    c. Teach bedtime relaxation techniques

        (1) Relaxation exercises

        (2) Hot baths

        (3) Back rub

        (4) Soft music

    d. Provide rest periods for manic clients

    e. Decrease environmental stimuli

    f. Limit intake of caffeinated drinks

    g. Administer sedatives hs prn

3. Alteration in elimination

    a. Monitor intake and output

    b. Promote fluid intake

    c. Promote high fiber diet

    d. Promote exercise

    e. Administer laxatives prn

    f. Catheterize prn

4. Alterations in Hygiene

    a. Matter-of-factly assist with bathing, dressing, grooming as needed

    b. Promote independence in activities of daily living (ADLs)

    c. Set limits on neglect of self-care

    d. Positively reinforce self-care behaviors

- Psychotherapeutic Interventions

    1. Intervening in Uncomplicated Grief Reaction

        a. Objective to assist individuals experiencing loss resolve grieving and prevent dysfunctional coping

        b. Self-awareness necessary to understand own feelings and responses to loss

        c. Communicate open and directly but respect need for denial

        d. Assess prior losses and coping patterns to determine:

            (1) Stresses previously experienced

            (2) Coping style/resources

            (3) Support systems

            (4) Nature of current relationship

            (5) Persons at high risk for dysfunctional coping behaviors

        e. Provide anticipatory guidance prior to loss

            (1) Discuss impending loss

            (2) Review and analyze significance of past losses and responses in relation to impending loss

            (3) Teach about mourning process

            (4) Assist family in formulation of coping strategies

        f. Support patient and family

            (1) Consider cultural, religious and social customs of mourning

            (2) Provide private place for expression of feelings

            (3) Do not leave alone until a support system is available

        g. Assist in grief work

            (1) Help patient experience and express feelings of loss

            (2) Normalize intensity of feelings

            (3) Non-judgmentally accept hostility, anger, guilt, ambivalence, crying, testing and withdrawal

      (4) Respond empathetically yet communicate hope for future

      (5) Initially, assist in immediate decision-making if necessary

      (6) Initially, support defenses such as denial, dependence, reaction formation, over-identification, etc.

      (7) Encourage exploration and analysis of dysfunctional coping patterns

      (8) Support and reinforce development of functional coping patterns, gradual release of attachment bonds, and eventual investment in new relationships and interests

      (9) Promote social network support

         (a) Family

         (b) Friends

         (c) Clergy

         (d) Community agency

         (e) Self-help groups

2. Cognitive interventions

    a. Objectives

      (1) Increase client's sense of control over his/her goals/behavior

      (2) Increase self-esteem

      (3) Assist client in modifying negative expectations

    b. Assist in exploring feelings to elicit patient's view of problem(s)

    c. Assist client in identifying negative thoughts

    d. Accept client perceptions, not conclusions

    e. Teach thought interruption or substitution

    f. Encourage client to increase realistic thinking by appraising personal assets, strengths, accomplishments, and opportunities

    g. Encourage formulation of realistic versus unrealistic goals

3. Behavioral interventions

   a. Objectives

      (1) Activating clients in a realistic goal-directed way

      (2) Develop alternative problem-solving and coping strategies

      (3) Increase self-esteem

      (4) Instill hope

      (5) Increase client responsibility for change

      (6) Gradual redirection of self-preoccupation to interests in outside world

   b. Assess client strengths and weaknesses and personal and environmental factors that maintain depression

   c. Work with client to develop a structured daily program of activities which:

      (1) Considers probability of succeeding

      (2) Considers attention span, distractibility and motivation

      (3) Contains realistic goals and expectations

      (4) Provides opportunities for performance-based positive reinforcement

   d. Involve clients in:

      (1) Assertiveness training

      (2) Role playing

      (3) Social skills training

      (4) Stress management

         (a) Relaxation exercises

         (b) Meditation

         (c) Physical fitness/exercise

   e. Increase client's present versus past or future orientation.

4. Interpersonal interventions

   a. Objectives

       (1)   Increase appropriate expression of thoughts and feelings

       (2)   Increase self-esteem

       (3)   Increase social interaction

b.   Facilitate expression of feelings

       (1)   Acknowledge client pain and despair

       (2)   Reinforce that depression is self-limiting

       (3)   Convey hope for future

       (4)   Do not give false reassurance

       (5)   Engage in active listening

       (6)   Demonstrate acceptance of thoughts and feelings

       (7)   Facilitate expression of positive and negative thoughts and feelings

       (8)   Assist client in identifying strategies for expressing and coping with negative feelings (anger, guilt, aggressiveness, etc.)

       (9)   Provide objective feedback and positive reinforcement

c.   Increasing Self-Esteem

       (1)   Schedule regular sessions with client

       (2)   Accept negativism without judgement

       (3)   Minimize time focused on real or perceived failures

       (4)   Focus on identifying strengths and accomplishments

       (5)   Collaborate with client in identifying factors maintaining low self-esteem

          (a)   Interpersonal deficits

          (b)   Role transitions

          (c)   Role disputes

          (d)   Marital conflict

          (e)   Grief

       (6)   Collaborate with client in areas to change

       (7)   Collaborate on goals and problem-solving strategies

(8) Involve in activities that produce immediate success

(9) Provide realistic positive feedback

(10) See Cognitive and Behavioral Interventions

- Family Interventions

  1. Objectives

     a. Family participation in discharge planning

     b. Increased functional family interaction patterns

     c. Increase family effectiveness in coping with grief, loss, stress

  2. Assess family functioning

  3. Family education including:

     a. Client's diagnosis and treatment plan, including medications

     b. Relapse signs and symptoms and what to do should they reappear

     c. Community resources (medical, social, vocational, support groups)

     d. Positive support and knowledge to anticipate and avoid problems

     e. Resocialization issues

  4. Explore dysfunctional family interaction patterns that maintain depressive or manic symptoms

     a. Dependency/codependency

     b. Dysfunctional communication patterns

     c. Unrealistic expectations

     d. Reinforcement of secondary gains of depressive or manic behavior

     e. Dysfunctional role patterns/strain

     f. Stress and grief coping patterns

     g. Sources of conflict

        (1) Demandingness

        (2) Manipulation

(3) Testing

(4) Impulsivity

(5) Underfunctioning/overfunctioning

5. Refer to or conduct family therapy sessions

6. Family intervention when suicide is attempted or completed

   a. Explore family response to stress

   b. Explore family relationships re: isolation, scapegoating, estrangement

   c. Explore family communication patterns

   d. Promote grief rituals and customs

   e. Facilitate open expression of feelings (guilt, anger, sadness, helplessness, etc.)

   f. Refer to or conduct family therapy; refer to support groups

- Group Interventions

  1. Objectives

     a. Increase self-esteem through identification with group

     b. Increase awareness of personal strengths

     c. Increase social support

     d. Increase shared humanness

     e. Modify dysfunctional communication and interaction patterns

     f. Learn functional ways to cope with stress

     g. Decrease social withdrawal

  2. Gradually involve clients in:

     a. Psychotherapy groups

     b. Assertiveness training groups

     c. Social skills training groups

     d. Occupational therapy

     e. Art therapy

     f. Activity groups

3. Group interventions

   a. Devise a structured plan of therapeutic activities that considers client's level of depression or mania

   b. Encourage attendance at group sessions and activities

   c. Accept non-verbal participation

   d. Set limits on disruptive behavior

   e. Positively reinforce appropriate participation

   f. Encourage sharing of common feelings, thoughts, behaviors, life experiences among clients

   g. Promote problem-solving within group

   h. Promote modification of dysfunctional expectations of self and others

   i. Teach stress management strategies

   j. Instruct and model social skills

   k. Use role playing and rehearsal of social interactions

   l. Encourage initiation of socialization in an expanded social environment

- Milieu Interventions

  1. Objectives

     a. Maintain client safety

     b. Decrease manipulation

     c. Increase self-responsibility

  2. Interventions to maintain client safety

     a. Complete assessment of suicidal risk

     b. Determine level of precautions

        (1) Level of observation

        (2) Removal of dangerous objects

        (3) Limits in freedom and activity

     c. Initiate no harm contract with client

     d.   Establish rapport and communicate expectations related to safety issues

     e.   Use seclusion and restraints as last resort to maintain safety

3.   Interventions to decrease manipulation

     a.   Develop coordinated limit setting plan that presents a united front

     b.   Set consistent, realistic limits and consequences

     c.   Set expectations for personal responsibility

        (1)   Obeying rules

        (2)   Cleaning room

        (3)   Dressing modestly, etc.

     d.   Give positive feedback for appropriate behavior

     e.   Avoid defensive personal responses

     f.   Explore purpose and meaning of behavior with client

     g.   Engage client in learning how to make decisions and accept responsibility

4.   Structuring the environment

     a.   Establish a structured daily program of activities

     b.   Monitor environmental stimuli

     c.   Involve client in unit activities appropriate to level of functioning

     d.   Provide appropriate positive reinforcement

     e.   Avoid reinforcing negative or inappropriate behavior

     f.   Set agreed upon limits on manipulative, demanding and testing behaviors

     g.   Engage client in developing functional coping strategies

        (1)   Stress management

           (a)   Exercise

           (b)   Relaxation response

           (c)   Meditation

    (d) Nutritional diet

    (e) Adequate sleep

    (f) Differentiating normal mood response and stress from illness symptoms

- Community Resources
    1. Objectives
        a. Facilitate reintegration of client in community through coordination of services
        b. Increase use of support systems
        c. Expand social interactions
        d. Maximum independent functioning
    2. Interventions
        a. Collaborate discharge planning to include:
            (1) Appropriate living arrangements
                (a) Family
                (b) Solo
                (c) Halfway house
                (d) Group home
            (2) Employment/vocational planning
            (3) Referral to psychoeducation programs
                (a) Vocational rehabilitation
                (b) Social skills training
                (c) Mental health education programs
            (4) Referral to day treatment programs
            (5) Referral to support/self help groups
                (a) National Alliance for the Mentally Ill (NAMI)
                (b) Manic-Depressive and Depressive Association
                (c) Recovery, Inc.

b. Professional involvement in advocacy groups, community and professional organizations, self-help groups, political coalitions lobbying for mental health resources and rights

Questions
Select the best answer

1. Susan Z, age 20, was at a bar in the town where she went to college. Always an outgoing, life-of-the-party type, Susan became loud and abusive to people at the bar, jumped on the bar and began doing a strip dance, singing loudly, knocking over everything in sight. The police were called and at the station house, Susan loudly rambled on about how all the women in her family were life-of-the-party types. The community mental health nurse interviewing Susan understands that:

    a. Bipolar disorder does not have a higher rate in families with relatives who have the disorder.
    b. Bipolar disorder does have a higher rate in families with relatives who have the disorder.
    c. Bipolar disorder is inherited.
    d. Bipolar disorder is not recurring.

2. People at highest risk for suicide are:

    a. Married, white males below age 60
    b. Single, white males above age 60
    c. Black males
    d. Males below age 24 and above age 50

3. What percentage of the annual suicides are associated with depression?

    a. 20%
    b. 30%
    c. 50%
    d. 80%

4. Mr. B. has experienced depressed mood and difficulty sleeping over the past six weeks. He reports having no appetite and has lost 15 pounds during this time. Mr. B. describes a loss of interest in most of the activities he used to find pleasurable and a diminished ability to concentrate. Although this is the first time he has felt this way, Mr. B. states that he frequently thinks about taking his life. The Clinical Nurse Specialist would probably give him which of the following diagnoses?

    a. Bipolar disorder, depressed
    b. Major depression, recurrent
    c. Major depression
    d. Seasonal affective disorder

5. Mrs. C., age 42 calls the Mental Health Center with the following complaint. I've been taking venlafaxine 75 mg bid for depression and now I can't sleep, am running around getting all distracted, and talking a mile a minute. The clinical nurse specialist must rule out:

   a. The emergence of hypomania
   b. Non-compliance with venlafaxine dosing
   c. No relationship of symptoms with venlafaxine
   d. The need for electroconvulsive therapy

6. In addition to assessment for specific signs and symptoms of major depressive disorder, it is essential for the Clinical Nurse Specialist to assess the patient's _____ in order to make an accurate differential diagnosis.

   a. prior episodes of unipolar depression or bipolar disorder
   b. risk for suicide
   c. concurrent substance abuse
   d. non-psychiatric physical health problems

7. A priority feature of the assessment process with the depressed patient is:

   a. Assessment of family history
   b. Assessment of suicide risk
   c. Assessment of concurrent substance abuse
   d. Assessment of stressful life events

8. When assessing the depressed patient, a frequently used patient self report questionnaire is:

   a. The Beck Depression Inventory
   b. Hamilton Rating Scale for Depression
   c. Schedule for Affective Disorders and Schizophrenia
   d. Minnesota Multiphasic Personality Inventory

9. An experimental laboratory test to assess levels of norepinephrine in depressed patients prior to initiating pharmacotherapy is:

   a. CBC test
   b. Urinary MHPG test
   c. TRH stimulation test
   d. Dexamethasone suppression test

10. Which laboratory test is proposed to differentiate unipolar depression from bipolar disorder?

    a. Urinary MHPG test
    b. Dexamethasone suppression test
    c. TRH and CRH stimulation test
    d. SMAC test

11. At an appointment with the Clinical Nurse Specialist in private practice, Edward K. reports that for the past 3 or 4 years he becomes depressed in October after golf season is finished, begins to feel better in April, and feels totally normal and happy again by May. He says to the nurse, "Maybe I need other meaningful things in my life." The CNS would probably give him which of the following diagnoses?

    a. Major depression, recurrent
    b. Major depression
    c. Bereavement
    d. Seasonal Affective Disorder

12. Marcia S., age 53, describes herself as being depressed for as long as she can remember. She describes it as "living under a gray cloud." Three weeks ago, Marcia describes waking up feeling like the gray cloud turned black. She feels sad, hopeless, worthless, guilty about something she cannot identify, and pessimistic about things getting better for her. The nurse would probably give her which of the following diagnoses?

    a. Dysthymia
    b. Double depression
    c. Depression, recurrent type
    d. Depression, melancholic type

13. Karen K. called the office of the Clinical Specialist in private practice saying she had to have an appointment now or she was going to fall apart. During the assessment interview, Karen described herself as becoming increasingly depressed following the birth of her first child nine months ago in April. At first she felt blue, then increasingly despondent, sleeping a lot, hardly able to get out of a chair, crying all the time. She is now fearful that she might hurt the baby if she doesn't get some help. The CNS would probably give her which diagnosis?

a. Major depression
b. Major depression, melancholic type
c. Major depression, psychotic type
d. Major depression, postpartum type

14. Carl W., 60 years old, has been hospitalized on a medical unit for various aches and pains he has been experiencing for several weeks. He feels depressed, tense and unable to sleep at night. In talking to the nurse, he reveals that his wife died 8 months ago and he has not adjusted to the loss. To maximize the opportunity to determine the extent of Mr. W's bereavement versus depression, the nurse should:

    a. Ask the internist for a psychiatric consultation for Mr. W. as soon as possible
    b. Continue the discussion about his wife's death
    c. Explore his ambivalence toward his wife
    d. Inform the head nurse about Mr. W's feelings

15. D, age 33, is brought to the local hospital by her husband who tells the nurse that she has been involved in a whirl wind of activity that began several months ago when she quit her job to write the "Great American Novel." At the same time, she began painting her house. When he tried to get her to slow down, her activity just increased, taking little time to sleep or eat, and began spending huge amounts of money. Her husband brought her to the hospital following a call from the bank informing him that she had just tried to cash a check for $500,000. On admission, D. is agitated, speaking loudly and challenging the nurse.
    The nurse would probably give D. which of the following diagnoses?

    a. Bipolar Disorder: Depressed Phase
    b. Bipolar Disorder: Manic Phase
    c. Bipolar Disorder: Hypomanic Phase
    d. Bipolar Disorder: Recurrent Type

16. Two days ago, G. arrived on the psychiatric unit in a manic episode, exhibiting extreme excitement, disorientation, incoherent speech, agitation, frantic, aimless physical activity, and grandiose delusions. Which assessment finding is most characteristic of this stage of mania?

    a. Expansive mood
    b. Depressed mood
    c. Hypersomnia
    d. Low self-esteem

17. Jason King, age 55, is admitted to the psychiatric unit of the general hospital. His wife states that he has gradually become withdrawn over the last month, refusing to bathe or change clothes, eating little, failing to go to work and sleeping only 3 to 4 hours per night. This evening Mrs. King heard a shot from the basement and found Mr. King bleeding from a superficial chest wound.
To assess Mr. King's current potential for suicide, the nurse should:

    a. Ask Mr. King why he feels like killing himself
    b. Observe Mr. King for scars on his wrists or other signs of previous attempts
    c. Ask Mrs. King about any previous suicide attempts or threats by Mr. King.
    d. Determine if there is a family history of suicide

18. To further assess Mr. King's suicide potential, the CNS should be particularly alert to his expression of:

    a. Frustration and impatience
    b. Anger and resentment
    c. Anxiety and loneliness
    d. Helplessness and hopelessness

19. The neurotransmitter hypothesis proposes that depression occurs as a result of:

    a. Depletion of dopamine at the post-synaptic receptor site
    b. Imbalance of norepinephrine at the post-synaptic receptor site
    c. Disturbance in regulation of biological rhythms
    d. Shift in melatonin production and secretion

20. The kindling hypothesis proposes that in bipolar disorder, manic phase, patients have daily subthreshold electrical stimulation producing seizure like activity including all of the following, except:

    a. Tonic movements
    b. Auras
    c. Irritability
    d. Rapid mood swing

21. The circadian rhythm hypothesis proposes that people with unipolar depression may:

    a. Be in a chronic state of sleep satiety
    b. Have chronic hypo arousal
    c. Have REM phase delay

    d. Be in an acute state of hypersomnia

22. The circadian rhythm hypothesis proposes that people with unipolar depression may:

    a. Be in a chronic state of somnolence
    b. Have a disturbance in regulation of biological rhythms
    c. Have circadian rhythms that occur at a time late for sleep onset
    d. Be in a chronic state of under arousal

23. Based on an understanding of the psychoanalytic theory of depression, the nurse can best help a patient develop more healthy coping mechanisms by:

    a. Promoting interpersonal relationships with peers
    b. Allowing her to assume responsibility for her decisions
    c. Promoting the external expression of anger
    d. Setting realistic limits on her maladaptive behavior

24. When assessing a depressed person's premorbid personality characteristics, the nurse would expect that he/she demonstrated:

    a. Vulnerability to loss
    b. Overmeticulousness
    c. Stubbornness
    d. Vulnerability to anger

25. Blanche, 26 years old, is admitted to the psychiatric unit with a diagnosis of bi-polar disorder, manic episode. She is brought in by her husband, who states that she was fine until 3 days before admission. At that time she decided to plan a huge high school reunion and began calling all her classmates. Her speech became louder, more rapid, and insulting when the idea was not greeted with enthusiasm. Yesterday she went on a shopping spree and charged clothing worth $7000. This morning she went into her husband's office and began reor-ganizing his files. She became quite agitated, and her husband brought her to the emergency room.
In assessing Blanche, the nurse is aware that the manic episode is in reality an:

    a. Attempt to block unconscious feelings of depression
    b. Incorrect interpretation of environmental stimuli
    c. Exaggerated response to an elating situation
    d. Uncontrolled acting out of uncensored id drives

26. Laurie M., age 32, is married and is a very successful attorney. She and her

husband have a Victorian house they have restored. They ski, play tennis and have an active social life. Yet Laurie reports feeling depressed all the time. She perceives her self as "never measuring up." Despite having friends, she thinks they are only nice to her because they like her husband. She never enjoys the sports she does, because she never performs as well as she thinks she should. According to cognitive theory, Laurie's symptoms are most likely related to:

   a. Logical errors
   b. Negative feedback
   c. Developmental trauma
   d. Distorted self-concept

27. Laurie's cognitive, affective, and behavior patterns are maintained by irrational beliefs and rules called:

   a. Logical errors
   b. Silent assumptions
   c. Cognitive distortions
   d. Developmental trauma

28. Ted H., age 26, dropped out of college once, failed out twice, and currently works nights as a janitor in a factory. Both Ted and his family regard him as the family disappointment. Ted calls the mental health clinic because he feels depressed and very worried that he is going to lose his job. He states that his company is laying people off, and despite good evaluations, he knows that he will, as usual, be one of the unlucky who get fired.
According to the Hopelessness Theory of Depression, the Clinical Nurse Specialist understands that Ted's symptoms are most likely to occur when negative life events are perceived to be:

   a. Stable, global, important
   b. Unstable, global, important
   c. Stable, specific, important
   d. Unstable, global, important

29. Ted's ability to affect the outcome of potentially negative life events, like losing his job, is perceived by him to be:

   a. Nonexistent
   b. Low
   c. Moderate
   d. High

30. Fran S., age 57, is brought to the hospital Emergency Department by her daughter. She sits crying in a chair saying, "how much can a person take? I cannot take anymore." Her daughter reports that Mrs. S's husband was killed in a car accident 3 years ago and her 80-year-old mother was diagnosed with Alzheimers last year. Six months ago, her son revealed that he is homosexual and last week told the family that he has been HIV positive for 3 years and was just diagnosed as having Kaposi's sarcoma. Since that time, Fran has been mute other than when she is crying and muttering. She refuses to eat, bathe, or change her clothes. She has not slept more than 3 hours a night and says she just wants to crawl under a cover and not come out.
The Clinical Nurse Specialist understands that Fran's depression may be precipitated by:

   a. Cluster stress events
   b. Anniversary reaction
   c. Stress reaction
   d. Lack of social support

31. If Fran S. began to feel depressed around the time of year when her husband was killed, this would be called a(n):

   a. Nodal event
   b. Stress reaction
   c. Anniversary reaction
   d. Life cycle stressor

32. Bipolar patients frequently report family relationship patterns that consist of:

   a. Open communication patterns
   b. Realistic expectations
   c. Closed communication patterns
   d. Unrealistic expectations

33. When a manic patient exhibits extreme excitement, disorientation, frantic, aimless physical activity and grandiose delusions, which nursing diagnostic category would hold the highest priority?

   a. Ineffective individual coping
   b. Hopelessness
   c. Potential for self-harm
   d. Personal identity disturbance

34. Carl W., age 70, is hospitalized for depression. His wife died one year ago. He

has felt sad and tense ever since. He has lost 40 pounds this year, has difficulty getting up in the morning, has missed numerous days of work and says to the nurse, ''What's the use of talking? I'd rather be dead. I can't go on without my wife.''

The Clinical Nurse Specialist makes the nursing diagnosis of dysfunctional grieving associated with the loss of his wife. She makes this nursing diagnosis because of Mr. W's:

 a. Prolonged period of grief and mourning after his wife's death
 b. Difficulty expressing his loss
 c. Inability to talk about his loss
 d. Inability to sleep and symptoms of depression

35. Which of the following is not an initial objective of pharmacological intervention in unipolar depression or bipolar disorder:

 a. Symptom reduction
 b. Improved function
 c. Recurrence prevention
 d. Seizure prevention

36. The role of the nurse in pharmacological interventions that facilitates post discharge compliance with the medication regimen is:

 a. Collection of assessment data
 b. Coordination of treatment modalities
 c. Monitoring of side effects
 d. Patient education

37. M., a depressed patient, is started on imipramine (Tofranil) 75 mg orally at bedtime. The nurse should tell the patient that:

 a. The medication may be habit forming, so it will be discontinued as soon as she feels better.
 b. The medication has no serious side effects.
 c. She should avoid eating such foods as aged cheese, yogurt and red wine while taking the medication.
 d. The medication may initially cause some tiredness, which should become less bothersome over time.

38. M., a depressed patient, will be started on a tricyclic antidepressant. The Clinical Nurse Specialist understands that this type of medication:

 a. Decreases reuptake of neurotransmitters

  b. Increases reuptake of neurotransmitters
  c. Increases metabolism of neurotransmitters
  d. Regulates the frontal cortex where norepinephrine is made

39. D., a severely depressed patient, has not responded to tricyclic antidepressants. Prior to beginning ECT, a decision is made to initiate a trial of another antidepressant. The drug family of choice would be:

  a. Heterocyclics
  b. Monoamine oxidase inhibitors (MAOIs)
  c. Selective Serotonin Reuptake Inhibitors (SSRIs)
  d. Lithium

40. The physician orders tranylcypromine sulfate (Parnate) for D. The nurse would be aware that D. understood the teaching about the drug when the patient states, ''While taking the medicine, I should avoid eating'':

  a. Fish
  b. Red meat
  c. Citrus fruit
  d. Processed cheese

41. The nurse should teach a depressed patient on MAOIs that failure to adhere to dietary restrictions can result in:

  a. Hyperglycemic episodes
  b. Bradycardia
  c. Hypertensive crisis
  d. Snycope

42. A Clinical Nurse Specialist orders lithium carbonate 300 mg four times a day and chlorpromazine 100 mg four times a day for a manic patient who has just been admitted to the inpatient psychiatric unit exhibiting extreme excitement, disorientation, frantic, aimless activity, and grandiose delusions. Which statement best explains the reason for ordering chlorpromazine?

  a. A lower dose of lithium can be given
  b. Chlorpromazine helps control the manic symptoms until the lithium takes effect
  c. Joint administration makes both drugs more effective
  d. Joint administration decreases the risk of lithium toxicity

43. The physician plans to order lithium carbonate for a manic patient. Before beginning the lithium treatment regimen, the nurse performs a physical assessment. She is aware that lithium is contraindicated when a patient exhibits dysfunction of the:

    a. Renal system
    b. Reproductive system
    c. Endocrine system
    d. Respiratory system

44. Early signs of lithium toxicity include:

    a. Coarse tremors, ataxia, drowsiness, diarrhea
    b. Ataxia, confusion, and seizures
    c. Elevated white blood cell count and orthostatic hypotension
    d. Restlessness, shuffling gait, and involuntary muscle movements

45. One week after a manic patient begins taking lithium, this nurse notes that his serum lithium level is 1 mEq/liter. How should the nurse respond?

    a. Call the physician immediately to report the laboratory results
    b. Observe the patient closely for signs of lithium toxicity
    c. Withhold the next dose and repeat the blood work
    d. Continue administering the medication as ordered

46. An alternative first-line pharmacologic treatment modality for mood stabilization of bipolar disorder is:

    a. Clonazepam
    b. Risperidone
    c. Valproate
    d. Serentil

47. Two weeks after a manic patient begins taking carbamezapine (Tegretol), the nurse notes that her serum Tegretol level is 14 mg/l. How should the Clinical Nurse Specialist respond?

    a. Call the physician immediately to report the laboratory results
    b. Observe the patient closely for signs of toxicity
    c. Withhold the next dose and notify the physician
    d. Continue administering the medication as ordered

48. M., a patient with severe depression, does not respond to several trials of antidepressant medications. At a team conference, a decision is made to initiate a

series of electro convulsive therapy (ECT) treatments. When should nursing intervention begin?

   a. As soon as the patient and family are presented with this treatment alternative
   b. The night before ECT is scheduled
   c. Immediately after ECT is administered
   d. When the patient returns to the unit after ECT therapy

49. The interdisciplinary team is considering electro convulsive therapy (ECT) treatments for M., a patient with severe depression. The Clinical Nurse Specialist knows that which of the following are not appropriate indications for ECT as a treatment approach:

   a. Emergency therapy for suicidal patients
   b. Patients who are unresponsive to antidepressants
   c. Use during time lag between initiation of pharmacotherapy and onset of effectiveness
   d. Effectiveness in treatment of relatives

50. The most distressing side effect of ECT is:

   a. Memory loss
   b. Ataxia
   c. Hypotension
   d. Hyponatremia

51. The most serious side effect of ECT is:

   a. Memory loss
   b. Cardiac arrhythmias
   c. Hypotension
   d. Agitation

52. The most effective approach to meeting a manic patient's hydration and nutrition needs would be to:

   a. Leave finger foods and liquids in her room and let her eat and drink as she moves about
   b. Bring her to the dining room and encourage her to sit and eat with calm, quiet companions
   c. Explain mealtime routines and allow her to make her own decisions about eating
   d. Provide essential nutrition through high-calorie tube feedings

53. A depressed patient has difficulty sleeping at night. She reports feeling fatigued and unrefreshed. The nurse should NOT encourage the patient to:

 a. Limit intake of caffeinated drinks
 b. Take sedatives hs
 c. Take daytime naps
 d. Receive back rubs

54. The nursing staff request a consultation with the Clinical Nurse Specialist about a manic patient who demonstrates resistive behavior in relation to hygiene activities. He refuses to bathe, brush his teeth, or change his clothes. The CNS suggests which of the following interventions?

 a. Matter of factly assist with hygiene activities
 b. Ignore the behavior
 c. Confront the patient about his behavior
 d. Suggest that his medication be augmented with a neuroleptic

55. Andrew M., age 42, is brought to the psychiatric unit by his parents and a sister who states, "He's just not himself since his wife died two years ago. He has no interests and doesn't care for himself any more, just sitting alone when he's not working. The nurse discusses the plan of care with Andrew. The nurse recognizes that it would be most helpful to:

 a. Involve him in outdoor group games each day
 b. Encourage him to do relaxation exercises
 c. Encourage him to talk about and plan for the future
 d. Talk with him about his wife and the details of her death

56. Andrew attends group therapy in which the Clinical Nurse Specialist is the leader. During one session, another client talks about his wife leaving and his feeling of abandonment. When the members are leaving the session, the CNS notices that tears are running down Andrew's face.
Considering his problems, the CNS should:

 a. Ask the group members to return and discuss Andrew's feelings
 b. Observe Andrew's behavior carefully over the next few hours
 c. Go to Andrew's room and ask him to discuss his thoughts and feelings
 d. Ask another patient to stay and spend time talking with Andrew

57. In planning activities for Mr. R., a depressed patient, the nurse finds him very resistive and complaining about his inadequacies and worthlessness. The best approach by the nurse would be to:

> a. Involve Mr. R. in activities in which he will be assured of success
> b. Listen to Mr. R. and delay the planned activity for another time
> c. Schedule activities that Mr. R. can complete independently
> d. Encourage Mr. R. to select an activity in which he has some interest

58. Which of the following responses reflects a cognitive approach to dealing with low self-esteem?

     a. For each negative trait you list about yourself, I will ask you to give me a positive trait
     b. Can you recall six positive things about yourself?
     c. What do you think interferes with your ability to view yourself in a positive manner?
     d. What do you think would enable you to see yourself in a positive way?

59. D., age 33, was brought to the hospital by her husband following a call from the bank informing him that she had just tried to cash a check for $500,000 in an account that had a $5 balance. D.'s husband states that she has hardly slept or eaten in the past two weeks. On admission, D. is agitated, speaking loudly and challenging the nurse. Which approach would be most therapeutic in working with D.?

     a. Teaching the patient about banking procedures
     b. Confronting the patient about her unappropriate behavior
     c. Kindly but firmly guiding the patient into such activities as bathing and eating
     d. Showing the patient that she is in a controlled environment

60. When developing a standardized care plan for manic clients which of the following are *NOT* important to consider when designing behavioral interventions:

     a. Attention span
     b. Distractability
     c. Unit resources
     d. Medication supply

61. Ms. W. is admitted to the psychiatric unit with a diagnosis of severe depression. One morning, Ms. W. said to the nurse, "God is punishing me for my past sins." The nurse's best response is:

     a. "God is punishing you for your sins, Ms. W.?"

b. ''Why do you think that, Ms. W.?''
c. ''You really seem upset about this''
d. ''What sins would he be punishing you for?''

62. Ms. W. tells the nurse that she has an unhappy marriage and has had several affairs. Although she feels that her husband ignores her, she blames herself for having had these affairs. The most appropriate response to assist Ms. W. in exploring her thoughts and feelings is:

   a. ''Help me to understand how these affairs are all your fault?''
   b. ''Tell me why the affairs are your fault.''
   c. ''It sounds like your husband ignores you. Who could blame you for having an affair?''
   d. ''Tell me about your husband.''

63. James R., a manic patient, is approaching discharge. He is to be discharged on lithium carbonate. In the family teaching plan for discharge, the nurse should stress the importance of:

   a. Watching his diet to avoid aged cheese, yogurt, and caffeinated beverages
   b. Taking the pills with milk
   c. Having a CBC done once a month
   d. Having his blood levels checked as ordered

64. The Clinical Nurse Specialist is meeting with a group of recurrent bipolar patients and their families. A key preventive intervention designed to maintain family function is:

   a. Recognition of relapse signs and symptoms
   b. Referral for family therapy
   c. Referral to NAMI
   d. Recognition of early signs of lithium toxicity

65. Mrs. K. is admitted to the psychiatric unit following a suicide attempt. Mrs. K. does not answer any of the nurses' questions. To assess Mrs. K's current potential for suicide, the nurse should:

   a. Ask Mrs. K. why she feels like killing herself
   b. Observe Mrs. K. for scars on her wrists or other signs of previous attempts
   c. Ask Mr. K. about any previous suicide attempts or threats by Mrs. K.
   d. Determine if there is a family history of suicide

66. In teaching an orientation group about nursing care of the suicidal patient, the Clinical Nurse Specialist teaches that the suicidal risk for a depressed patient is often greatest:

    a. When the depression is most severe
    b. Before any kind of somatic treatment is started
    c. When the patient begins to express anger
    d. When the patient makes a sudden and dramatic improvement

67. A manic patient is assigned to a private room that is somewhat removed from the nurse's station. The primary reason for this room assignment is:

    a. Decreased environmental stimuli
    b. Prevent the patient's excessive activity from disturbing others
    c. Deter the patient from disturbing the nurses
    d. Provide the patient with a quiet environment for thinking about his problems

68. On the unit, a manic patient is elated and sarcastic. She is constantly cursing and using foul language. She has the other clients on the units terrified. The Clinical Nurse Specialist, who has been asked to consult in the management of this patient, advises the staff to:

    a. Demand that she stop what she is doing
    b. Firmly tell her that her behavior is unacceptable
    c. Ask her what is bothering her
    d. Increase her medication or have additional medication ordered

69. Mr. M., a 50 year old man who has been treated for double-depression during the past two years, states to the Clinical Nurse Specialist 'They've tried every medicine, nothing works, even the ones you can't eat cheese with. In reviewing his history, the CNS notes the distinct absence of which of the essential laboratory tests that may explain his lack of response to pharmacological agents:

    a. Blood gases
    b. Cardiac enzymes
    c. Free thyroxine
    d. White blood cell count

Answers

1. b	24. a	47. c
2. b	25. a	48. a
3. c	26. a	49. d
4. c	27. b	50. a
5. a	28. a	51. b
6. b	29. a	52. a
7. b	30. a	53. c
8. a	31. c	54. a
9. b	32. d	55. d
10. c	33. c	56. c
11. d	34. d	57. a
12. a	35. d	58. a
13. d	36. d	59. c
14. b	37. d	60. d
15. b	38. a	61. c
16. a	39. b	62. a
17. c	40. d	63. d
18. d	41. c	64. a
19. b	42. b	65. c
20. a	43. a	66. d
21. a	44. a	67. a
22. b	45. d	68. b
23. c	46. c	69. c

Bibliography

Agency for Healthcare Policy and Research (1993). *Depression in primary care,* Rockville, MD: U.S. Department of Health and Human Services. AHCPR Publication No. 93-0551.

American Psychiatric Association. (1994). *Diagnostic and statistical manual of mental disorders* (4th ed.). Washington, DC: Author.

Antai-Otong, D. (1995). *Psychiatric nursing: Biological and behavioral concepts.* Philadelphia: W. B. Saunders Company.

Arana, G. W., & Hyman, S. E. (1991). *Handbook of psychiatric drug therapy* (2nd ed.). Toronto, Canada: Little, Brown and Company.

Bertrus, P. A., & Elmore, S. K. (1991). Seasonal affective disorder, part I: A review of the neural mechanisms for psychosocial nurses. *Archives of Psychiatric Nursing.* 5(6), 357–364.

Bezchlibnyk-Butler, K. Z., & Jeffries, J. J. (1996). *Clinical handbook of psychotropic drugs* (5th ed.). Lewiston, NY: Hogrefe & Huber Publishers.

Gold, P. W., Goodwin, F. K., & Chrousos, G. P. (1988). Clinical and biochemical manifestations of depression—part one. *New England Journal of Medicine.* 319, 348–353.

Goodwin, F. K., & Jamison, K. R. (1990). *Manic-depressive illness.* New York: Oxford University Press.

Haber, J., Krainovich-Miller, B., Leach-McMahon, A. & Price-Hoskins, P. (1997). *Comprehensive psychiatric nursing* (5th ed.). St Louis: C.V. Mosby Co.

Moller, M.D., & Murphy, M. F. (1998). Recovering from psychosis: A wellness approach. Nine Mile Falls, WA: Psychiatric Rehabilitation Nurses, Inc.

Simmons-Alling, S. (1987). New approaches to managing affective disorders. *Archives of Psychiatric Nursing.* 1(4), 219–224.

Smith, P. F., & Darlington, C. L. (1996). *Clinical pharmacology: A primer.* NJ: Lawrence Erlbaum Associates.

Stuart, G. W., & Sundeen, S.J. (1995). *Principles and practice of psychiatric nursing* (5th ed.). St. Louis: C. V. Mosby Co.

Ugarriza, D. N. (1992). Postpartum affective disorders. *Journal of Psychosocial Nursing.* 30(5), 29–31.

The author and editor would like to express appreciation to Dr. Judith Haber for authoring this chapter in the first edition of this review book. Her original contribution served as a very strong foundation for rewriting this Chaper for the second edition.

Behavioral Syndromes and Disorders of Adult Personality

Richardean Benjamin-Coleman

Eating Disorders

Fear of obesity and the pursuit of thinness represent the driving force in both Anorexia and Bulimia Nervosa, two of the most common eating disorders (Stuart & Sundeen, 1995).

Anorexia Nervosa

- Definition/Symptoms
  1. Refusal to eat
  2. Intense fear of gaining weight or becoming fat
  3. Weight less than 85% of expected weight
  4. Distorted body image
  5. At least 3 consecutive missed menstrual periods
  6. Excessive exercising
  7. Preoccupation with food
  8. Bodily changes
     a. Emaciated appearance
     b. Lanugo growth on face, extremities and trunk
     c. Bradycardia, hypotension, arrhythmias
     d. Delayed gastric motility
     e. Dry skin, dry and falling hair
  9. Laboratory changes
     a. Leukopenia
     b. Mild anemia
     c. Low serum potassium
     d. Elevated blood urea nitrogen
     e. High serum calcium levels that may indicate that osteoporosis is occurring, and renal calculi may result
- Mental status variations
  1. Mood and affect
     a. Dysphoric mood with crying spells

     b.   Emotionally labile

     c.   Anxiety

     d.   Low self-esteem

2.   Sleep disturbance (insomnia or hypersomnia)

3.   Thought processes

     a.   Distorted body image

     b.   Delusional thinking about body size

     c.   Concrete thinking

     d.   Overpowering fear of losing control

     e.   Hypochondriasis

     f.   Obsession with food and cooking

     g.   Decreased concentration

4.   Appearance—emaciated

5.   Defense mechanisms

     a.   Repression

     b.   Regression

     c.   Denial

     d.   Manipulation—untruthful about food intake and methods of losing weight

6.   Impaired judgment related to food

7.   Impaired insight

     a.   Intellectualization

     b.   Perfectionistic

8.   Behavior

     a.   Ritualistic

     b.   Compulsive

• Psychotherapeutic interventions

1.   Individual psychotherapy

     a.   Establish realistic thinking process

       b.   Increase self-esteem

       c.   Establish a healthy sense of control and autonomy

       d.   Deal with underlying psychologic conflicts

  2. Cognitive/behavior therapy

       a.   Establish contract

       b.   Describe expected behaviors

       c.   Eliminate power struggle

       d.   Initiate consistency from staff to coordinate treatment

  3. Teach relaxation.

- Family dynamics

  1. Overly strict and disagreement concerning discipline

  2. Power and control issues

  3. High value placed on perfectionism

  4. Parental criticism promotes perfectionistic and obsessive behavior in child

  5. Feelings of helplessness and ambivalence

  6. Perceived loss of control in life

  7. Family unable to resolve problems which arise with the family

  8. Need ''sick'' member to enable the other family members to communicate with each other

  9. Less understanding and nurturant and more belittling, blaming, rejecting and neglectful

- Milieu approaches

  1. Provide for safety and physical needs

  2. Sit with and observe during and 60 minutes after meals

  3. Counteract effects of starvation by promoting weight gain and restoring normal nutritional balance

  4. Include dietitian in treatment plan

  5. Encourage client to share feelings with staff

  6. Maintain consistency among staff members

7. Document intake and output

8. Avoid discussing food or eating with client once protocol established

9. Use behavioral reinforcement

10. Provide group interaction with peers

11. Address adolescent development issues

- Treatment objectives

  1. Increase weight to normal range

  2. Help client re-establish normal eating behavior, avoid excessive exercise, self-induced vomiting or laxative abuse

  3. Explain physical symptoms in a way which is understood by the client

  4. In hospital, give client opportunity to be responsible for own weight gain and reward for conforming to treatment regimen

Bulimia Nervosa

- Symptoms

  1. Recurrent episodes of binge eating

  2. Self-induced vomiting or abuses laxatives/diuretics

  3. Dieting/fasting or excessive exercise to control weight

  4. Weight usually within normal range

  5. Dehydration, electrolyte imbalance

  6. Gastric acid in vomitus contributes to erosion of tooth enamel

  7. Psychoactive substance abuse/dependence

  8. Perceived inability to control binging

  9. Average of at least 2 binges a week for at least 3 months

  10. Depressed mood and self-deprecatory thoughts following binges

  11. Exaggerated concern about body shape and weight

  12. Enlargement of face and cheeks due to swelling of salivary glands

  13. Changes in EKG—cardiac arrhythmias leading to renal problems

- Mental status variations

  1. Judgment and insight

     a. Recognizes eating behavior is abnormal

     b. Problems with impulse control (stealing, drug and/or alcohol abuse, self-mutilation, suicide attempt)

     c. Manipulative and untruthful

     d. Difficulty identifying and dealing with emotions

  2. Thought processes

     a. Overly concerned with body shape and weight

     b. Obsessional ideas

  3. Mood—depressed (feels sad and lonely, empty and isolated with self-criticism and guilt feelings)

  4. Orientation—lethargy and confusion due to extreme dehydration caused by self-induced vomiting and excessive use of laxatives

- Psychotherapeutic interventions

  1. Cognitive Behavior therapy—see anorexia

  2. Family therapy—see Family dynamics, anorexia

  3. Relaxation

  4. Supportive psychotherapy

  5. Behavior therapy

     a. Positive reinforcement

     b. Informational feedback

     c. Progressive desensitization focusing on feelings prior to an episode of binge eating

- Family dynamics

  1. Family environment chaotic, conflictual with marital discord and hostility

  2. Sexual abuse

- Milieu interventions

  1. Behavioral diaries

2. Express feelings—gain insight into eating behavior

3. Reinforce healthy coping

4. Teach to recognize cues for hunger and satiation

5. Limit exercising in treatment

6. Avoid keeping food records, weighing frequently, constantly counting calories, cooking for others and reading recipes

- Differential Diagnoses for Anorexia and Bulimia

    1. Depressive disorders

        a. Absence of distorted body image

        b. Absence of intense fear of obesity

        c. True loss of appetite

    2. Obsessive-compulsive disorder

    3. Schizophrenic disorders

        a. Bizarre eating patterns present without eating disorder syndrome or concern with the caloric content of food

        b. Refusal to eat

    4. Somatization disorder

        a. Absence of fear of becoming overweight

        b. Amenorrhea for 3 months or more is unusual

    5. Medical illnesses

        a. Hyperthyroidism

        b. Neoplasms

        c. Anemia

        d. Diabetes mellitus

        e. Crohn's disease

        f. Neurological diseases

    6. Borderline personality disorder

- Nursing Diagnoses for Anorexia and Bulimia (Townsend, 1997)

    1. Body image disturbance

2. Fluid volume deficit—high risk

3. Anxiety (moderate to severe)

4. Altered nutrition—less than body requirements

   a. Nursing interventions

      (1) Implement behavioral modification protocol for gradual weight gain

      (2) Supervise meals to ensure adequate intake of nutrients

      (3) In collaboration with dietitian, determine number of calories required to provide adequate nutrition and weight gain

      (4) Sit with client during mealtime for support and to observe amount ingested

      (5) Strictly document intake and output

      (6) Weigh client daily upon arising

      (7) Once nutritional status is stable explore with client feelings associated with fears

      (8) Observe weighing activity to assure that client is not secreting weights to falsify data

   b. Outcome criteria

      (1) Client has achieved and maintained at least 85 percent of expected body weight.

      (2) Vital signs, blood pressure, and laboratory serum studies are within normal limits.

      (3) Client verbalizes importance of adequate nutrition.

- Genetic/Biological Theories for Anorexia and Bulimia

   1. Decreased hypothalamic norepinephrine activation

   2. Dysfunction of lateral hypothalamus

   3. Abnormal dexamethasone suppression test findings

   4. Bulimics may have a low serum serotonin level

   5. Hereditary predisposition

    6. Excess endorphins shutting down the feeding system and inhibiting release initiating amenorrhea

    7. Chronic deficit of endorphins initiating feeding to stimulate this down regulated system

- Biochemical Approaches for Anorexia and Bulimia

    1. No specific medications for anorexia

    2. Medications may be given for associated symptoms such as depression or anxiety

    3. Bulimia with Depression—Parnate 30 to 40mg/day

- Intrapersonal Theories for Anorexia and Bulimia

    1. Unresolved conflicts during childhood

    2. Inconsistent parental response to child's needs

    3. Disturbance of self-esteem

    4. Food serves as a means to express feelings

    5. Anorexia—separation, individuation, and control issues

    6. Independence/dependence struggle between woman and parent(s)

    7. Avoidance of sexuality

- Group Approaches for Anorexia and Bulimia

    1. Types

        a. Supportive

        b. Self-help

        c. Small group therapy

        d. Support group for parents

        e. Outpatient

    2. Group functions

        a. Foster self-esteem

        b. Gain insight

        c. Share concerns

        d. Provide constructive support from peers

- Family therapy for Anorexia and Bulimia
    1. Education of members about the disorder
    2. Support family as they deal with guilt and stigma of having member with disorder
    3. Focus on fostering open, healthy interaction patterns
- Community resources for Anorexia and Bulimia
    1. Eating disorder groups
    2. Family support groups
    3. Twelve-step programs

Sexual and Gender Identity Disorders

Paraphilias

Repetitive or preferred sexual fantasies or behaviors that involve giving or receiving pain, or activity with a nonconsenting partner, to experience full sexual arousal and satisfaction (Wilson & Kneisl, 1996)

- Definitions
    1. Fetishism—uses clothing as source of sexual arousal
    2. Exhibitionism—exposes genitals in public
    3. Frotteurism—body contact with strangers in public places
    4. Pedophilia—sexual contact with prepubescent child
    5. Sexual masochism—receives physical/mental pain from sexual partner
    6. Sexual sadism—inflicts physical/mental pain on sexual partner
    7. Transvestic fetishism—recurrent cross-dressing by heterosexual male
    8. Voyeurism—watching others undressing/engaged in sexual activity
- Differential diagnoses
    1. Nonpathogenic sexual experimentation
    2. Rule out public urination
    3. Rule out exposure as prelude to sexual activity with child

   4. Rule out poor judgment due to:

      a. Mental retardation

      b. Organic personality syndrome

      c. Alcohol intoxication

      d. Schizophrenia

- Mental status variations

   1. Inadequate social skills

   2. Depressed mood and anxiety accompany the behaviors

   3. Poor judgement and impulse control

- Genetic/biological theories

   1. Limbic system or temporal lobe abnormalities

   2. Abnormal levels of androgens

- Biochemical approaches

   1. Antiandrogenics—Medroxyprogesterone—5mg to 10mg/day induces a reversible chemical castration

- Intrapersonal theories

   1. Unresolved Oedipal Complex leading to identification with opposite gender parent or object for libido cathexis

   2. Castration anxiety

- Psychotherapeutic interventions

   1. Psychodynamic psychotherapy

      a. Explore thoughts, feelings, and behavior that precede paraphiliac behavior in order to control occurrences

      b. Eliminate anxiety or depression that accompanies behavior

   2. Behavior therapy

      a. Systematic desensitization

      b. Aversive techniques

      c. Assertiveness training

   3. Combination of psychodynamic and behavioral techniques

- Milieu approaches—nurse's role is primarily associated with prevention of problems, which focuses on the development of adaptive coping strategies to deal with stressful life events.

Gender Identity Disorder

- Definition: Persistent discomfort with one's assigned gender and a feeling that it is inappropriate or inaccurate (Sugar, 1995)

- Signs and Symptoms—DSM-IV Criteria (APA, 1994)

    1. A strong and persistent cross-gender identification (not merely a desire for any perceived cultural advantages of being the other sex)

        a. In children, manifested by at least four of the following:

            (1) Repeatedly stated desire to be, or insistence that he or she is, the other sex

            (2) In boys, preference for cross-dressing or simulating female attire; in girls, insistence on wearing only stereotypical masculine clothing

            (3) Strong and persistent preferences for cross-sex roles in make-believe play or persistent fantasies of being the other sex

            (4) Intense desire to participate in the stereotypical games and pastimes of the other sex

            (5) Strong preference for playmates of the other sex

        b. In adolescents and adults, manifested by symptoms such as

            (1) Stated desire to be the other sex

            (2) Frequent passing as the other sex

            (3) Desire to live or be treated as the other sex

            (4) The conviction that one has the typical feelings and reactions of the other sex

    2. Persistent discomfort with one's sex or sense of inappropriateness in the gender role of that sex.

        a. In children, manifested by any of the following:

            (1) In boys, assertion that his penis or testes are disgusting

or will disappear or assertion that it would be better not to have a penis

 (2) Aversion toward rough-and-tumble play and rejection of male stereotypical toys, games, and activities

 (3) In girls, rejection of urinating in a sitting position or assertion that she does not want to grow breasts or menstruate, or marked aversion toward normative feminine clothing.

 b. In adolescents and adults, manifested by symptoms such as preoccupation with getting rid of one's primary and secondary sex characteristics (e.g., request for hormones, surgery, or other procedures to alter physical sexual characteristics to simulate the other sex) or belief that one was born the wrong sex.

 3. Not concurrent with a physical intersex condition (e.g., androgen insensitivity syndrome or congenital hyperplasia)

 4. Clinically significant distress or impairment in social, occupational, or other important areas of functioning.

- Differential diagnoses

 1. Schizophrenia—rarely develop delusion that focuses on sex change; may have hallucinations or ideas of reference.

 2. Late adolescents who are uncomfortable with own bodies but feel guilty because of attraction to members of own sex. May feel homosexuality is worse than transsexualism and want sex reassignment to lead normal heterosexual lives.

 3. Nonconformity to stereotypical sex role behavior—cross gender wishes due to nonconforming

 4. Transvestic fetishism—cross dressing behavior is for sexual excitement

- Mental status variations

 1. Dysphoric mood

 2. Anxiety

- Genetic/biological theories

 1. Prenatal estrogen and androgen levels favor development of the disorder

2. Chromosomal abnormalities

- Intrapersonal theories

    1. In boys

        a. Physical or psychological loss of the mother that results in separation anxiety in the child

        b. Severe disruption or distortion in mother-son relationship that results in the mother's withdrawal which leads to separation anxiety and feminine behavior

        c. Feminine behavior and/or identification caused by excessive closeness to mother

    2. In girls

        a. Mother lacks self-esteem as a woman and derogates femininity as inferior. Mother rejects girl who turns to father who nurtures and protects from the aggressive mother.

    3. In both boys and girls—separation threats and behavior as defense against separation

- Psychotherapeutic interventions

    1. Psychotherapy

        a. Assist to individuate from mother

        b. Aid in developing diverse perceptions of women and femaleness

        c. Work through loss of the attachment figure

    2. Behavioral therapy

        a. Systematically arrange that rewards follow sex-appropriate behaviors

        b. Target behaviors, such as selection of toys and dress-up play, exclusive affiliation with opposite sex, and mannerism

        c. Enhance behavior deficiencies such as poor athletic ability

        d. Focus on overt sex-type behaviors rather than gender identity or gender dysphoria

        e. Provide social attention or social reinforcement

      f.   Encourage self-monitoring procedures.

- Family dynamics

  1. Strong interest in opposite-gender role behavior and weak reinforcement of normative gender-role behavior by parents

  2. Extreme physical and psychological closeness with son by the mother

  3. Parental encouragement of cross-gender behavior—mothers of feminine boys themselves had gender identity conflicts as children which led them to devalue men and masculinity.

  4. Father is physically absent or psychologically peripheral—no counterforce to pathogenic mother-son relationship

Sexual Dysfunctions

- Definitions (APA, 1994)

  1. Male Erectile Disorder—persistent or recurrent inability to maintain an erection until completion of sexual activity

  2. Female Sexual Arousal Disorder—persistent or recurrent inability to attain or maintain an adequate lubrication-swelling response of sexual excitement until completion of the sexual activity

  3. Dyspareunia—pain before, during, and after sexual intercourse

  4. Vaginismus—recurrent or persistent involuntary spasm of the musculature of the outer third of the vagina that interferes with sexual intercourse

  5. Orgasmic Disorder—persistent or recurrent delay in, or absence of, orgasm following a normal sexual excitement phase

  6. Premature Ejaculation—persistent or recurrent ejaculation with minimal sexual stimulation before, upon, or shortly after penetration and before the person wishes it

  7. Hypoactive Sexual Desire Disorder—persistently or recurrently deficient (or absent) sexual fantasies and desire for sexual activity

  8. Sexual Aversion Disorder—persistent or recurrent extreme aversion to and avoidance of all (or almost all), genital sexual contact with a sexual partner

- Differential diagnoses

1. Central nervous system tumors

2. Mood disorder

3. Rape trauma syndrome

4. Neuroendocrine disorders

5. Penile, prostate, or testicular cancer

6. End-stage renal disease

- Mental status variations—affect may be sad, depressed, or anxious
- Genetic/biological theories

   1. Decreased levels of serum testosterone

   2. Elevated levels of prolactin

   3. Physical changes due to:

      a. Surgery, aging, or trauma

      b. Drug abuse or medication side effects

      c. Neurological disorders

      d. Infection and poor hygiene

- Intrapersonal theories

   1. Religious orthodoxy

   2. Gender identity or sexual preference

   3. Sexual phobias

   4. Depression

   5. Fear of becoming pregnant

   6. Traumatic sexual experiences in childhood

   7. Negative conditioning that sex is dirty

- Psychotherapeutic interventions

   1. Cognitive therapy—change maladaptive beliefs

   2. Psychodynamic therapy—resolve intrapsychic conflicts

   3. Behavioral therapy

      a. Systematic desensitization

      b. Sensate focus exercises

     c.   Masturbatory training

     d.   "Squeeze" technique for premature ejaculation

  4. Marital/sex therapy to treat dysfunctions of sexual response cycle

  5. Hypnotherapy

- Milieu approaches

  1. Use nondirective approach in completing assessment

  2. Use language that is understandable to the client

  3. Convey attitude of warmth, openness, honesty and objectivity

  4. Remain nonjudgmental

- Nursing Diagnoses for Sexual and Gender Identity Disorders (Wilson & Kneisl, 1996)

  1. Altered sexuality patterns

  2. Personal identity disturbance

  3. Sexual dysfunction

     a.   Nursing interventions

        (1) Encourage partners to express feelings

        (2) Help client and partner to learn means of clear and open communication (primary intervention)

        (3) Explore with couple information about sex positions or habits

        (4) Assist to identify relationship problems

        (5) Contract to work on problems

        (6) Provide information about sexual techniques

        (7) Refer for sex therapy with trained counselor

     b.   Outcome criteria

        (1) Client identifies conflicts that contribute to loss of sexual desire

        (2) Client resumes sexual activity at level satisfactory to self and partner

- Family Therapy—Couples/Marital Therapy for Sexual and Identity Disorders
    1. Homework assignments or exercises
    2. Observing and responding to homework
- Group Approaches for Sexual and Identity Disorders
    1. Discussion of problems and concerns
    2. Homework for individual and couple exploration
    3. Group support and reassurance
- Community Resources for Sexual and Identity Disorders
    1. Sex Addicts Anonymous
    2. American Association of Sex Educators, Counselors, and Therapists (AASECT)

Personality Disorders

An enduring pattern of perceiving, relating to, and thinking about the environment and oneself to the extent that it leads to inflexible and maladaptive and either significant functional impairment or subjective distress (APA, 1994)

Antisocial Personality Disorder

- Symptoms
    1. More common in men
    2. History of irresponsibility and impulsiveness
    3. Lacks remorse for actions
    4. Exploits and manipulates others
    5. Self-centered
    6. Anger that leads to hostile outbursts
- Differential diagnoses
    1. Conduct disorder—if person younger than 18 years with characteristic features present

2. Psychoactive substance abuse—episodic behavior associated with alcohol/drug intake

3. Mental retardation—may exhibit remorse due to actions or behavior

4. Schizophrenia—presence of prolonged psychotic episodes

5. Manic episode—mood changes

6. Cyclothymic disorder—periods with hypomanic symptoms and depressive symptoms

7. Borderline—fear of abandonment, substance abuse

- Mental status variations
    1. Absence of anxiety or depression
    2. Suicide threats and somatic preoccupation
    3. Absence of delusions or other signs of irrational thinking
    4. Highly manipulative and untrustworthy
    5. Lacks remorse
    6. . Compulsive recklessness
    7. Impulsivity
- Genetic/biological theories
    1. Hereditary predisposition
    2. Low cortical arousal and reduced level of inhibitory anxiety may play a role
    3. Biochemical approaches (Kaplan & Sadock, 1995)
        a. Lithium carbonate—900mg to 1200mg/day
        b. Inderal—160mg to 240mg/day
        c. Side effects—medications are seldom prescribed outside a structured setting because of high risk of abuse by clients with antisocial personality disorder
- Intrapersonal theories—arrest in normal psychological development with failure to integrate ambivalent feelings originally aroused against the primary caretaker
- Psychotherapeutic interventions
    1. Confrontation of inappropriate behavior

2. Individual psychotherapy

3. Structured living with supervision

4. Outpatient supportive therapy

- Family dynamics

    1. Chaotic home environment

    2. Parental deprivation during the first 5 years of life

    3. Presence of intermittent appearance of inconsistent, impulsive parents

    4. Traumatic abandonment experiences

    5. Physical and sexual abuse

- Group therapy

    1. Help client assume responsibility for behaviors

    2. Confront inappropriate and manipulative behaviors

    3. Allow client to receive parenting not previously received

    4. Allow client to tolerate feelings of emptiness, depression, and anxiety

    5. Develop socially appropriate behavioral responses

- Community resources

    1. Alcoholics Anonymous

    2. Emotions Anonymous

    3. Narcotics Anonymous

Borderline Personality Disorder

- Symptoms

    1. Two-thirds of those diagnosed are female

    2. Self-mutilation, labile mood

    3. Impulsivity

    4. Outbursts of intense anger and rage

    5. Unstable relationships

    6.   Identity confusion

    7.   Frantic efforts to avoid real or imagined abandonment

- Differential diagnoses

    1.   Cyclothymia—presence of hypomania

    2.   Schizophrenia—presence of prolonged psychotic episodes, thought disorder or other signs

    3.   Paranoid personalities—extreme suspiciousness

    4.   Schizotypes—show marked peculiarities of thinking, strange ideation, and recurrent ideas of reference

- Mental status variations

    1.   Affect—mood swings, anxious, depressed

    2.   Thought processes

        a.   Difficulty concentrating

        b.   Suicidal gestures and attempts

    3.   Insight lacking—poor judgment

    4.   Defense mechanisms

        a.   Manipulation

        b.   Splitting

        c.   Projection

        d.   Denial

        e.   Rationalization

        f.   Idealization

        g.   Devaluation

    5.   Memory—recent memory disturbance

- Intrapersonal theories

    1.   Inconsistent and unpredictable parenting

    2.   Unmet need for love

    3.   Separation/individuation phase not accomplished

- Psychotherapeutic interventions

1. Reality oriented therapy favored over in-depth unconscious interpretations

2. Long-term psychotherapy with supportive modifications to develop trust

3. Behavioral therapy—structured living under supervision

- Biochemical approaches

    1. Anticonvulsants—Carbamazepine—200mg bid with food

    2. Antidepressants—Parnate—10-20mg/day maintenance dose

    3. Anti-anxiety—Prozac—20mg/day not to exceed 80mg/day

    4. Antipsychotic

        a. Chlorpromazine 150-500mg/day

        b. Haloperidol 7-12mg/day

- Family dynamics

    1. Parent may be critical and rejecting, or

    2. Parent may be suffocating and smothering and interferes with optimal progression of attachment-separation sequences

- Community resources

    1. Day hospital programs

    2. Halfway houses

- Milieu Approaches for Borderline and Antisocial Personality Disorders

    1. Staff develops self-awareness to avoid negative counter-transference

    2. Establish trusting relationship with client

    3. Institute safety precautions

    4. Provide structured supportive and consistent environment

    5. Apply behavioral limits judiciously

    6. Assist client in taking responsibility for consequences of actions

    7. Assist the client in identifying feelings and in learning how to express them in a socially acceptable manner

    8. Enhance the client's self-esteem and sense of self-worth

- Nursing Diagnoses for Borderline and Antisocial Personality Disorders (Townsend, 1997)

  1. Impaired social interaction

  2. High risk for violence—directed at others

  3. High risk for self-directed violence

     a. Nursing interventions

        (1) Observe client for unsafe behavior

        (2) Determine suicidal potential

        (3) Obtain contract not to harm self or others

        (4) Assist client to recognize and accept consequence of own behavior

        (5) Act as role model for appropriate expression of feelings

        (6) Remove all dangerous objects from client's environment

        (7) Provide physical outlets to redirect anger

        (8) Provide restrictive measures (e.g., medication, restraints to ensure client safety)

     b. Outcome criteria

        (1) Anxiety level maintained to avoid aggressive acts

        (2) Client recognizes, verbalizes and accepts consequences of own behavior

The following personality disorders will be individually defined and then discussed as a group (Kaplan & Sadock, 1995).

- Definitions

  1. Paranoid Personality Disorder—characterized by long-standing suspiciousness and mistrust of people in general

     a. Differential diagnoses

        (1) Paranoid schizophrenia—characterized by persistent psychotic symptoms (hallucinations and bizarre delusions)

        (2) Delusional disorder, paranoid type—characterized by prominent and persistent delusions of persecution

(3) Schizotypal personality disorder—cognitive and perceptual distortions

2. Schizoid Personality Disorder—diagnosed in patients who display a lifelong pattern of social withdrawal; often described as eccentric

   a. Differential diagnoses

      (1) Schizotypal personality disorder—cognitive and perceptual distortions

      (2) Paranoid personality disorder—characterized by suspiciousness and paranoid ideation

      (3) Avoidant personality disorder—involves social isolation but strongly desire relationships with others

      (4) Obsessive-compulsive personality disorder—characterized by social detachment due to excessive devotion to work and difficulty expressing emotions rather than lack of desire or capacity for intimacy

3. Schizotypal Personality Disorder—individuals are strikingly odd or strange, even to laypersons; magical thinking, peculiar ideas, ideas of reference illusions, and derealization are part of their everyday world

   a. Differential diagnoses

      (1) Schizophrenia—has enduring psychosis

      (2) Paranoid and schizoid personality disorders—characterized by cognitive and perceptual distortion, marked eccentricity or oddness and profound social discomfort

      (3) Avoidant personality disorder—desire relationships

      (4) Borderline—engages in social isolation as a result of having intentionally driven others away

4. Histrionic Personality Disorder—characterized by colorful, dramatic, extroverted behavior in excitable, emotional persons; accompanying their flamboyant presentation, however, is often an inability to maintain deep, long-lasting attachments

   a. Differential diagnoses

      (1) Borderline personality disorder—may have rapidly shifting emotions and less capacity for ambivalence

(2) Borderline and antisocial personality disorder—may crave excitement and become frustrated by delayed gratification; more likely to behave impulsively and violate the rights of others

(3) Narcissistic personality disorder—craves attention but wants to be admired for superiority rather than weakness or being dependent

(4) Manic and hypomanic states—episodic in nature and present with other classic symptoms of mania or hypomania

5. Narcissistic Personality Disorder—characterized by a heightened sense of self-importance and grandiose feelings that they are unique in some way

   a. Differential diagnoses

      (1) Other personality disorders—absence of grandiosity

      (2) Borderline personality—unstable self-image, self-destructiveness, impulsivity and abandonment fears

      (3) Antisocial—insensitive and exploitive, exhibits impulsivity and more materialistic

      (4) Schizotypal and paranoid—suspiciousness, social withdrawal and alienation

      (5) Manic or hypomanic episodes—presence of grandiosity

6. Avoidant Personality Disorder—persons show extreme sensitivity to rejection, which may lead to a socially withdrawn life; behavior is due to shyness rather than desire to be asocial

   a. Differential diagnoses

      (1) Schizoid personality disorder—social isolation due to interpersonal indifference, insensitive to social interactions, lacks self-consciousness and indifferent to criticism

      (2) Dependent personality disorder—strong desire for relationships, low self-confidence and interpersonal insecurity, but more secure when relating to and clinging to others, fear of interpersonal loss

(3) Social phobia—involves prominent anxiety in social setting, consisting only of fear of performing in social settings

7. Dependent Personality Disorder—persons with the disorder subordinate their own needs to those of others, get others to assume responsibility for major areas in their lives, lack of confidence, and may experience intense discomfort when alone for more than a brief period of time

   a. Differential diagnoses

      (1) Borderline personality disorder—characterized by intense attachments, need others to alleviate a sense of emptiness or to provide them with a sense of identity

      (2) Avoidant personality disorder—so strongly fear hurt and rejection that they will withdraw from relationships, not as likely to cling to others

      (3) Histrionic personality disorder—excessive need for reassurances and approval motivated by a need for praise and desire to be the center of attention

8. Obsessive-Compulsive Personality Disorder—characterized by emotional constriction, orderliness, perseverance, stubbornness, and indecisiveness

   a. Differential diagnoses

      (1) Narcissistic personality disorder—attempt to be perfect primarily as a means of sustaining their grandiosity rather than avoiding mistakes; not as critical of self as they are of others

      (2) Antisocial personality disorder

      (3) Dependent personality disorder—indecisiveness due to need for help and reassurance rather than to a self-inflicted fear of being inaccurate

      (4) Obsessive-compulsive disorder—characterized by repetitive unwanted thoughts and ritualistic behaviors rather than personality traits

9. Passive—Aggressive Personality Disorder

   a. Differential diagnoses

    (1)   Oppositional defiant disorder of childhood

    (2)   Borderline personality disorder

    (3)   Depressive personality disorder—more likely to inhibit the expression of aggression; mood consistently gloomy and unhappy, rather than erratically hostile and moody

- Genetic/biological theories

  1. Hereditary—Cluster A (paranoid, schizotypal, schizoid)—family history of psychiatric disorders such as alcoholism, drug addiction or schizophrenia

  2. Schizotypal—more often have first-degree biological relatives diagnosed with schizophrenia

  3. Imbalance in dopamine and serotonin neurotransmitter of persons with schizotypal personality disorder

  4. High anxiety in avoidant personality disorder found due to increased cortisol and sympathetic arousal

  5. Cluster B illnesses (borderline, histrionic, narcissistic, antisocial)—related to history of mood disorders, alcoholism and somatization disorders among family members

  6. Obsessive-compulsive personality disorder found with basal ganglia and frontal cortex dysfunctions

  7. Children with high innate submissiveness and low activity and persistence may elicit parental responses that promote dependent personality disorder

  8. Avoidant personality disorder—genetically based, temperamental predisposition to social avoidance or an inability to perform flexibly in new situations

- Biochemical approaches—used to treat anxiety, depression and psychotic-like symptoms

  1. MAOIs—social anxiety, social phobia and depressive symptoms

  2. Navane—schizotypal; decreases illusions, ideas of reference, obsessive symptoms and phobic disorder

  3. Haldol—paranoid thinking, anxiety and hostility

4. No evidence of significant role in treatment of narcissistic personality disorder, dependent personality disorder, and passive-aggressive personality disorder

- Intrapersonal theories

    1. Contradictory and inconsistent training methods as major factors related to development of passive-aggressive personality disorder

    2. Schizoid personality disorder—grossly inadequate, cold, or neglectful early parenting which creates expectation that the relationship would not be gratifying and leads to subsequent defensive withdrawal from others

    3. Obsessive-compulsive personality disorder—excessive parental disapproval and control, which may cause the child to stifle emotional expression (especially anger), and focus on the details of childhood tasks, and attempt to be perfect as a way to win the approval of critical, over controlling, and perhaps obsessional parents

    4. Histrionic personality disorder—fixation at the phallic phase leads to seeking sexual involvement with opposite-sex parent and leads to a conflictual relationship with the same-sex parent

    5. Paranoid—recipient of irrational and overwhelming parental rage may lead to an identification with that rage and its projection onto others

    6. Dependent personality disorder—develops from underindulgence and ongoing reinforcement patterns during the oral stage; family environments which inhibit expressions of feelings and exhibit high control; excessive dependence may represent a reaction formation against the expression of hostility or assertiveness; cultural and social factors contribute to excessive dependence in women and minorities

    7. Narcissistic personality disorder—results from ongoing childhood experiences of having fears, failures, dependence, or other signs of vulnerability that is responded to with criticism, disdain, or neglect

    8. Avoidant personality disorder—children who are rejected, belittled, and censured by their parents may develop feelings of self-depreciation and social alienation

    9. Depressive personality disorder—disturbance of early object relations, which lead to an excessively severe superego, the inhibited expression of aggression, and excessive dependence on the love and acceptance of others

- Psychotherapeutic interventions

    1. Psychotherapy—treatment of choice, focus on the client's feelings rather than intellectualized thoughts

    2. Cognitive therapy—to address faulty thinking

    3. Behavioral therapy

        a. Narcissistic personality disorder—no evidence of success

        b. Obsessive-compulsive personality disorder—maybe useful

    4. Assertiveness training

- Family dynamics

    1. Cluster A (paranoid, schizotypal, schizoid)—subjected to parental antagonism by serving as scapegoats for displaced parental aggression

    2. Cluster C (avoidant, passive-aggressive, dependent, obsessive-compulsive disorders)—families are over-controlling, child expected to live up to impossible standards and then condemned when fails

- Nursing diagnoses (Wilson & Kneisal, 1996)

    1. Defensive coping related to guardedness and secretiveness

        a. Nursing interventions

            (1) Respect client's privacy

            (2) Give feedback based on observed nonverbal cues of responsiveness, such as eye movements, posturing, voice tones

            (3) Point out inconsistent behaviors such as affect and verbalizations

            (4) Provide a daily schedule of activities and inform client of changes as needed

            (5) Help client identify adaptive diversionary activities (leisure, recreation) in one-to-one sessions and groups

            (6) Use role playing to help client identify feelings, thoughts, and responses brought on by stressful situations

        b. Outcome criteria

            (1) Responds to feedback without rationalizing, projecting, or intellectualizing

        (2)   Demonstrates decreased suspicion by interacting with the nurse at least once per day

  2.   Impaired thought processes related to suspiciousness and distortions of reality

     a.   Nursing intervention

        (1)   Say firmly and kindly that you do not share client's interpretations of an event but do acknowledge client's feelings

        (2)   Follow through on commitments made to client; respond honestly at all times

        (3)   Give positive reinforcement for successes in a matter-of-fact manner

        (4)   Refocus conversation to reality-based topics, and set limits on duration and frequency of suspicious concerns during one-to-one session and groups

        (5)   Help client identify and verbalize feelings

        (6)   Include client in formulating treatment plan

     b.   Outcome criteria

        (1)   Focuses on ideas that are reality based

        (2)   Accepts positive feedback without questioning motives or hidden meanings

        (3)   Accepts responsibility for own feelings and thoughts without attributing them to others; makes "I" statements

- Group approaches

  1.   Schizoid personality disorder—to increase comfort in social situations

  2.   Obsessive-compulsive personality disorder—focus on current life situations and confrontation

  3.   Paranoid personality disorder—may not be good due to excessive suspiciousness

  4.   Dependent personality disorder—to encourage autonomy and increase social self-confidence

5. Avoidant—social skills training

- Community Resources

  1. Obsessive-compulsive disorder support group

  2. Assertiveness training groups and seminars

Sleep Disorders
Primary Insomnia

- Definition: The inability to initiate or maintain adequate sleep not due to any other cause (e.g., psychiatric illness, medical illness, or drug use)

- Differential diagnoses

  1. Physical conditions

  2. Medication—withdrawal from CNS stimulants

  3. Dysthymia—mood disturbance

  4. Cyclothymia—insomnia due to hypomania

  5. Normal aging—changes in sleep pattern

  6. Psychiatric disorder

  7. Constant pain

  8. Obstructive lung disease

  9. Neurological diseases

- Mental status variations

  1. Anxiety

  2. Depression

  3. Appears tired (e.g., sleepy, dark circles under eyes)

  4. Difficulty concentrating

- Nursing diagnoses

  1. Ineffective individual coping

  2. Sleep pattern disturbance

     a. Nursing Interventions

        (1) Discuss reasons for disturbance

        (2) Provide a comfortable safe environment

(3) Encourage expression of emotions that may affect sleep

(4) Provide a variety of stimuli during waking hours

b. Outcome criteria

(1) Express anxieties, worries, and stress

(2) Accept that minor interruptions to sleep may exist and not dwell on them.

(3) Learn techniques to reduce tension.

- Genetic/biological theories

1. Increased autonomic activity

2. Increased physiologic activation as evidenced by increased heart rate, core body temperature, skin conductance

3. Increased levels of stress

4. Other psychopathology

   a. Mood disorders

   b. Psychoactive substance abuse disorder

5. Physical disorders that cause pain/discomfort such as arthritis, angina

6. Hormonal disturbances

7. Lifestyle that includes frequent changes or irregular sleep-wake patterns

8. Febrile illness in childhood associated with sleep terror disorder and sleep walking disorder

- Biochemical approaches

1. Benzodiazepines

   a. Triazolam—.25mg to 0.5mg at hs

   b. Temazepam—15mg to 30mg at hs

   c. Estazolam—1 mg at hs

2. Side effects of benzodiazepines

   a. Drowsiness, sedation

   b. Ataxia, dizziness

   c. Feelings of detachment

       d.   Increased irritability or hostility

       e.   Antegrade amnesia

       f.   Dependency

       g.   Rebound insomnia/anxiety

3. Barbiturates—Secobarbital 100 to 200mg at hs

4. Nonbenzodiazepine—Meprobamate 800mg at hs

5. Nonbarbiturates—Buspirone 15 to 25mg at hs

6. Chloral derivatives—Chloral hydrate 500 to 1000mg at hs

7. Side effects of Chloral Hydrate

       a.   Daytime sedation and drowsiness

       b.   Decrease in mental and physical responsiveness and efficiency

       c.   Dizziness

       d.   Fatigue

       e.   Light-headedness

       f.   Incoordination

       g.   Impaired motor performance, judgment and attention

       h.   Paradoxical excitement

       i.   Antegrade amnesia

       j.   Headache, blurred vision, nausea and vomiting, epigastric distress and diarrhea, or weight gain

8. Antidepressants—Trazodone 50–200mg at hs

- Intrapersonal theories

1. Higher levels of depressed mood and anxiety than normal individuals

2. Increased cognitive activity for clients without medical or psychiatric disorder other than anxiety caused by stress

- Psychotherapeutic interventions (Williams, Karacan, Moore & Hirshkowitz, 1995)

1. Sleep hygiene training

2. Stimulus control instructions

3. Sleep restriction

4. Chronotherapy

5. Bright light therapy

6. Relaxation, meditation, biofeedback

7. Cognitive therapy

    a. Alter view of sleep problem

    b. Paradoxical intention with thought stopping and identification of irrational beliefs about sleep

- Family dynamics/family therapy—none described

- Group approaches

    1. Self-hypnosis

    2. Autogenic training

    3. Share concerns

    4. Gain insight

- Milieu approaches

    1. Decrease caffeine and alcohol intake during afternoon and evening

    2. Increase exercise during morning and afternoon

    3. Encourage use of relaxation techniques

    4. Discourage daytime naps

    5. Encourage expression of emotion that might affect sleep

    6. Eliminate or diminish environmental factors that may disturb sleep

    7. Encourage client to get out of bed for alternative activities when unable to fall asleep

- Community resources

    1. Stress management training

    2. Biofeedback training

    3. Yoga classes

- Definitions only will be provided for the following sleep disorders (APA, 1994):

1. Narcolepsy—excessive daytime sleepiness and abnormal manifestations of REM sleep

2. Breathing-related Sleep Disorder—sleep disturbance due to sleep-related breathing difficulties (e.g., sleep apnea or central alveolar hypoventilation syndrome)

3. Circadian Rhythm Sleep Disorder (Sleep-Wake schedule Disorder)—sleep disruption due to mismatch between the sleep-wake schedule required by a person's environment and his/her circadian sleep-wake pattern

4. Sleep Terror Disorder—recurrent episodes of abrupt awakening from sleep without dream recall

5. Sleepwalking Disorder—repeated episodes of arising from bed during sleep and walking about

6. Primary Hypersomnia—excessive sleepiness that results in impairment in social, occupational, or other important areas of functioning

Impulse Control Disorders

Characterized by the failure to resist an impulse, drive or temptation to perform some act that is harmful to the person or others. There is increasing tension or arousal before committing the act and pleasure, gratification or relief during the act (Kaplan & Sadock, 1995).

Intermittent Explosive Disorder

- Definition: Those individuals who have discrete episodes of losing control of aggressive impulses resulting in serious assault or the destruction of property

- Differential diagnoses

  1. Psychotic disorders—violent behavior may result in response to delusions and hallucinations, and there is gross impairment of reality testing.

  2. Organic mental disorder—violent behavior results from confusion or medical condition.

  3. Antisocial or borderline personality disorder—aggressiveness and impulsivity are part of the client's character and are present between outbursts.

4. Conduct disorder—presents with a repetitive and resistant pattern of behavior as opposed to an episodic pattern

5. Intoxication with a psychoactive substance

6. Bipolar disorder—manic behavior present

- Mental status variation
  1. Uncontrolled anger
  2. Impulsivity
  3. Poor judgment
  4. Emotional instability
  5. Paranoia
- Genetic/biological theories
  1. Prenatal trauma, infantile seizures, head trauma, encephalitis, and hyperactivity
  2. Disordered brain physiology in the limbic system
  3. Hereditary predisposition
  4. Abnormalities of serotonergic metabolism
  5. Frontal and temporal abnormalities
- Biochemical approaches
  1. Lithium—300mg tid—qid
  2. Carbamazepine—200mg bid with food
  3. Oxazepam—10 to 30mg tid or qid
  4. Propranolol—60 to 640mg/day
- Nursing diagnoses for impulse control disorders
  1. Ineffective individual coping
  2. High risk for violence directed toward others
     a. Nursing interventions
        (1) Convey an accepting attitude toward the client
        (2) Maintain low level of stimuli in client's environment (low lighting, few people, simple decor, low noise level)

          (3)   Help client recognize the signs that tension is increasing and ways in which violence can be averted

          (4)   Explain to client that should explosive behavior occur, staff will intervene in whatever way is required (e.g., tranquilizing medication, restraints, isolation) to protect the client and others

          (5)   Help client identify the true object of his/her hostility

    b. Outcome criteria

          (1)   Client will not cause harm to self or others

          (2)   Able to verbalize the symptoms of increasing tension

          (3)   Able to verbalize strategies to avoid becoming violent

- Intrapersonal theories—early frustration, oppression and hostility as predisposing factors

- Psychotherapeutic interventions—individual psychotherapies have met with little success.

- Family dynamics

    1. Early chaotic and violent family environment with heavy drinking, by one or both parents

    2. Parental brutality, child abuse, and emotional and physical unavailability of a father figure

    3. Family therapy helpful when client is adolescent or young adult

- Group approaches/group therapy

    1. Foster group loyalty

    2. Peer pressure to reinforce expectations and provide confrontation

- Milieu approaches

    1. Provide structured outlets for the energy of anger

    2. Encourage physical activity that allows large muscle involvement

        a. Punching bag

        b. Jogging, swimming, weight lifting

    3. External controls

        a. Physical restraints

    (1) Monitor frequently

    (2) Remove dangerous articles

    (3) Provide fluids and food

  b. Indications for use

    (1) Physical assault—self, others, and environment

    (2) Physical and verbal threats

 4. Teach appropriate expression of anger

 5. Reduce sources of undue anxiety or high levels of anxiety to prevent angry outbursts

- Community resources—mental health centers

Pathological Gambling

- Definition: Chronic and progressive failure to resist impulses to gamble and gambling behavior that compromises, disrupts, or damages personal, family or vocational pursuits (Kaplan & Sadock, 1995)

- Differential diagnoses

 1. Social gambling—associated with gambling with friends, on special occasions, and with predetermined acceptable and tolerable losses

 2. Manic episode—history of marked mood change and loss of judgment preceding the gambling

 3. Antisocial personality disorder—marked mood changes and loss of judgment preceding the gambling

- Mental status variations

 1. Anxious

 2. Impulsive

 3. Lacks insight

- Genetic/biological theories

 1. Fathers of men and mothers of women more likely to have the disorder than the general population

 2. Noradrenergic deficits

- Biochemical approaches—none recommended

- Intrapersonal theories

    1. Unconscious desire to lose and gamble to relieve unconscious psychic guilt

    2. Learned maladaptive behavior

- Psychotherapeutic interventions

    1. Psychodynamic psychotherapy to confront sense of omnipotence

    2. Behavior therapy—imaginal desensitization (relaxation paired with visualization of avoidance of gambling)

- Family dynamics

    1. Absent, inconsistent, or harsh discipline

    2. Substance abusing parent

- Group approaches

    1. Inspirational group therapy

    2. Public confession

    3. Peer pressure

    4. Reformed gamblers as sponsors to help individuals resist the impulse of gambling

- Milieu approaches—remove client from the environment in order to assist them to gain insight into the problem

- Community resources—Gamblers Anonymous

- Definitions only will be provided for the following impulse control disorders:

    1. Kleptomania—recurrent inability to resist the impulse to steal objects not needed for personal use or their monetary value; without premeditation and little thought of legal consequences

    2. Pyromania—the deliberate and purposeful fire setting on more than one occasion; tension or an affective arousal before setting the fires; and intense pleasure, gratification, or relief when setting the fires or seeing the fires burn

    3. Trichotillomania—recurrent failure to resist impulses to pull out one's own hair; onset usually occurring before age 17 and affects females more often

Questions

1. Which of the following characteristics are most typical of bulimia?

   a. Unsuccessful efforts to control weight normally
   b. Persistent overconcern with body shape and weight combined with periods of strict dieting
   c. Self-induced vomiting alternating with periods of normal eating
   d. Episodes of binge eating and self-induced vomiting or other severe weight control methods

2. The clinical nurse specialist is giving an inservice on Bulimia Nervosa. Which of the following would be valid information to present? Families with a member with Bulimia Nervosa are:

   a. Rigid and inflexible
   b. Chaotic
   c. Overprotective
   d. Abusive

3. In order to assess a client's eating patterns, which of the following might the nurse use?

   a. "Do you often feel fat?"
   b. "Who plans the family meals?"
   c. "What do you eat in a typical day?"
   d. "What do you think about your present weight?"

4. Based on the client's response to the question above, what nursing diagnosis is most likely? Alteration in nutrition: less than body requirement related to:

   a. Abuse of laxative as evidenced by electrolyte imbalances
   b. Physical exertion in excess of energy produced through caloric intake as evidenced by weight loss
   c. Self-induced vomiting as evidenced by swollen glands
   d. Refusal to eat as evidenced by loss of 15% of body weight

5. When the clinical nurse specialist engages the family of a client with a diagnosis of Anorexia Nervosa in family therapy, what type of family dynamics might she/he expect to see:

   a. Overly strict and disagreement about discipline
   b. Overprotective, abusive, rigid

    c. Impulsive, rigid, perfectionistic

    d. Controlling, impulsive, abusive

6. Which of the following would *NOT* be an area for milieu management of Bulimia Nervosa

    a. Maintain behavioral diary

    b. Promote exercise

    c. Promote expression of feelings

    d. Develop adaptive coping

7. While conducting an initial assessment the nurse gathered the following sex history; pain before, during and after sexual intercourse. Which of the following nursing diagnoses would be most appropriate for the data described?

    a. Transvestic fetishism

    b. Sexual Arousal Disorder

    c. Sexual Dysfunction

    d. Altered Sexuality Patterns

8. According to the premise of cognitive therapy, which of the following would represent an example of cognitive restructuring in the treatment of the client with a Sexual Dysfunction?

    a. Maintain a diary of all stressful events

    b. Asks someone else to validate negative thoughts

    c. Identify irrational thoughts and counter thoughts with rational explanations

    d. Practice affirmations

9. In psychosocial development models, the term ''gender identity'' refers to the:

    a. Personal perception of being male or female

    b. Outward expression of socially accepted masculine or feminine traits

    c. Sexual classification assigned at birth

    d. Congruence of hormone levels and sexual behavior

10. Which of the following is true about a person with Paraphilia?

    a. Paraphilia is a sexual dysfunction

    b. Persons with Paraphilia do not have normal sexual habits

    c. Erotic pleasure is received from the activity

    d. The Paraphilia tends to be obsessional in nature

11. The first intervention in assessment at the initiation of sex therapy is:

    a. Clarification of each member's perceptions of the other
    b. Exploration of each member's beliefs about sexuality
    c. Separate assessments to enhance free expression
    d. Assessment of the couple's communication patterns

12. The nurse is assessing a client's sexual problem. In order to assess the client's feelings and attitudes about sex, the nurse might ask:

    a. The client's beliefs about alternative sexuality
    b. How the client's religion views sex
    c. For a description of the client's earliest sexual experiences
    d. The client's perception of his/her parent's relationship

13. As the nurse plans treatment for a sexual problem, it is important to focus the interventions toward?

    a. The couple
    b. The identified client
    c. Each member individually
    d. The partner

14. The primary intervention by the nurse in sex therapy is:

    a. Activities for the couple
    b. Homework assignments
    c. Communication clarification
    d. Values clarification

15. Which of the following mental status variations would the nurse expect to see in a patient with a medical diagnosis of gender identity disorder?

    a. Dysphoric mood
    b. Poor insight
    c. Hallucinations
    d. Memory loss

16. Which of the following is a manifestation of gender identity disorder?

    a. Fetishism
    b. Cross-dressing
    c. Sexual sadism
    d. Masochism

17. Mr. Cartwright tells the nurse that his sexual functioning is normal when his wife wears gold pumps. He states, "Without the gold pumps. I'm not interested in sex." The clinical nurse specialist assesses this as:

    a. Pedophilia
    b. Exhibitionism
    c. Voyeurism
    d. Fetishism

18. Which of the following would be best to use when the nurse assesses a client's sexual functioning?

    a. "Have you recently experienced a change in your self-esteem."
    b. Has anything such as illness, pregnancy, or a health problem interfered with your role as a wife/husband."
    c. "Has anything such as a heart attack or surgery changed the way you feel about yourself as a man/woman?"
    d. "Has anything such as surgery or disease changed your body's ability to function sexually?"

19. A new nurse tells the clinical nurse specialist "I'm unsure about my role when clients bring up sexual problems." The clinical nurse specialist should give clarification by saying:

    a. "All nurses qualify as sexual counselors because of their knowledge about biopsychosocial aspects of sexuality throughout the life cycle."
    b. "All nurses should be able to screen for sexual dysfunction and give limited information about sexual feelings, behaviors, and myths."
    c. "All nurses should defer questions about sex to other health care professionals because of their limited knowledge."
    d. "All nurses who are interested in sexual dysfunction can provide sex therapy for individuals and couples."

20. The nurse is caring for a client who presents with a medical diagnosis of Antisocial Personality Disorder. Which of the following nursing diagnoses would be most appropriate?

    a. Ineffective family coping
    b. Impaired social interaction
    c. Anxiety
    d. Altered sensory perception

21. Joan, who has a history of conflictual relationships, expresses the desire for friends but acts in alienating ways with people who befriend her. Which of the following would be an important nursing intervention for Joan?

    a. Help her find friends who are patient and extra caring
    b. Establish a therapeutic relationship in which role-modeling and role-playing may occur
    c. Accept her as she is, because she can't change
    d. Point out her difficulties in relationships and suggested areas for improvement

22. Mr. Grady constantly bends rules to meet his needs and then gets angry when other patients and staff confront him on his behavior. He threatens patients and manipulates staff to get what he wants. Which is the best nursing approach to use with Mr. Grady?

    a. Administer p.r.n. medication every time Mr. Bradley does not follow the rules
    b. Ignore his behavior and privately tell the other patients to let Mr. Grady switch the television channels as much as he wants
    c. Encourage the other staff to take turns watching Mr. Grady
    d. Set firm limits for Mr. Grady and be consistent in confronting behaviors and enforcing unit rules

23. The affect most commonly found in the client with Borderline Personality Disorder is one of:

    a. Happiness and elation
    b. Apathy and flatness
    c. Sadness and depression
    d. Anger and hostility

24. The action by the nurse that would be most appropriate when Mr. Smith states, *"I'm no good, I'm better off dead."* would be:

    a. Stating, "I will stay with you until you are less depressed."
    b. Stating, "I think you are a good person, who should think about living."
    c. Alerting all staff to provide 24-hour observation of the client
    d. Removing all articles that may be potentially dangerous

25. Limit setting is an intervention strategy to be utilized with which of the following behaviors?

    a. Manipulation

    b. Repression

    c. Reaction formation

    d. Projection

26. Conrad, 29 years old, is admitted for psychiatric observation after being arrested for breaking windows in the home of his former girlfriend, who refuses to see him. His history reveals abuse as a child by a punitive step-father, torturing family pets, and one arrest for disorderly conduct. Which nursing diagnosis should be considered?

    a. Impaired social interaction

    b. Altered thought processes

    c. High risk for trauma

    d. High risk for violence directed at others

27. Under which of the following circumstances is restraint appropriate?

    a. To encourage adherence to unit rules.

    b. To control difficult interpersonal situations.

    c. To establish the consequence of behaviors.

    d. To prevent harm to self and others.

28. Which of the following mental status variations would the nurse expect to see in a client with a diagnosis of Borderline Personality Disorder:

    a. Euphoria

    b. Good insight and judgment

    c. Mood lability

    d. Hallucinations

29. While you are caring for Jennifer she tells you that she's afraid her husband will leave her because she has no interest in sex anymore. Jennifer asks the nurse if anything can be done about her lack of interest in sex. The most appropriate referral by the nurse for this client is:

    a. Marriage counselor

    b. Psychiatrist

    c. Psychoanalyst

    d. Sex therapist

30. The psychiatric nurse clinical specialist is asked to assess a 24-year-old female who reports that she is unable to have intercourse because of involuntary contractions of her vagina. The term is described as:

a. Arousal disorder
b. Dyspareunia
c. Orgasmic dysfunction
d. Vaginismus

31. The nurse is evaluating the outcome of measures to promote sleep. Which of the following would indicate that these measures have been successful?

a. Client able to sleep at least 4 hours each night
b. Client states he felt rested the next day
c. Client accepts minor interruptions to sleep as normal
d. Client able to verbalize anxieties

32. The sleeping disorder that can be described as excessive daytime sleepiness is which of the following disorders

a. Sleep Terror Disorder
b. Primary Hypersomnia
c. Circadian rhythm sleep disorder
d. Narcolepsy

33. The nurse is admitting a client with a diagnosis of Primary Insomnia. Which of the following assessment findings would be essential to confirm the diagnosis?

a. Inability to obtain sleep not due to any other cause
b. Inability to obtain sleep due to a medical disorder
c. Disturbance of sleep-wake cycle
d. Excessive daytime sleepiness

34. You are the psychiatric clinical specialist on a sleep disorder unit. Which of the following is the key aspect of a psychotherapeutic intervention program:

a. Verbalize feelings
b. Gain insight
c. Thought stopping
d. Sleep hygiene training

35. Which of the following nursing diagnosis is most appropriate for a client with a sleep disorder?

a. Perceptual disturbances
b. Impaired thought processes
c. Sleep pattern disturbance
d. Ineffective family coping

36. Which of the following would *NOT* be examples of milieu approaches for Primary Insomnia?

    a. Decrease alcohol and caffeine intake during afternoon and evening
    b. Thought stopping
    c. Discourage daytime naps
    d. Increase exercise during morning and afternoon

37. Which of the following phenomena would most likely accompany a diagnosis of Primary Insomnia?

    a. Medication withdrawal
    b. Situational/Environmental changes
    c. Normal aging
    d. Mood disorders

38. The clinical specialist is implementing a behavior modification plan with a client with a diagnosis of pathological gambling. Which of the following family dynamics might he/she expect to observe?

    a. Absent, inconsistent or harsh discipline
    b. Chaotic and violent environment
    c. Rigid and overprotective parents
    d. Heavy drinking

39. Ferman, a 15 year-old female has complained of an intense impulse to pull her hair out, followed by a sense of relief at having carried out the act. Which of the following medical diagnoses would be most appropriate for the clinical nurse specialist to make?

    a. Obsessive-Compulsive Personality Disorder
    b. Tinea capitis
    c. Trichotillomania
    d. Autism

40. Which of the following would *NOT* be a mental status variation for the client with a diagnosis of pathological gambling?

    a. Anxiety
    b. Impulsivity
    c. Sadness
    d. Poor insight

41. Johnson C. Smith is diagnosed with Pyromania. Which of the following behaviors would the nurse expect to observe in Mr. Smith?

    a. Aggressiveness
    b. Sadness
    c. Obsessive-compulsiveness
    d. Intense pleasure when watching fires

42. John is pacing the hall near the nurses station swearing loudly. An appropriate initial intervention for the nurse would be to say

    a. "John, please quiet down."
    b. "Hey, John, what's up?"
    c. "John, you seem pretty upset. Tell me about it."
    d. "John, you need to go to your room to get control of yourself."

43. Which of the following interventions is *NOT* appropriate for the nurse to use in the above situation?

    a. Telling the client that violence is not acceptable
    b. Speaking in a loud, urgent tone of voice
    c. Standing with arms relaxed at sides
    d. Listening attentively to the client

44. It becomes necessary to give an intramuscular injection of psychotropic medication to a client who is becoming increasingly more aggressive. The client is in the television room. The nurse should

    a. Enter the room; say, "Would you like to come to your room and take some medication your doctor has ordered for you?"
    b. Take three staff members with you to the room as a show of solidarity; say, "Mr. Summer, please come to your room so I can give you some medication that will help you feel more comfortable."
    c. Take a male staff member to the television room; tell Mr. Summer, "Mr. Summer, you can come to your room willingly to take your shot or Mr. Crinshaw and I will take you there."
    d. Enter the television room; place Mr. Summer in a basket hold; say, "I'm going to take you to your room to give you an injection of medication to calm you."

45. Following an incident in which staff intervention was required to control a client's aggressive behavior, which of the following data would be least important to the staff's evaluation of the intervention?

a. The client's behavior preceding and during the incident
b. Intervention techniques used
c. The environment
d. The staff's views about theories of the etiology of aggression

46. Based on the client's potential for violence toward others and inability to cope with anger, which short-term goal would be most appropriate? The client will

   a. Acknowledge his angry feelings.
   b. Describe situations that provoke angry feelings.
   c. List how he's handled his anger in the past.
   d. Practice expressing anger

47. The impulse control disorder that is characterized as the deliberate and purposeful setting of fires is which of the following

   a. Pyromania
   b. Kleptomania
   c. Trichotillomania
   d. Intermittent explosive disorder

48. The impulse control disorder that is characterized as the inability to resist the impulse to steal objects is which one of the following

   a. Pyromania
   b. Kleptomania
   c. Trichotillomania
   d. Intermittent explosive disorder

Answers

1. d	17. d	33. a
2. b	18. d	34. d
3. c	19. b	35. c
4. d	20. b	36. b
5. a	21. b	37. b
6. b	22. d	38. a
7. c	23. c	39. c
8. c	24. c	40. c
9. a	25. a	41. d
10. c	26. d	42. c
11. d	27. d	43. b
12. b	28. c	44. b
13. a	29. d	45. d
14. c	30. d	46. b
15. a	31. c	47. a
16. b	32. d	48. b

Bibliography

American Psychiatric Association. (1994). *Diagnostic and statistical manual of mental disorders* (4th ed.). Washington, DC: Author.

Beemer, B. R. (1996). Gender dysphoria update. *Journal of Psychosocial Nursing, 34*(4), 12-19.

Blair, D. T. (1996). Integration and synthesis cognitive behavioral therapies within the biological paradigm. *Journal of Psychosocial Nursing, 34*(12), 26-31.

Burgess, A. W. (1997). *Psychiatric nursing promoting mental health.* St. Louis: Mosby.

DeCaria, C. M., Hollander, E., Grossman, R., Wong, C. M., Mosovich, S. A., & Cherkasky, S. (1996). Diagnosis, neurobiology and treatment of pathological gambling. *Journal of Clinical Psychiatry, 57*(suppl 8), 80-84.

Fichter, M. M., Kruger, R., Rief, W., Holland, R., & Dohne, J. (1996). Fluvoxamine in prevention of relapse in bulimia nervosa: Effects on eating specific psychopathology. *Journal of Clinical Psychopharmacology, 16*(1), 9-19.

Fisher, M., Golden, N. H., Katzman, D. K., Kreipe, R. E., Rees, J., Schebendach, J., Sigman, G., Ammerman, S., & Hoberman, H. M. (1995). Eating disorders in adolescents: A background paper. *Journal of Adolescent Health, 16*, 420-437.

Greene, H., & Ugarriza, D. N. (1995). Borderline personality disorder: History, theory and nursing intervention. *Journal of Psychosocial Nursing, 33*(12), 26-30.

Gorman, L. M., Sultan, D. F., & Raines, M. L. (1996). *Davis's manual of psychosocial nursing for general patient care.* Philadelphia: F. A. Davis Co.

Gunderson, J. G., & Phillips, K. A. (1995). Personality disorder. In H. L. Kaplan & B. J. Sadock (Eds.), *Comprehensive textbook of psychiatry* (pp. 1425-1461). Baltimore, MD: Williams & Wilkins Co.

Kaplan, H. I., & Sadock, B. J. (1995). *Comprehensive textbook of psychiatry.* Baltimore, MD: Williams & Wilkins.

Linehan, M. M., Oldham, J. M. & Silk, K. (1995). Diagnosis: Personality . . . now what. *Patient Care, 6*, 75-91.

McGowan, A., & Whitebread, J. (1996). Out of control—the most effective way to help the binge-eating patient. *Journal of Psychosocial Nursing, 34*(1), 30-37.

Stuart, G. W., & Sundeen, S. J. (1995). *principles and practice of psychiatric nursing.* St. Louis: Mosby.

Sugar, M. C. (1995). A clinical approach to childhood gender identity disorder. *American Journal of Psychotherapy, 49*(2), 260-281.

Townsend, M. C. (1997). *Nursing diagnoses in psychiatric nursing.* Philadelphia: F. A. Davis.

Williams, R. L., Karacan, I., Moore, C. A., & Hirshkiwitz, M. (1995). Sleep disorders. In Kaplan & Sadock (Eds.). *Comprehensive textbook of psychiatry.* Baltimore, MD: Williams & Wilkins Co.

Wilson, H. S., & Kneisl, C. R. (1996). *Psychiatric nursing*, NY: Addison-Wesley Nursing.

Cognitive Mental Disorders

Jane Bryant Neese
Anita Thompson-Heisterman
Ivo L. Abraham

Cognitive Mental Disorders are associated with or caused by disturbance in the physiological functioning of brain tissue—structural, hormonal, biochemical, electrical, etc.—which causes cognitive deficits; ranges along continuum from acute (delirium) to chronic (Dementia of the Alzheimer's type).

Delirium

- Definition: A transient, reversible, confusional state resulting from a gross disruption in brain physiology and developing from a wide variety of factors (Lipowski, 1992); although symptoms are similar in their disturbance of consciousness and cognition, the delirium disorders are differentiated on etiology (*Delirium Due to a General Medical Condition, Substance-Induced Delirium, Delirium Due to Multiple Etiologies,* and *Delirium Not Otherwise Specified*) (APA, 1994); can progress to permanent dementia if identifying causes are not diagnosed and treated.

- Signs and Symptoms

    1. Disturbance of consciousness

    2. Change in cognition (memory deficit)

    3. Disturbance in sleep-wake cycle and level of psychomotor activity

    4. Disorientation to time, place, or persons

    5. Reduced ability to focus, shift, or maintain attention

    6. Disorganization of thinking (may manifest as irrelevant, rambling, or incoherent speech)

    7. Perceptual disturbances resulting in illusions and hallucinations;

    8. Emotional disturbances constituting lability of affect

    9. Transient, occurs abruptly, and fluctuates throughout the day (APA, 1994; Lipowski, 1992)

- Differential Diagnosis

    1. Schizophrenia—due to perceptual, affective, and behavioral similarities

    2. Schizophreniform Disorder and other psychotic disorders

Table 1

Differentiation of Symptoms

Factors	Delirium	Dementia
Level of consciousness	Fluctuates throughout the day	Alert; clear sensorium
Mood/affect	Irritable; fluctuates; can be volatile or depressed	Depends on situation
EEG	Diffusely abnormal, slowing	Focal points lower range of normal
Onset	Rapid; abrupt	Insidious; slow
24 Hour Course	Fluctuates	Stable
Duration	Short—from less than a week to no more than a month	long term; years
Behavior	Agitated; lethargic; fluctuating	"sundowning"; more confused at night
Thought processes	Thoughts may be slow or accelerated; somewhat dreamlike; presence of hallucinations (illusions); sometimes delusions, but they are poorly organized	Slow thought processes; impoverished; Delusions may be present but often absent
Orientation	Usually impaired, especially to time and place, but not usually to person	May be impaired or intact; may tend to confabulate
Memory	Recent and remote impaired; common knowledge intact	Recent memory impaired; remote memory may be intact; loss of common knowledge
Perceptions	Misperceptions often, especially visual	Misperceptions are absent
Speech	Slow or rapid, often incoherent	Normal
Involuntary movements	Asterixis or course tremor often present	Absent
Physical illness or drug toxicity	One or both are present	Often absent

Note. From "Depression in the General Hospital" by J. B. Neese, 1991, *Nursing Clinics of North America, 26*(3), p. 615. Copyright 1991 by W. B. Saunders. Adapted from "Transient cognitive disorders (delirium, acute confusion states) in the elderly" by Z. J. L. Lipowski, 1983. *American Journal of Psychiatry, 140,* p. 432. Copyright 1991 by W. B. Saunders. Adapted by permission.

3. Dementia—onset of delirium is abrupt and duration is shorter than dementia with symptoms lasting a day to no longer than one month (Breitner & Welsh, 1995; Lipowski, 1992). Refer to Table 1 for differentation of symptoms.

4. Depression—sluggishness and depressed affect when delirious, similar to major depressive episode or an adjustment disorder with depressed mood, however, depression is not the underlying pathology

5. Anxiety Disorder—due to affective and behavioral similarities

6. Definitive diagnosis based on constellation of findings, rapidity of onset, and associated medical and environmental risk factors (Breintner & Welsh, 1995)

7. Delirium Due to a General Medical Condition—etiology primarily from a physical disorder such as cancer, head trauma, lupus, etc. (APA, 1994)

8. Delirium Due to Multiple Etiologies—etiology from two different causes such as a substance abuse and a physical/medical disorder (i.e. congestive heart disease, chronic obstructive pulmonary disorder, etc.) (APA, 1994)

9 Substance Intoxication Delirium, Substance Withdrawal Delirium, and Substance-Induced Delirium—etiology from an ingestion or withdrawal of medications, toxins or substances such as alcohol, narcotics, barbiturates, steroids, etc. (APA, 1994)

10. Cognitive Disorder Not Otherwise Specified—not all symptoms of delirium are present, however, symptoms may signal the onset of delirium although a physical disorder has not been diagnosed at the time (APA, 1994)

- Mental Status

    1. Fluctuating cognitive impairment with lucid intervals

    2. Inability to maintain attention or engage in goal-directed behavior; difficulty following questions upon examination and may perseverate in response to earlier questions

    3. Disorganization of thought—difficulty maintaining coherent stream of thought, easily distracted; speech rambling, inconsequential, or illogical; faulty reasoning and lack of goal-directed behavior

    4. Perceptual disturbances—illusions, hallucinations, delusions may be present, but they generally are poorly organized; can suffer acute paranoid delusions accompanied by fear, anxiety, attempts to escape or destructive rage episodes

    5. Impairment in the level of consciousness—the client falls asleep during the interview

    6. Disturbed sleep-wake cycle—hypervigilant during the night and sleeps during the day

    7. Abnormally increased or decreased psychomotor activity; may pick at the bed linen or be sluggish, resembling catatonia-like movements; three clinical patterns (Lipowski,1992)

        a. Hypoalert-hypoactive client who is lethargic and drowsy

b. Hyperalert-hyperactive client who is restless and agitated

c. Mixed variant who shifts between lethargy and agitation

8. Disorientation in all spheres (place, time, and/or person); disorientation to place and time is very common; however, disorientation to person is rare

9. Memory impairment—usually short-term memory is impaired and both anterograde (memory for events just prior to onset of delirium) and retrograde (memory for events just after the episode) amnesia are present

10. Emotional lability ranging from depressive to rage affects

- Nursing Diagnoses

  1. Alteration in thought processes is the major NANDA-approved nursing diagnosis for delirium (NANDA, 1994).

  2. Others include communication, impaired verbal; sensory/perceptual alterations (specify which one is disturbed); fatigue; high risk for injury; altered nutrition; altered role performance; self-care deficit; and sleep pattern disturbance.

  3. Anxiety—acute anxiety, fear, and hypervigilant behavior may accompany delusions as a result of the delirium

- Biological Theories: Usually delirium can be attributed to a wide range of physical disorders ranging from metabolic disturbances to withdrawal from substances such as alcohol or sedative-hypnotic agents (APA, 1994; Lipowski, 1992; St. Pierre, 1996; Tune, Carr, Hoag, & Cooper, 1992). Medication intoxication is the most common cause in the elderly.

  1. Risk factors associated with delirium:

     a. Severity of illness—the more severe the illness, the more likely delirium will occur

     b. Age—the older the patient, the more likely delirium will occur (Brietner & Welsh, 1995); persons over age 80 most vulnerable

     c. Impairment in cognition (Schor, Levoff, Lipsitz, Reily, Cleary, Rowe, & Evans, 1992) or physical functioning, such as confinement in a restricted space or bed

d. Presence of dementia—approximately 25% to 50% of patients diagnosed with dementia have been found to have delirium superimposed upon the dementia (Lipowski, 1992)

e. Chronic lesions on neuroimaging studies (Lipowski, 1992)

f. Chronic brain diseases such as Parkinsonism (Lipowski, 1992) or metastases to the brain

g. Systemic infection (Schor et al., 1992)

h. Narcotic use (Schor et al., 1992)

i. Disruption of the sleep cycle

j. Relocation—especially if rapid, sudden and unplanned

k. Pain

l. Hearing or visual impairment

m. Amnesia as a result of drugs, surgery, or trauma

n. Environment—sensory overload or deprivation such as critical care unit (St. Pierre, 1996)

2. The following disorders have been credited with causing delirium:

a. Primary intracranial diseases (Barry, 1996; Lipowski, 1992)

b. Systemic infections or diseases that secondarily affect the brain—in the elderly, most often the causes of delirium are related to other illnesses such as cancer, congestive heart failure, myocardial infarction, uremia, diabetes, hypoglycemia, malnutrition, dehydration, sodium depletion, hypokalemia, stroke, and epilepsy (Barry, 1996; Lipowski, 1992).

c. Metabolic disorders (hypoxia, hypercarbia, hypoglycemia, electrolyte imbalance, hepatic or renal disease, or thiamine deficiency (Inaba-Roland & Maricle, 1992)

d. Post-operative states

e. Cerebrovascular events—thrombotic, embolitic, hemorrhagic (Inaba-Roland & Maricle, 1992)

f. Postictal activity (Lipowski, 1992)

g. Post head trauma (Lipowski, 1992)

h. Substance intoxication and withdrawal (Barry, 1996; Lipowski, 1992) (Refer to Table 2 for drugs causing delirium.)

Table 2

Drugs Causing Psychiatric Symptoms

Drug Classification	Generic Drug Name	Reactions Similar in Symptomatology to Various Cognitive Mental Disorders
Antiviral agents	Acyclovir, Amantadine	Visual hallucinations, depersonalization, confusion, insomnia, depression
B-2 Antagonist	Albuterol	Hallucinations
Antianxiety	Alprazolam, Diazepam	Manic symptoms, insomnia, anxiety, paranoia, hallucinations, depression, suicidal thoughts
Antibiotics	Amoxicillin, Chloramphenicol, Cephalosporins, Dapsone, Erythromycin, Gentamicin, Penicillin G procaine	Confusion, auditory hallucinations, hyperactivity, disorientation, paranoia, insomnia
Stimulants	Amphetamines, caffeine, cocaine, Methylphenidate, and similar anorectic agents	Hallucinations, paranoia, anxiety, restlessness, confusion, paranoid delusions
Antineoplastics	Asparaginase, Cisplatin, Chorambucil, Vincristine, Vinblastine	Confusion, depression, paranoia, disorientation, hallucinations
Antihypertensives	Atenolol, Captopril, Methyldopa, Prazosin, Propranolol, Timolol	Confusion, disorientation, hallucinations, insomnia, severe depression, paranoia, hyperactivity
Relaxants	Baclofen, Cyclobenzeprine	Hallucinations, paranoia, depression, anxiety, confusion, manic psychosis, delusions, hyperactivity
Sedative/Hypnotics	Barbiturates, Triazolam, Ethchlorvynol	Excitement, hyperactivity, visual hallucinations, depression, paranoia, anterograde amnesia, anxiety
Dopamine agonist	Bromocriptine	Delusions, visual or auditory hallucinations, paranoia, depression, anxiety
Antimalarial	Chloroquine, Hydroxychloroquine	Confusion, delusions, hallucinations, difficulty concentrating
Anticonvulsant	Clonazepam	Hallucinations, paranoia
Narcotics	Codeine, Methadone, Morphine, Pentazocine, Propoxyphene	Psychosis, disorientation, dysphoria, agitation, euphoria, nightmares, paranoia, depression, auditory hallucinations, confusion
Steroids	Corticosteroids, Oxymetazoline	Depression, confusion, paranoia, hallucinations, anxiety
Antituberculars	Cycloserine, Ethionamide, isoniazid	Anxiety, depression, confusion, disorientation, hallucinations, paranoia
Immunosuppressant	Cyclosporine	Hallucinations, depression
Antidysrhythmics	Digitalis glycosides, Disopyramide, Quinidine, Lidocaine, Tocainide	Confusion, delusions, amnesia, visual or auditory hallucinations, paranoia, depression, disorientation
Adrenergics	Ephedrine, Pseudoephedrine	Hallucinations, paranoia

	Table 2 — Continued	
Drug Classification	*Generic Drug Name*	*Reactions Similar in Symptomatology to Various Organic Mental Disorders*
Nonsteroidals	Ibuprofen, Indomethacin, Naproxen, Sulindac	Paranoia, depression, inability to concentrate, confusion, hallucinations, disorientation, personality change
Antidepressants	Isocarboxazid, Phenelzine	Insomnia, anxiety, paranoid delusions, hyperactivity
Serotonin antagonist	Methysergide	Depersonalization, hallucinations
Cholinergic	Metoclopramide	Severe depression
Amebicides	Metronidazole, Pargyline	Depression, disorientation, manic psychosis, hallucinations
Urinary tract anti-infectives	Nalidixic acid, Trimethoprim sulfamethoxazole	Confusion, depression, hallucinations, psychosis
Calcium channel blocker	Nifedipine	Hyperexcitability, depression
Nasal decongestant	Phenylephrine	Depression, hallucinations, paranoia
Keratolytic	Podophyllin	Delirium, paranoia
Diuretics	Polythiazide, Trichlormethiazide	Depression, suicidal ideation
Local anesthetic	Procainamide	Paranoia, hallucinations
Nonnarcotic analgesic	Salicylates	Hallucinations, paranoia
Spasmolytic	Theophylline	Hyperactivity
Antihelmintic	Thiabendazole	Hallucinations
Hormone	Thyroid hormones	Depression, hallucinations, paranoia

Note. From "Drugs that Cause Psychiatric Symptoms" by M. Abramowiez, 1993, *The Medical Letter, 535*(901), pp. 65–70. Copyright 1986 by The Medical Letter Inc. Adapted by permission.

- Biochemical Interventions

  1. Dependent on determination of identifying causes which entails:

     a. Complete physical examination

     b. Complete neurological examination

     c. Complete battery of laboratory tests including but not limited to: SMA12, complete blood count, complete urine drug screen, electroencephalogram (EEG), B12 levels, thyroid profile, CT scan and MRI (Lipowski, 1992; St. Pierre, 1996)

  2. Treatment of the underlying cause(s)

     a. Restore adequate fluid and electrolyte balance, nutrition, and vitamin supply (Lipowski, 1992; St. Pierre, 1996).

     b. Eliminate medication(s) suspected to affect mental status. Due to changes in pharmacodynamics and pharmacokinetics in later life, careful consideration and individualization in drug therapy is essential in caring for the elderly. Drug reactions occur two to three times more often in the elderly than in young adults (CMA, 1993). (Table 2 lists medications associated with causing delirium.)

    (1)   If toxicity from cimetidine or ranitidine is suspected, the use of physostigmine reverses the delirium for "15 to 60 minutes following a 1 to 2 mg intravenous dose" (Francis, 1992, p. 836).

    (2)   Caution, however, should be taken when administering physostigmine for antidepressant overdoses due to the potentiation action of physostigmine with antidepressants.

  c.   The following are physiological changes in old age that affect absorption and elimination of medications:

    (1)   Multiple chronic diseases that are associated with reduced serum albumin levels (Ferrini & Ferrini, 1992)

    (2)   Hepatic functioning that decreases with normal aging; drugs have been shown to have a longer half-life and decrease plasma clearance. Drugs that require a high rate of hepatic extraction should be used judiciously (i.e., major tranquilizers, tricyclic antidepressants, and antiarrhythmic agents (Ferrini & Ferrini, 1992)

    (3)   Decline in renal functioning due to the glomerular filtration and tubular secretion rates; creatinine clearance is an indicator of adequate renal drug elimination in the elderly. Lithium, digoxin, procainamide, chlorpropamide, cimetidine and amantadine are drugs that are primarily eliminated by the kidneys.

    (4)   General decline in nutritional status that includes protein and vitamin intake is common.

    (5)   Cigarette smoking affects hepatic functioning.

    (6)   The central nervous system is more sensitive in the elderly; therefore, smaller doses of benzodiazepines are indicated to produce similar amount of sedation as in younger adults (Gorbien, Bishop, Beers, et al., 1992).

(7) The elderly are prone to postural hypotension, urinary retention, sedation, and falls associated with psychoactive medications; therefore, beginning dosages should be lower than in young adults and close observation is indicated to protect the safety of this population (Gorbien et al., 1992).

d. Treat withdrawal from substances

(1) Alcohol withdrawal delirium develops after recent cessation or reduction of alcohol consumption. Marked autonomic activity occurs, usually within one week. The condition is also called ''delirium tremens.''

(2) Management of acute withdrawal with benzodiazepines is indicated. Chlordiazepoxide (Librium) 25 mgm prn for withdrawal symptoms is often chosen. It is important to monitor the withdrawal carefully, checking vital signs and mental status.

(3) Need to replace thiamine and other vitamins to prevent permanent organic disorder due to deficiency.

e. If client becomes agitated and restless, pharmacologic restraint may be necessary.

(1) Haloperidol—most commonly used sedative because of low anticholinergic side effects, quick sedation, and low incidence of orthostatic hypotension (Tune & Ross, 1994; Lipowski, 1992); potential for extrapyramidal symptoms such as ''cog-wheel'' rigidity in joints (can be seen in flexing and extending the elbow) and excessive salivation, and dystonic reactions such as torticollis (extreme turning of head to one side with the inability to correct posture). A low dose of 0.25 to 0.5 mg tid prn given by mouth in liquid suspension or intramuscularly usually diminishes agitation.

(2) Droperidol—has a more rapid onset of sedation and can be given in the same dosages as haloperidol; hypotension is side effect

- Psychosocial Approaches

1. Be attentive to the client's concerns and fears, which may be expressed in the hallucinations and/or delusions (Lipowski, 1992).

2. Reorient the client to reality, especially when illusions are present.

3. Reduce fear and anxiety by providing a calm reassuring manner, assuring the client that you will be sure he is safe.

4. Explain all procedures to allay anxiety.

5. If client is extremely agitated, the use of physical restraints is not recommended as they may increase fear and agitation along with increasing the risk of problems associated with immobility. The use of "sitters" or enlisting the family's help is more efficacious.

- Family Dynamics/Family Therapy

   1. Involve the family in assessment, planning, intervention, and evaluation of the nursing care plan.

   2. Family can provide useful information as to the clients premorbid cognitive status, the possible causative factor of the delirium, history of the client and other critical data.

   3. Family can assist in planning psychosocial interventions which are likely to be most successful.

   4. Family can assist in interventions by helping to orient and reassure the client.

   5. Family needs to be provided with information and reassurance along with referral information for use post delirium.

   6. Family members may exhibit grief reactions such as anger, hostility, bargaining, depression, guilt, avoidance, denial, and ambivalence (Barry, 1996).

- Group Approaches: For delirious clients, group intervention, of any kind, is contraindicated.

- Milieu Approaches

   1. Aimed at providing safety, support, and structure

   2. Environmental interventions help reestablish orientation by placing clock, calendar, and familiar belongings in the client's room.

   3. Encourage family visits to assist patient with orientation.

   4. Correct any sensory deficit that the patient may have by having eyeglasses or hearing aid made available and within close reach.

5. Place the client in a room with windows to help orient to day and night.

6. Keep outside, distracting noises to a minimum and keep a low light on at night.

7. Reduce, but don't eliminate stimulation, as sensory deprivation also contributes to delirium.

- Community Resources: Not indicated during the acute episode but may be chosen as a referral for aftercare based on:

  1. Etiology of the delirium (i.e., Alcoholics Anonymous; Narcotics Anonymous; social support such as senior center, case management or home health services)

  2. Need for the client and/or family to resolve the emotional trauma associated with the acute episode of delirium through participation in individual, group, or family counseling/therapy.

Dementia

- Definition

  1. Development of multiple cognitive deficits which cause significant impairment in social or occupational functioning, represent a significant decline from a previous level of functioning, do not occur during the course of a delirium, and are judged to be related to a causative factor (APA, 1994).

  2. Etiology

     a. Hereditary factors

     b. Cerebrovascular disease—in particular, stroke and cerebral blood flow problems

     c. Cerebral oxygenation problems

     d. Infectious diseases of, or affecting, the central nervous system

     e. Brain trauma

     f. Toxins

     g. Metabolic disturbances

     h. Hypoglycemia

     i. Normal pressure hydrocephalus

      j. Degenerative neurologic diseases

      k. Medications (See Table 2)

      l. AIDS

  3. Criteria for severity of Dementia

      a. Mild—although work or social activities are significantly impaired, the capacity for independent living remains, with adequate personal hygiene and relatively intact judgment.

      b. Moderate—independent living is hazardous, and some degree of supervision is necessary.

      c. Severe—activities of daily living are so impaired that continual supervision is required, (e.g., unable to maintain minimal personal hygiene; largely incoherent or mute.)

- Differential Diagnosis:

  1. Dementia of the Alzheimer's Type

  2. Vascular Dementia

  3. Dementia Due to HIV Disease

  4. Delirium

  5. Dementia Due to Parkinson's Disease

  6. Dementia Due to Huntington's Disease

  7. Dementia Due to Pick's Disease

  8. Dementia Due to Creutzfeldt-Jakob Disease

  9. Dementia Due to Other General Medical Conditions

  10. Dementia Due to Multiple Etiologies

  11. Substance-Induced Persisting Dementia

  12. Dementia Not Otherwise Specified

  13. Dementia Due to Head Trauma

  14. Schizophrenia

  15. Major Depressive Disorder

  16. Malingering and Factitious Disorder

Dementia of the Alzheimer's Type

- Definition
    1. This type of dementia is characterized by a gradual and insidious onset and a generally progressive deteriorating course for which all other specific causes have been excluded by the history, physical examination, and laboratory tests (APA, 1994). It is the most prevalent of the dementias.
    2. This disease can occur with the following variations:
        a. Senile or presenile onset, depending on whether after or before age 65
        b. Within senile and presenile variants, disease can be with delirium, with delusions, with depression or uncomplicated.

- Signs and Symptoms
    1. Characterized by multifaceted loss of intellectual abilities, such as memory, judgment, abstract thought, and other higher cortical functions, changes in personality and behavior, and significant decline and impairment in social and occupational functioning (APA, 1994)

    2. The clinical aspects of Alzheimer's disease are summarized in Table 3.

- Differential Diagnosis

    Exclusion of all alternative specific causes of dementia by complete history, physical examination, and laboratory tests

    1. Benign forgetfulness, common phenomenon among older adults
    2. Subdural hematoma
    3. Normal pressure hydrocephalus
    4. Brain tumors
    5. Parkinson's disease
    6. Vitamin B_{12} deficiency
    7. Hypothyroidism
    8. Delirium
    9. Acute psychotic episode

Table 3

Clinical Aspects of Alzheimer's Disease

Symptom Category	*Signs and Symptoms*
Memory	Recent memory deficits
	Remote memory deficits
	Disorientation
	Forgetfulness
	Confusion
	Dementia
Concentration	Short attention span
	Inability to acquire new information
Language and Speech	Word finding deficits
	Agnosia
	Anomia
	Paraphrasia
	Aphasia
	Echolalia
	Paralalia
	Logoclia
	Mutism
Praxis	Inability to conceptualize
	Difficulty with complex tasks
	Inability to write
Thought Content	Simple delusions
	Persecutory delusions
	Suicidal ideation
Lability	Fear and fearfulness
	Anxiety
	Anger
	Irritability
	Crying spells
	Catastrophic reactions
Depressed Mood	Sadness
	Hopelessness
	Helplessness
	Feelings of worthlessness
	Guilt
	Depression
	Suicidality
Mania	Busy behaviors
	Meddlesome
	Interference in affairs of others
	Destructive behavior
	Violence

Table 3 — Continued	
Symptom Category	*Signs and Symptoms*
Related to Personality Change	Stubbornness
	Angry outburst
	Verbal abuse
	Restlessness
	Combativeness
	Agitation
	Resistance to care
	Assaultive and violent behaviors
	Wandering
	Roaming through rooms
	Regressive behaviors
	Hiding and hoarding things
Related to Vegetative Disorders	Sleep disturbance
	Urinary incontinence
	Dietary changes: (binge eating, pica)
	Sexual disinhibition
Related to Neuromotor Dysfunction	Apraxia
	Ataxia
	Gait disorder
	Tremors
	Seizures
	Flexional contracture
	Primitive reflexes
Sensory Distortion	Misidentification of people
	Misidentification of places
	Confusion of people and places
	Inability to recognize mirror image
	Treating TV events/people as real illusions
Sensory Deception	Visual hallucinations
	Auditory hallucinations
	Olfactory hallucinations
Social Withdrawal	Withdrawal from family
	Withdrawal from close social groups
	Withdrawal from complex groups
Personal	Increased self-preoccupation
	Personal isolation
Activities of Daily Living	Instrumental ADLs
	Physical ADLs
Self-Care	Nutrition
	Sleep/Rest
	Medication behavior

Note. From "Alzheimer's Disease and Nursing: New Scientific and Clinical Insights" by E. S. Yi, I. L. Abraham amd S. Holroyd, 1994, *Nursing Clinics of North America, 29*(1), pp. 88–89. Copyright by W. B. Saunders. Adapted by permission.

10. Major depressive episode

11. Multi-infarct dementia (see below)

12. Medication interactions

13. AIDS dementia complex (ADC)

- Mental Status: Manifestations include:

   1. Recent and remote memory deficits

   2. Short attention span and inability to concentrate

   3. Impairment in abstract thinking and judgment

   4. Other disturbances of higher cortical functioning, such as agnosia, apraxia, aphasia, and constructional difficulty

   5. Affective lability

   6. Perceptual disturbances such as hallucination

   7. Depressed mood

- Genetic/Biological Theories: According to APA (1994) and Yi, Abraham & Holroyd (1994):

   1. Cause(s) of disease still unknown

   2. Hereditary factors

      a. Familial patterns exist

      b. Genetic markers on chromosomes 1, 14, 19 and 21

      c. People with one variant of the gene for the cholesterol carrying protein apolipoprotein E (The Apo E gene) are at increased risk for late-onset Alzheimer's Disease.

      d. Alzheimer's type lesions occur around age 40 in most if not all people with Down's Syndrome

Vascular Dementia

- Definition: Direct consequence of cerebrovascular disease, characterized by the often abrupt onset of a stepwise deterioration in intellectual functioning that, early in the course, leaves some intellectual functions relatively intact (patchy deterioration) (APA, 1994)

- Signs and Symptoms

  1. Multiple cognitive deficits manifested by memory impairment and disturbance in executive functioning (i.e., planning, organizing, sequencing, abstracting), aphasia, apraxia, and/or agnosia (APA, 1994)

  2. A stepwise deteriorating course with "patchy" distribution of deficits (affecting some functions, but not others) early in the course (APA, 1994)

  3. Since the cause is cerebrovascular disease, focal neurologic signs and symptoms (e.g., exaggeration of deep tendon reflexes are an important diagnostic determinant)

     a. "Weaknesses in the limbs, reflex asymmetries, extensor plantar responses, dysarthria, and small-stepped gait" (APA, 1994).

     b. Can present with delirium, delusions, or depression pseudobulbar palsy, gait abnormalities, weakness of an extremity

  4. Evidence of significant cerebrovascular disease that is judged to be etiologically related to the disturbance

- Differential Diagnosis (APA, 1994; and Abraham et al., 1994):

  1. General differential diagnosis of Dementia due to Other General Medical Conditions and Dementia of the Alzheimer's Type (see above)

  2. Impairment due to single stroke

- Mental Status: Is differentiated from other primary dementias only by the fact that the cognitive manifestations may wax and wan, showing patchy or stepwise deterioration

- Biological Theories: Cerebrovascular diseases, commonly referred to as "mini-strokes"

- Nursing Diagnoses

  1. Alteration in thought processes—a state in which an individual experiences a disruption in cognitive operations and activities is the most common nursing diagnosis approved by NANDA that applies to dementia (Rawlins et al., 1993, pp. 659–660)

a. Defining characteristics include physical, emotional, and intellectual.

b. Physical dimensions include altered sleep pattern and hyperactivity.

c. Emotional dimensions include inappropriate or labile affect and anxiety.

d. Intellectual dimensions include altered states of consciousness (disorientation to time, place, person), impaired memory, confabulation, distractibility, disturbed thought flow, disturbed thought content, impaired problem solving, impaired judgment, inability to follow conversation, alteration in perception, cognitive disturbance, suicidal/homicidal ideation, attention deficit, egocentricity, inappropriate/non-reality based thinking (Rawlins et al., 1993).

2. Numerous other nursing diagnoses can also apply to clients with dementia due to the complexity of the illness and the level of care required.

a. Self-care deficit—feeding, bathing, toileting

b. Impaired verbal communication; sensory/perceptual alterations; anxiety; fear.

c. High risk for fluid volume deficit; high risk for injury; altered nutrition

d. Sleep pattern disturbance; fatigue

e. Personal identity disturbance; altered role performance; social interaction—impaired; social isolation

f. Ineffective coping—individual and family; caregiver role strain.

- Biochemical Interventions

1. Initially these depend on the etiologic factor causing the dementia as the need is to treat the underlying cause of the disturbance (e.g., treat diabetes with insulin, hypothyroidism with thyroid replacement, thiamine deficiency with replacement, and iatrogenic disorders by eliminating the causative drug).

2. If biochemical intervention is indicated for control of agitation or hallucination associated with dementia, drug treatment should be

used cautiously, beginning with the lowest possible dose and tapering upward as needed. Haloperidol is the drug of choice for controlling agitation in dementias due to lower anticholinergic effects. Low dosage of 0.25 mg should be initiated. Side effects include dystonias (rigidity in joints and torticollis) and excessive salivation. Orthostatic blood pressures should be monitored and the client and his caregiver(s) should be taught the side effects.

3. Short-acting benzodiazepines such as oxazepam (Serax) or Lorazepam (Ativan) are used to treat behavioral agitation, but are not as useful as low dose neuroleptics (Coccaro, Kramer, Zemishlany, Thorne, Rice, et al., 1990). Must be used with extreme caution as side effects can increase confusion in elderly organically impaired clients while controlling agitation and irritability. May cause dizziness and drowsiness. Need to check orthostatic blood pressure (sitting and standing) and monitor mental status. Need to monitor withdrawal symptoms and assess for suicide if depressed.

4. No treatment available to stop or reverse the progression of Alzheimer's disease. Several drugs are used for management of symptoms of the disorder. Depression is often a feature of dementia, although it may be difficult to detect. It has multiple adverse effects on the demented patient, including aggravation of behavioral symptoms. The following medications can be used to treat depression occurring with dementia.

    a. Tricyclic antidepressants. All cause orthostatic hypotension, sedation, and anticholinergic effects. Nortriptyline (Aventyl) 25-150 mg per day or Desipramine (Norpramine) 25 mg per day as an initial dose are the tricyclics of choice in elderly patients since they have fewer side effects (Yi, Abraham & Holroyd, 1994). Serum levels of tricyclic antidepressants should be closely monitored. All antidepressants should be given at the lowest possible effective dose in the elderly or those with compromised medical conditions.

    b. Selective serotonin re-uptake inhibitors (SSRIs). A new class of antidepressants including fluoxetine (Prozac) and sertraline (Zoloft). The most common side effects in the elderly are nausea, weight loss, nervousness, and agitation (Yi, et al, 1994). Usual fluoxetine dose is 20 mg daily, although it can be given 10 mg per day in the elderly. Sertraline dose is generally 50 mg per day.

c. Trazodone—a serotonin uptake blocker well tolerated in the elderly due to low anticholinergic effects. It can be very sedating, which may be a desired outcome if sleep disturbance exists. Use trazodone with extreme caution because of high orthostatic hypotensive side effects. Need to monitor orthostatic blood pressure. Other side effects include dry mouth, insomnia, headache, tremor, nausea, and rash (Yi et al., 1994). Trazodone (Desyrel) is usually given at 150 mg per day in divided doses.

5. In vascular dementia biochemical approaches are directed at treating the cardiovascular factor causing the dementia in addition to managing behavioral symptoms. Multi-infarct dementia is managed like thrombotic stroke or transient ischemic attacks with appropriate doses of ASA for the anticoagulant effect.

6. Anticonvulsants such as carbamazepine (Tegretol) or phenytoin (Dilantin) may be used to control seizures. Phenobarbital may be avoided due to potential for abuse by alcoholic. Phenytoin is given in three divided doses of 100 mg each for seizure prophylaxis. Side effects include agranulocytosis, leukopenia, aplastic anemia, drowsiness, dizziness, nausea, and vomiting. Need to assess blood levels, assess mental status, teach client not to d/c the drug abruptly, since seizures may occur and to use good oral hygiene to prevent gingival hyperplasia.

- Psychosocial Approaches

  1. Based on careful nursing assessment of the patient.

  2. Adaptations to interviewing techniques needed with cognitively impaired clients include; need to allow more time, speak slowly and clearly, and provide an environment free of distractions (Thompson-Heisterman, Smullen & Abraham, 1992).

  3. Goal of nursing care regardless of the setting is to help the client maintain the highest possible level of independence. Skill training can assist the client to reach his/her potential (Tappen, 1994).

  4. Use warm, caring, respectful approach.

  5. Use clear, simple and direct communication.

  6. Keep tasks within the client's abilities, using sequencing and cuing (i.e., laying out the client's clothing in the order in which he/she needs to put it on.)

7. Avoid over- or under-stimulation.

8. Provide adequate rest and nutrition.

9. If the dementia is vascular, provide information to the client regarding managing risk factors associated with cardiovascular disease (diet, exercise, decrease stress, medication, signs of impending stroke, etc.).

- Family Dynamics/Family Therapy

    1. Family needs to be included in the assessment as well as the intervention phase of treatment with cognitively impaired clients as they can provide much useful information regarding how to best care for their loved one.

    2. Family members are often the hidden victims of the illness, especially when the dementia is chronic rather than reversible.

    3. Family interventions always include providing support and education, and in some cases, such as when the dementia is due to substance abuse, counseling or therapy may be indicated.

    4. Family interventions also include assisting the family with anticipatory grief that usually is a deep sadness that occurs before the anticipated future loss. Symptoms of anticipatory grief are depression, an increased preoccupation with the affected family member, an analysis of all the possible problems that may occur during the course of the disease, and anticipation how each family member will need to readjust to care for the affected family member (Barry, 1996). In addition to anticipatory grief, family members also may experience the bereavement stages proposed by Kubler-Ross (1969): denial, anger, bargaining, depression, and acceptance.

- Group Approaches: In selecting elder group participants, as with young adults, extreme paranoia and severe cognitive impairment is usually contraindicated for effective group work. Therefore, elders who are experiencing the latter stages of Alzheimer's Disease or other dementias, will not benefit from most of the following groups while those with mild cognitive impairment can and do benefit from group therapy.

    1. Reminiscence groups aim to increase self-esteem through positive affiliations and interactions with others (Ashton, 1993). These groups may be helpful for elders and individuals with mild cognitive disorders and depression.

    2. Cognitive-behavioral groups assist clients in correcting negative

thoughts and attitudes, as well as maladaptive ways in which clients process information (Hitch, 1994). This type of group can be helpful to elders who suffer from mild cognitive impairment with superimposed depression or who have one of the above disorders.

3. Educational groups seek to inform and emphasize learning and discussion instead of therapy (Neese & Abraham, 1992). For elders who have mild cognitive impairment and their families, educational groups addressing the various types of dementias are an excellent method to help alleviate the isolation that clients and families feel when faced with a chronic disorder.

4. Validation Groups developed by Feil (1989) to benefit even severely impaired clients. The goals of validation are to stimulate communication in order to prevent withdrawal inward, to restore well-being, to facilitate the resolution of unresolved issues to prepare for death, and to reduce caregiver burnout by teaching empathy skills (Bleatheman & Morton, 1996; Fine & Rouse-Bane, 1995).

5. Activity, movement, and sensory stimulation groups also enhance functioning in cognitively impaired older adults (Arno & Frank, 1994).

- Milieu Approaches

  1. Milieu interventions are a critical factor in the treatment of both acute and chronic dementias whether the client is at home or in an institution.

  2. Provide safety, structure, and support.

  3. Provide consistency of routine.

  4. Provide orientation and environmental cues.

  5. Explain procedures in clear, direct language to enhance understanding and allay anxiety.

  6. Provide for adequate rest, nutrition, and elimination.

  7. Disruptive behavior in demented clients often occurs in response to an environmental trigger. Therefore, it is very important to assess and modify the environment (Whall, 1995). Disruptive behavior often occurred as the client's responses to pain, need for control, need to feel safe, need for stimulation, and need to decrease stress.

  8. Boehm, Whall, Cosgrove, Locke & Schlenic (1995) caution regarding the need to avoid chemical and physical restraints through

modification of the environment. Federal mandates, specified in the Omnibus Budget Reconciliation Act (OBRA) passed by Congress in 1989, stipulate that if neuroleptic drugs are used in nursing homes, there must be a specific medical reason. They cannot be used solely for chemical restraint. Both types of restraints have many complications including increasing agitation and confusion.

- Community Resources

    1. Potential resources for clients and caregivers are extensive depending on the etiology, duration, and level of cognitive and functional impairment associated with the dementia.

    2. Organizations related to organic factors causing the disorder would include Alcoholics Anonymous, The American Cancer, Diabetes, Lung Association, and the Alzheimer's Disease and Related Disorders Foundation.

    3. A wide array of community services that may be needed to maintain the client and family, including home health agencies, social services, outreach programs, homebound meals, church support, day care, respite care, hospice, nursing homes, and others.

Dementia Due to HIV Disease

- Definition: This type of dementia presents with similar symptoms of other dementia in a client with the diagnosis of HIV disease or AIDS. Most often this type of dementia is known as AIDS dementia complex (ADC). Other nomenclature includes AIDS neurocognitive disorder, HIV encephalopathy, and HIV subcortical dementia. ADC usually occurs later in the progress of HIV disease as the CD4 lymphocyte count decreases (Griepp, Landau-Stanton, & Clements, 1993).

- Signs and Symptoms: Characterized by memory changes with slowing and loss of precision; difficulty performing cognitive tasks; confusion, changes in mood (apathy or agitation), decreased attention and concentration, and psychomotor activity changes (hyperreflexia, tremor, ataxic gait, and dysarthric speech). Deterioration in handwriting may be the first symptom that appears (Griepp, Landau-Stanton, & Clements, 1993; Hollander & Katz, 1997).

- Etiology

    1. Approximately 31–65% of HIV infected people will exhibit some form of neurological abnormalities during the course of their illness

with the highest percentage of neurological deficits occurring at the later stages of the disease (Griepp, Landau-Stanton, & Clements, 1993).

2. The exact mechanism of how HIV causes neurological deficits is not known. Some related factors are the metabolic changes that usually occur in HIV such as hypoglycemia, hyponatremia, hypoxia, and medication usage and/or abuse. Other infectious causes are progressive multi-focal leukoencephalopathy, nocardia, tuberculosis, cytomegalovirus, syphilis, and herpes simplex encephalitis (Griepp, Landau-Stanton, & Clements, 1993; Hollander & Katz, 1997).

3. No specific diagnostic test to determine ADC; cerebrospinal fluid (CSF) findings can be inconclusive and not grow the HIV virus; other diagnostic tests to confirm ADC are: CT, MRI (look for fornical enhancement), Trails A & B, Finger Tap, Wisconsin Card Sort (Griepp, Landau-Stanton, & Clements, 1993)

- Biochemical Interventions

  1. Medication for ADC: Zidovudine has been effective in decreasing the dementia symptoms in early and late stages (Hollander & Katz, 1997).

  2. Treatment of other opportunistic viral infections with AZT.

  3. In the case of acute agitation, judicious use of small doses of antispychotics such as Trilafon, Haldol and Thorazine are indicated (Griepp, Landau-Stanton, & Clements, 1993).

- Psychosocial Approaches

  1. Based on careful assessment of patient, partner, and family

  2. Maintain a consistent environment, living situation, and relationships

  3. Assist patient in preparing for their death and saying ''good-bye.'' Common feelings are sadness, depression, anger, and denial. Other issues that HIV patients may confront are confidentiality, secrets, organizing legal and financial affairs, dependency, and feelings of hope and hopelessness (Bor, Miller, & Goldman, 1992).

  4. As with most dementia patients, create a system to reinforce memory and orientation to reality using pictures, clocks, calendars, lists of activities of daily living, assist client to maintain diary of activities during the day, use friends and visitors to continue to relate to

the patient, and pause between sentences to allow patient enough time to react and interact (Griepp, Landau-Stanton, & Clements, 1993).

4. Use other psychosocial approaches listed under Vascular Dementia and Dementia of the Alzheimer's type.

- Family Interventions

  1. Maintain a realistic outlook and assist the family in accepting their normal feelings of fatigue, irritability, anger, fantasizing escape, or needing a break (respite) from caring for their loved one

  2. Encourage time off when possible including going into a separate room for a break, walking around the building, having a meal in a different place than the patient, etc.

  3. Assist family and/or partner to adapt to technology and the environment by suggesting pill boxes for daily or weekly medication schedule, use an alarm clock to alert family of medication times, use picture albums of family, friends, and/or partner for reminiscence, discussions, and reorientation.

  4. Assist family in problem solving difficult management problems such as disturbed behavior at night.

  5. As with other dementias, assist the family, friends, and partner in grieving their anticipated loss (Griepp, Landau-Stanton, & Clements, 1993).

Questions
Select the best answer

1. Ms. S, age 50, has been hospitalized for cholecystectomy. Two days postoperatively she develops pneumonia. The nurse notes that Ms. S. does not know where she is and that she is picking at the bedclothes. What is the most likely diagnosis?

   a. Hemorrhage
   b. Sensory deprivation
   c. Delirium
   d. Urinary tract infection

2. Ms. S is likely to be oriented to which of the following:

   a. The time of day
   b. The day of the week
   c. Her daughter
   d. The name of her medication

3. Which of the following is the hallmark indication of delirium?

   a. Fluctuation of sensorium and limited attention span
   b. Global cognitive impairment
   c. Severe agitation
   d. Dysphoria

4. What level of consciousness is Ms. S. likely to exhibit during delirium?

   a. Alert and oriented
   b. Hyper-vigilant
   c. Fluctuating
   d. Comatose

5. Ms. S is likely to *NOT* exhibit what type of perceptual disturbance?

   a. Poorly organized delusions
   b. Hallucinations
   c. Illusions
   d. Well organized delusions

6. The onset of delirium is characterized by:

   a. Onset occurring over several days

    b. Abrupt onset

    c. Occurrence within two days of exposure to a causative factor

    d. Fluctuating onset

7. Ms. S. has an EEG. The findings are likely to show which feature?

    a. Diffusely abnormal slowing

    b. Normal

    c. Focal points

    d. Lower range of normal

8. Ms. S's nurse needs to write a care plan. Which is the major nursing diagnosis she would use?

    a. Self-care deficit

    b. Alteration in thought processes

    c. High risk for violence

    d. Alteration in role performance

9. One of the ways in which delirium is differentiated from dementia is that delirium is:

    a. Characterized by sundowning

    b. A progressive deteriorating disease

    c. Characterized by fluctuating level of consciousness

    d. Chronic

10. Which of the following is *NOT* a risk factor for delirium?

    a. Use of narcotics

    b. Family dynamics

    c. Systemic illness

    d. Presence of dementia

11. Delirium is most common in which age group?

    a. Age 10–20

    b. Age 20–40

    c. Age 40–60

    d. Age 60–80

12. Which of the following physical disorders is least likely to cause delirium?

    a. Hypertension

b. Substance abuse and withdrawal
c. Metabolic disorders
d. Systemic infections

13. Ms. S was determined to have delirium. What intervention is most critical?

    a. Symptom management
    b. Treating the underlying cause
    c. Administering medication
    d. Education of the patient

14. Which intervention would be the second most important?

    a. Symptom management
    b. Treating the underlying cause
    c. Administering medication
    d. Education of the patient

15. Which of the following drugs would be least likely to further complicate Ms. S's delirium?

    a. Antibiotics
    b. Antihistamines
    c. Antihypertensives
    d. Vitamin B_{12}

16. Mr. D is a 65-year-old widowed white male. He is brought to the emergency room by his family because he has become agitated, disoriented, and has been hallucinating. Family reports that Mr. D takes ranitadine for ulcer disease. What is the most likely cause of his symptoms?

    a. His age
    b. His ulcer disease
    c. His medication
    d. An undetected organic factor

17. The most important initial nursing intervention for Mr. D is to:

    a. Interview Mr. D without his family present
    b. Use chemical restraints to protect Mr. D
    c. Provide the family with a list of support groups
    d. Institute measures to clear the medication from Mr. D's body

18. Which of the following medications could the nurse anticipate for Mr. D.?

    a. Chlordiazepoxide 25 mg po
    b. Physostigmine 2mg IV
    c. Chlorpromazine 100 mg IV
    d. Diazepam 10 mg IV

19. In administering physostigmine the nurse would be concerned about which of the following classes of medications potentiating the drug?

    a. Antiemetics
    b. Antianxiety
    c. Antidepressants
    d. Anticonvulsants

20. If Mr. D continues to be agitated, what other pharmacological agent is the physician likely to order?

    a. Haloperidol
    b. Chlorpromazine
    c. Thioridazine
    d. Lithium

21. The nurse would not anticipate which of the following side effects of haloperidol?

    a. Cogwheel rigidity
    b. Excessive salivation
    c. Dystonia
    d. Orthostatic hypertension

22. Which individual intervention would the nurse *NOT* use in caring for Mr. D.?

    a. Reorienting Mr. D to day, place, situation
    b. Being attentive to Mr. D's fears
    c. Telling Mr. D that he needs to eat to get better
    d. Offering fluids every 2 hours

23. Which of the following would *NOT* be an appropriate environmental intervention?

    a. Limiting family visits as these may be overstimulating
    b. Providing orientation devices (clocks, calendars) in Mr. D's room
    c. Keeping a low light on at night
    d. Having Mr. D wear his glasses during the day

24. Which of the following interventions is *NOT* indicated for Mr. D at this time?

    a. Individual
    b. Group
    c. Family
    d. Milieu

25. Which of the following is *NOT* a cognitive mental disorder?

    a. Affective disorders
    b. Dementia of the Alzheimer's Type
    c. Vascular Dementia
    d. Delirium

26. Ms. T, who is 85, is unable to perform several of her ADLs due to her inability to conceptualize and complete tasks. Her level of dementia is:

    a. Mild
    b. Moderate
    c. Severe
    d. Fluctuating

27. Ms. T.'s nurse notes that she has short-term memory loss. An example would be:

    a. Inability to remember what happened yesterday
    b. Inability to remember current president
    c. Inability to remember three objects after five minutes
    d. Inability to remember an anniversary

28. A disorder of language is also noted. What would it be called?

    a. Agnosia
    b. Anhedonia
    c. Apraxia
    d. Aphasia

29. Ms. B., a 68-year-old African American, has a B/P of 220/110. She has had several episodes of dizziness and temporary loss of consciousness. Her family notes that she has had difficulty remembering in the past few months. The most likely diagnosis would be:

    a. Dementia of Alzheimer's type
    b. Delirium

c. Vascular Dementia

d. Mood Disorder due to General Medical Condition

30. Mr. A is an 82-year-old white married male. He has been diagnosed as having probable Dementia of the Alzheimer's type. He has withdrawn from his activities at the senior center but continues to perform his ADLs. The level of severity of his dementia could be characterized as:

a. Mild

b. Moderate

c. Severe

d. Nonexistent

31. Which one of the following is *NOT* needed to make a diagnosis of dementia?

a. Impairment in short-term memory

b. Transient confusion

c. Impairment in long-term memory

d. Significant changes in social relationships

32. Which nursing diagnosis would be used for Mr. A's condition?

a. Self-care deficit

b. Social isolation

c. Sensory/perceptual alterations

d. Alteration in thought processes

33. Various types of dementias will not have symptoms similar to which of the following?

a. Acute psychotic episode

b. Delirium

c. Major depressive episode

d. Adjustment disorder

34. Which one of the etiologic factors is *NOT* a factor in dementia?

a. Heredity and degenerative neurologic disease

b. Cerebral vascular disease and normal pressure hydrocephalus

c. Lack of education, social isolation

d. Toxins and metabolic disturbances

35. Mr. W is a 68-year-old widowed white male with a history of alcohol abuse. On interview he is able to remember in detail an incident which occurred 20 years ago but cannot remember 3 objects after 5 minutes on the mental status exam. He has no change in personality and his judgment is good. Mr. W's condition is probably caused by:

    a. A deficiency of thiamine
    b. Heredity
    c. Situational stress
    d. A tumor

36. Ms. C is a 70-year-old widowed female. Recently she has become very suspicious about her neighbor, whom she believes is an FBI agent. On a recent CT scan a right cerebral lesion was discovered. Her suspiciousness is most likely related to:

    a. Her neighborhood
    b. Her family relationships
    c. Her cerebral tumor
    d. A grief reaction

37. Ms. C is brought to the emergency room by the police after locking herself in her apartment and making threatening phone calls to her neighbor. The best initial nursing response to her is:

    a. Tell her not to worry, her neighbor is not an FBI agent
    b. Take measures to allay her anxiety and protect her from harm
    c. Agree that the FBI does intrude into our lives
    d. Conduct a complete nursing assessment including physical examination

38. Which one of the following nursing diagnoses for Ms. C would *NOT* be included?

    a. Altered thought processes
    b. Fear related to persecutory delusions
    c. High risk for violence
    d. Knowledge deficit

39. Which is always associated with dementia?

    a. Ataxic gait
    b. Impaired memory and judgement
    c. Delusions
    d. Affective disturbances

40. Alzheimer's disease is primarily characterized by:

    a. Progressive memory decline
    b. Emotional distress
    c. Dysphoria
    d. Hallucinations

41. Assessment of Alzheimers disease is best done by a:

    a. Physician
    b. Nurse
    c. Multidisciplinary team
    d. Psychologist

42. Senile onset refers to:

    a. The development of the disease before age 65
    b. The development of the disease after the person is determined to be senile.
    c. The disease occurs after age 65
    d. The development of the disease before the person is determined to be senile

43. Mr. Y, an 80-year-old married male, has been diagnosed with Dementia of the Alzheimer's Type and placed on Haldol 10 mgm at night which is his only medication. He has become more agitated in the past week. His agitation is probably due to:

    a. His illness
    b. A change in his environment
    c. His medication
    d. A urinary tract infection

44. Mr. Y's wife, to whom he has been married for 50 years, dies 2 years after he is first diagnosed with dementia. Several months later he experiences weight loss, crying spells, and sleep disturbance. The most likely diagnosis would be:

    a. Dementia of the Alzheimer's Type with delusions
    b. Dementia of the Alzheimer's Type with depression
    c. Dementia of the Alzheimer's Type with delirium
    d. Dementia of the Alzheimer's Type with paranoia

45. Which affect would you *NOT* expect Mr. Y to have?

    a. Sadness
    b. Hopelessness
    c. Euphoria
    d. Helplessness

46. Which type of hallucination would you *NOT* expect Mr. Y to have?

    a. Tactile
    b. Visual
    c. Auditory
    d. Olfactory

47. Mr. Y develops praxis. This includes:

    a. Simple delusions
    b. Confusion
    c. Inability to write
    d. Short attention span

48. Which of the following medications would *NOT* be used to treat Mr. Y's depression?

    a. Prozac
    b. Zoloft
    c. Trazodone
    d. Haldol

49. Which of the following is classified as a selective serotonin re-uptake inhibitor (SSRI)?

    a. Trazodone
    b. Desipramine
    c. Fluoxetine
    d. Lithium

50. Alzheimer's disease is considered to result from:

    a. Aluminum intoxication
    b. Alcohol abuse
    c. Tumors
    d. Causes which are still unknown

51. Vascular dementia is characterized by which of the following:

    a. Stepwise and patchy deterioration in intellectual functioning
    b. Global cognitive impairments
    c. Retrograde amnesia
    d. Headaches and fainting spells

52. Which of the following are not causes of delirium?

    a. Medications
    b. Metabolic and endocrine imbalances
    c. Sensory deprivation
    d. Infectious diseases

53. Which of the following is the most prevalent form of dementia?

    a. AIDS Dementia Complex
    b. Amnestic disorder due to a General Medical Condition
    c. Dementia of the Alzheimer's type
    d. Vascular dementia

54. The second most prevalent dementia is:

    a. AIDS Dementia Complex
    b. Amnestic disorder due to a General Medical Condition
    c. Dementia of the Alzheimer's type
    d. Vascular dementia

55. Ms. T has dementia and resides in a nursing home. Which of the following individual interventions is not indicated to enhance her care?

    a. Provide balance between stimulation and rest
    b. Provide structure and support
    c. Provide clear and direct communication
    d. Provide intensive group therapy

56. Which of the following should be avoided in providing care to Ms. T.:

    a. The use of chemical and physical restraints
    b. Having family members visit
    c. Reminiscence groups as they would be too stimulating
    d. Orientation measures

57. The nurse is considering starting a group for residents of Ms. T's nursing home with mild cognitive impairment. Which type of group would be indicated?

    a. Reminiscence
    b. Jungian
    c. Psychoanalytic
    d. Gestalt

58. The primary purpose of cognitive behavioral group interventions is to:

    a. Increase self-esteem through positive affiliations with others
    b. Correct negative thoughts and attitudes
    c. Provide information
    d. Explore unconscious motivations of behavior

59. Mr. B, two days post admission for esophageal varices, develops delirium tremens. This state is most associated with which of the following conditions?

    a. Cocaine withdrawal
    b. Parkinson's disease
    c. Alcohol withdrawal
    d. Hypoxia

60. Which of the following community resources would be most helpful to Mr. B's family?

    a. Alanon
    b. Alzheimers Disease and Related Disorders Foundation
    c. American Heart Association
    d. Mental Health Association

61. Validation is a method to:

    a. Limit communication
    b. Restore well-being
    c. Facilitate avoidance of unresolved issues
    d. Teach sympathy skills

62. Dementia Due to HIV Disease is *NOT* called which of the following?

    a. AIDS Dementia Complex
    b. HIV vascular dementia
    c. HIV encephalopathy
    d. HIV subcortical dementia

Answers

1. c	22. c	43. c
2. c	23. a	44. b
3. a	24. b	45. c
4. c	25. a	46. a
5. d	26. c	47. c
6. b	27. c	48. d
7. a	28. d	49. c
8. b	29. c	50. d
9. c	30. a	51. a
10. b	31. b	52. c
11. d	32. d	53. c
12. a	33. d	54. d
13. b	34. c	55. d
14. a	35. a	56. a
15. d	36. c	57. a
16. c	37. b	58. b
17. d	38. d	59. c
18. b	39. b	60. a
19. c	40. a	61. b
20. a	41. c	62. b
21. d	42. c	

Bibliography

Abraham, I. L., Holroyd, S., Snustad, D. G., Manning, C. A., Brashear, H. R., Diamond, P., & Thompson-Heisterman, A. A. (1994). Multidisciplinary assessment of Alzheimer's disease. *Nursing Clinics of North America, 29*(1), 113–128.

Abraham, I. L., Niles, S. A., Thiel, B. P., Siarkowski, K. I., & Cowling, W. R. (1991). Therapeutic group work with depressed elderly. *Nursing Clinics of North America, 26*(3), 635–650.

Abramowiez, M. (1993). Drugs that cause psychiatric symptoms. *The Medical Letter on Drugs and Therapeutics, 35*(901), 65–70.

American Psychiatric Association. (1994). *Diagnostic and statistical manual of mental disorders (4th ed.).* Washington, DC: Author.

Arno, S., & Frank, D. L. (1994). A group for "wandering" institutionalized clients with primary degenerative dementia. *Perspectives in Psychiatric Care, 30*(3), 13–16.

Ashton, D. (1993). Therapeutic use of reminiscence with the elderly. *British Journal of Nursing, 2*(18), 894–898.

Barry, P. D. (1996). The physical cause of cognitive mental disorders. In P. D. Barry (Ed.), *Psychosocial nursing: Care of the physically ill patients and families (3rd ed. pp. 195–219).* Philadelphia: J. B. Lippincott.

Bleathman, C., & Morton, I. (1996). Validation therapy: A review of its contribution to dementia care. *British Journal of Nursing, 5*(4), 866–868.

Boehm, S., Whall, A. L., Cosgrove, K. L., Locke, J. D., & Schlenic, E. A. (1995). Behavioral analysis and nursing interventions for reducing disruptive behaviors of patients with dementia. *Applied Nursing Research, 8*(3), 118–122.

Bor, R., Miller, R., & Goldman, E. (1992). *Theory and practice of HIV counseling: A systematic approach.* New York: Brunner/Mazel.

Breitner, J. C., & Welsh, K. A. (1995). Diagnosis and management of memory loss and cognitive disorders among elderly persons. *Psychiatric Services, 46*(1), 29–35.

Canadian Medical Association (CNA). (1993). CMA policy summary: Medication use and the elderly. *Canadian Medical Association, 149*(8), 1152A–1152B.

Coccaro, E. F., Kramer, E., Zemishlany, Z., Thorne, A., Rice, C. M., Giordani, B., Duvvi, K., Bhupendra, M. P., Torres, J., Nora, R., Neufeld, R., Mohs, R. C., &

Davis, K. L. (1990). Pharmacologic treatment of noncognitive behavioral disturbances in elderly demented patients. *American Journal of Psychiatry, 147*(12), 1640–1645.

Feil, N. (1989). Validation: An empathetic approach to the care of dementia. *Clinical Gerontologist, 8*, 89–94.

Ferrini, A. F., & Ferrini, R. L. (1992). *Health in the Later Years* (2nd ed.). Madison: Brown & Benchmark.

Fine, I. L., & Rouse-Bane, D. (1995). Using validation techniques to improve communication with cognitively impaired older adults. *Journal of Gerontological Nursing, 21*(6), 39–45.

Francis, J. (1992). Delirium in older patients. *Journal of the American Geriatrics Society, 40*, 829–838.

Gorbien, M. J., Bishop, J., Beers, M. H., Norman, D., Osterweil, D., & Rubenstein, L. Z. (1992). Iatrogenic illness in hospitalized elderly people. *Journal of the American Geriatric Society, 40*, 1031–1042.

Griepp, A., Landau-Stanton, J., & Clementis, C. D. (1993). The neuropsychiatric aspects of HIV infection and patient care. In J. Landau-Stanton & C. D. Clements (Eds.), *AIDS health and mental health : A primary source book* (pp. 192–213). New York: Brunner/Mazel.

Hitch, S. (1994). Cognitive therapy as a tool for caring for the elderly confused person. *Journal of Clinical Nursing, 3*(1), 49–55.

Hollander, H., & Katz, M. H. (1997). HIV Infection. In L. M. Tierney, S. J. McPhee, & M. A. Papadakis (Eds.), *Current medical diagnosis & treatment* (36th ed., pp. 1178–1202). Stamford, CT: Appleton & Lange.

Inaba-Roland, K. E., & Maricle, R. A. (1992). Assessing delirium in acute care setting. *Heart and Lung, 21*(1), 48–55.

Kubler-Ross, E. (1969). *On death and dying*. New York: Macmillian.

Lipowski, Z. J. (1992). Update on delirium. *Psychiatric Clinics of North America, 15*(2), 335–346.

Neese, J. B. (1991). Depression in the general hospital. *Nursing Clinics of North America, 26*(3), 613–622.

Neese, J. B., & Abraham, I. L. (1992). Group interventions with the elderly. In K. C. Buckwalter (Ed.), *Geriatric mental health nursing: Current and future challenges* (pp.75–83). Thorofare, NJ: Slack

North American Nursing Diagnosis Association. (1994). *NANDA nursing diagnoses: Definition & classification.* St. Louis: Mosby.

Rawlins, R. P., Williams, S. R., & Beck, C. K. (1993). *Mental health-psychiatric nursing: A holistic life-cycle approach* (3rd ed., pp. 649–670). St. Louis: Mosby.

Schor, J. D., Levoff, S. E., Lipsitz, L. A., Reily, C. H., Cleary, P. D., Rowe, J. W., & Evans, D. A. (1992). Risk factors for delirium in hospitalized elderly. *JAMA, 267*(6), 827–831.

St. Pierre, J. (1996). Delirium in hospitalized elderly patients: Off track. *Critical Care Nursing Clinics of North America, 8*(1), 53–60.

Tappen, R. M. (1994). The effect of skill training on functional abilities of nursing home residents with dementia. *Research in Nursing and Health, 17*(3), 159–165.

Thompson-Heisterman, A. A., Smullen, D. E., & Abraham, I.L. (1992). Psychogeriatric nursing assessment. In K. C. Buckwalter (Ed.), *Geriatric mental health nursing: Current and future challenges* (pp. 17–26). Thorofare, NJ: Slack.

Tune, L., Carr, S., Hoag, E., & Cooper, T. (1992). Anticholinergic effects of drugs commonly prescribed for the elderly: Potential means for assessing risk of delirium. *American Journal of Psychiatry, 149*(10), 1393–1394.

Tune, L., & Ross, C. (1994). Delirium. In C. E. Coffey & J. L. Cummings (Eds.), *Textbook of geriatric neuropsychiatry* (p. 352–265). Washington, DC: American Psychiatric Press.

Whall, A. L. (1995). Disruptive behavior in late stage dementia: Using natural environments to decrease distress. *Journal of Gerontological Nursing, 21*(10), 56 - 57.

Yi, E. S., Abraham, I. L., & Holroyd, S. (1994). Alzheimer's disease and nursing: New scientific and clinical insights. *Nursing Clinics of North America, 29*(1), 85–99.

Behavioral and Emotional Disorders of Childhood and Adolescence

Michele L. Zimmerman

CHILD AND ADOLESCENT PSYCHIATRIC MENTAL HEALTH NURSING

Professional Standards

- Specialists in this area hold a master's or doctoral degree in child and adolescent psychiatric nursing and are certified as clinical specialists in child and adolescent psychiatric nursing by the American Nurses's Credentialing Center. They are recognized by their peers as Advanced Practice Registered Nurses.

- Standards for the child and adolescent psychiatric mental health nurse are set forth in *Statement on Psychiatric-Mental Health Clinical Nursing Practice and Standards of Psychiatric Nursing Practice* (1994).

Issues and Concerns

- Lifestyle and Environment

    1. 7.5 million children and adolescents, 12% of the total population, suffer a mental disorder; only 7%, the most disordered, receive help; there are high, and possibly increasing rates of psychiatric disorders in children and adolescents (Botz & Bidwell-Cerone, 1997; Zimmerman, 1997; Leaf, Algeria, Cohen, Goodman, Horwitz, Hoven, Narrow, Vaden-Kiernan & Regier, 1996).

        a. One in three children and adolescents do not receive care

        b. Many receive no treatment, or inappropriate treatment

        c. Negative outcomes increase progressively—if one risk factor for childhood mental illness is present, there is no greater incidence of childhood mental illness than no risk factors; but two risk factors increase the likelihood four times (Antai-Otong, 1995)

    2. The emotional, behavioral, and social baselines against which psychiatric conditions in children are identified and treated are more fluid than those of adults. Variations in behavior need close attention. Developmental assessment is critical.

    3. Medicine administered in childhood may alter normal psychological, behavioral and physiological development of children and adolescents. Because of that concern, children who would benefit from medicine may be denied treatment (Antai-Otong, 1995).

4. Increase in the prevalence of anxiety disorders, substance abuse, disruptive behavior disorders and serious depression

5. Suicide rate for youngsters age 15 to 19 has tripled since the 1960s.

6. All psychiatric disorders in adolescence appear to show some degree of comorbidity which leads to:

   a. Increased mental health service use

   b. Impaired role functioning

   c. Likelihood of suicidal behavior

   d. Academic problems

   e. Conflict with parents

7. Children and adolescents do not self-refer; impetus usually comes from adults such as parents and teachers (Journal of the American Academy of Child & Adolescent Psychiatry [JAACAP], 1997a)

- Cultural and Ethnic Considerations

  1. Cultural weaknesses

     a. Lack of acculturation means children of immigrants are at greater risk for depression and suicide (Hovey & King, 1996)

     b. Some folk medicine practices and child rearing practices may be perceived as abusive by Western cultural standards. The nurse needs to observe and educate parents about certain practices (Zimmerman, 1997), but needs to be aware of other cultural beliefs before imposing Western practices.

  2. Cultural strengths

     a. Strong loyalty to family, family cohesiveness and family ownership of children's problems in Native Americans, African-Americans, and Asian families

     b. Strong supportive extended family linkages and sharing in child care tasks by family, friends and neighbors in families of color

     c. Cultural emphasis on discipline, obedience to rules, and respect for elders who are sources of advice for child rearing in Asian families

    d.   Having bicultural competence preserves cultural identity while the child negotiates the dominant culture

    e.   Humor as a means of coping with adversity is a strength

    f.   Independence for children in Native American families; interdependence of siblings in Hispanic families

    g.   Strong religious values, customs, rituals and institutions that provide spiritual support and reinforce strong, ethical values for life decisions, and give meaning to life; churches provide group socialization activities and supplementary child care

    h.   Value placed on education of children, who are seen as the hope for the future by African-Americans and Asians

    i.   Strong ethnic community representatives and organizations that help people of color to bargain, negotiate, and obtain resources from larger societal systems (Gaudin,1993)

- Risk Factors For Mental And Emotional Disorders Are Increased In:

    1.   Children who live in poverty and in crowded, inner city environments (poverty increases intensity of all other risk factors)

    2.   Children of mentally ill and substance abusing parents

    3.   Children who are abused physically or sexually

    4.   Children of minority ethnic status (associated with poverty)

    5.   Children of teenage parents

    6.   Children in families with marital discord, parental conflict, divorce, instability in family environment, children in foster care

    7.   Children with chronic illness or disability

    8.   Children with prolonged parent child separation, multiple separations, frequent changes in primary caretaker

    9.   Homelessness (families with children are the fastest growing segment of the homeless population)

    10.   Native-American children from certain tribes whose suicide rates are 2-3 times that of the rest of the U.S. population for the same age

- Biological Or Genetic Insults That May Negatively Impact A Child's Mental Health Include:

1. Low birth weight

2. Developmental delay

3. Brain damage

4. Epilepsy

5. Addiction as a result of maternal substance abuse

6. Early difficulties in adjustment between infant and primary care-taker temperament styles

7. Mental retardation

8. Genetic defects

- Physical Illness And Impairments

  1. Illness often interferes with the acquisition of skills and negotiation of developmental milestones

  2. Children have fears and anxieties related to their developmental age, and the younger the child, the fewer coping strategies

  3. Regression occurs in the face of illness or disability

  4. Chronic illness may pose greater risk for psychological disturbance

  5. Children with AIDS are at particularly high risk

     a. Family dysfunction—extreme poverty, drug abuse, social isolation and/or homelessness

     b. Parental ill health or social stigmatization

  6. Circumstances that may decrease risk:

     a. Presence of primary attachment figure during the child's illness and or/hospitalization

     b. Family's functionality—stress management, coping, competence and ability to support child appropriately

     c. Community support and respite care for family

     d. Partnership of family and providers in assisting child to adapt to illness or impairment

     e. Attention to psychological and social needs along with physical and medical issues within the context of the child's developmental stage

       f. Assistance in achieving developmental milestones, realistic academic goals, self-esteem, mastery and social support (Johnson, 1995)

       g. Parents or caretakers who create an environment with non-threatening language, descriptive praise, play and related activity, mediated learning experiences and positive self talk (Johnson, 1995)

- Child Factors Which Reduce The Risk Of Psychopathology:

  1. Problem solving ability

  2. Social skills

  3. Warm, caring relationship with a supportive, consistent adult

  4. Compensatory experiences outside the home

  5. Personality characteristics such as perceived competence and social acceptance

  6. Normal intellectual development

  7. Social support from family, peers, and teachers (Johnson, 1997; Krauss, 1993)

- Family Constellations and Stressors: Child's functioning and well-being are dependent on the family and school setting in which he or she lives and studies (JAACAP, 1997a)

  1. Nuclear families

     a. Economic pressures on both parents to work

     b. Lack of adequate day care and the low priority given to child care

     c. Poor parenting skills

  2. Adoptive families

     a. Recent court rulings returning children to birth families

     b. Adopted children at higher risk for emotional mental disorders for a variety of complex reasons

  3. Separation and divorce

     a. Parental discord prior to a separation and divorce

    b.   Continuous discord regarding custody, visitation, child support and each parent's activities and friends

    c.   Children exposed to parental separation before school entry may show increased risk of later conduct or oppositional and mood disorders

    d.   Children exposed to parental separation after age 10 show increased risk of substance abuse

    e.   Children and adolescents in therapy may focus on parent's separation as a major event in their lives

4.   Blended families

    a.   Children must adjust to stepparents, stepsiblings and stepgrandparents

    b.   Visitation schedules often disrupt family routines; children often feel resentment, anger and a sense of abandonment

    c.   Loyalty conflicts and attachment problems are common and relate to child's developmental stages

5.   Alternative lifestyles

    a.   Children sense they are different or are teased

    b.   Adolescent peer pressure and developmental needs propel the youngster to fit in with the peer culture

6.   Foster families

    a.   Number of children in foster care increasing; 659,000 children served by the system in 1993, of which over 461,300 lived in foster care; 75% placed due to maltreatment or inadequate care (Rosen, 1998)

    b.   Fastest increase among infants and young children

    c.   Time in care is also increasing

    d.   Lack of permanency prevents the development of significant interpersonal relationships

    e.   Extremely high rate of psychopathology in children placed in out of home care, e.g., depression, conduct disorder, learning disabilities, and attention deficit disorder

      f.   Higher rates of developmental delay, educational problems, drug use, sexual activity and pregnancy

      g.   Highly elevated rates of physical health problems

      h.   Recommendations for mental health care followed less than half the time (Risley-Curtiss, 1996)

      i.   Crisis due to loyalty conflicts, loss of the foster parent, and/or impending return to a biological parent (Pilowsky & Kates, 1996)

- Access To Health Care

  1. Services for children are inadequate, inappropriate, or unavailable

  2. Over 12 million U.S. children lack health insurance

  3. Cutbacks in funding of mental health services have affected psychiatric care of children and adolescents

  4. Inadequate residential care is available

  5. In order to obtain services for their children, many parents must give custody to the state

  6. Inadequate numbers of mental health professionals are trained to provide the needed mental health services for children and adolescents

  7. Cost containment measures by managed care impact services

- Community Background

  1. Cultural context

  2. How family relates to neighborhood

  3. Religious and ethnic orientation

  4. Neighborhood resources and adverse circumstances

     a. Poverty

     b. Poor housing

     c. Crime or urban violence (JAACAP, 1997a)

Treatment Modalities in Childhood and Adolescence

- Individual Psychotherapy

  1. Supportive therapy

2. Play therapy—most commonly used modality with children; play therapy is an intervention defined as the purposeful use of toys and other equipment to assist child in communicating his or her perception of the world and to help him or her master environment (Zimmerman, 1997)

    a. Structured play encourages child to express the unconscious; therapist may encourage child to play or replay a scene

    b. Mutual story telling encourages children to express feelings or re-enact a trauma or loss, puppets may be used

    c. Nondirective play—children permitted to play without direction from the therapist

    d. Behavioral play—play to help child learn new ways of behaving

3. Behavioral modification—behavior therapists actively direct treatment:

    a. Most useful when implemented in home, classroom, and with individual child

    b. Parents taught behavioral management strategies

    c. Children and adolescents learn self-control and relaxation techniques

    d. Treatment goals are mutually set with child, therapist and parents

    e. Compatible with solution focused, short term approaches. (Zimmerman, 1997)

4. Cognitive therapy is beneficial for children aged 9 to 10 and older; cognitive therapy enables child and adolescent to utilize coping self-statements and to overcome dysfunctional cognitive distortions

5. Skills training has as its goal helping children achieve competence in mastering developmental tasks and to make use of environmental and personal resources to achieve a good outcome (Bloomquist, 1996)

- Group therapy

    1. Childhood

        a. Social skills groups

  b. Emotional expression

  c. Behavioral expression

  d. Protection from unsafe environment

  e. Coping with divorce, separation and blended families

  f. Recovery groups for children of substance abusing parents

  g. Art therapy groups for identification and expression of feelings

 2. Adolescence

  a. Peer relationships

  b. Substance abuse recovery/12 Step group

  c. Communication with parents

  d. Coping with divorce, separation and blended families

  e. Critical incident debriefing

  f. Decrease impulsive and high-risk behavior

- Family Therapy

 1. Helps family achieve healthy coping and interrupts behaviors that maintain child or adolescents symptoms

 2. Usually a mandatory component of a child's therapeutic environment; parental involvement is strong predictor of positive outcomes for child

 3. Problems treated:

  a. Communication and expression of feelings among family members

  b. Limit-setting skills

  c. Rules, consequences and rewards

  d. Dealing with separation dynamics

- Milieu Therapy

 1. Physical setting

  a. Age appropriate furniture that is mobile for arranging small conversation area

    b.   Games, puzzles, books and toys geared to developmental level of residents

    c.   Provision for safety

    d.   Sociopetal structure with all client rooms entering a central family room fosters interaction and supports safety

    e.   Warm, home like ambience with pictures, plants, padded furniture

    f.   Provision for privacy in sleeping, dressing and bathing while allowing necessary monitoring and supervision

    g.   Children and adolescents need own "space" for possessions, school work, writing, etc.

    h.   Provision of active orientation to treatment

        (1)   Bulletin boards with calendars, schedules, staff names

        (2)   Patient names, assignments, primary therapist and staff member, privilege level and point system

2.   Structured treatment programs

    a.   Philosophy—child and adolescent programs often based on a family systems model with developmental perspective

        (1)   Inpatient unit becomes a family that provides for expression of feelings, effective communication between members, development of coping skills and positive recreational experiences

        (2)   Family life simulated with meal preparation and other routine activities; birthdays and celebrations are planned and implemented

    b.   Rules, limit setting, and consequences

        (1)   Unit rule books

        (2)   Consistency in application of rules and consequences

        (3)   Peer or buddy system for older children and adolescents

        (4)   Positive reinforcement rather than punishment

        (5)   Point system for privileges with higher points indicating a higher level with more privileges

        (6)   Recognition in community meeting

(7) Limit setting is on a continuum with positive social interaction at one end and time out on the other

    (a) Positive social interaction such as smiles, nods, and encouragement

    (b) Extinction used for mildly inappropriate behaviors by withholding positive reinforcements or ignoring behavior; inappropriate behavior usually escalates after period of ignoring prior to extinguishing

    (c) Providing direction

    (d) Verbal reprimand or specific statements that point out consequences if inappropriate behavior continues

    (e) Privilege removal should be natural consequence to the behavior

    (f) Time out allows child to reflect and regain control and should equate to one minute per year of development (Johnson,1995; Antai-Otong, 1995)

  c. Treatment level system—organized, concrete way to show child's progress through treatment

    (1) Expectations and privileges increase with advance to next treatment level or phase

    (2) Child or adolescent may earn a set number of points each day; increased privileges are attached to higher levels

  3. School program must be provided as part of inpatient, partial or residential programs for children and adolescents

- Medication Management For Children

  1. Children differ in response to medication's main and side effects

  2. Children may metabolize and eliminate medications more rapidly

  3. When medicating children, start slow, titrate carefully, use lowest effective dose

  4. Final dose may be higher than in adults because of metabolic and organ differences

5. Clinical observations of effects are essential because of absence of carefully controlled studies of pharmacotherapy in children

6. Variation in dosing between adults and children considers difference in size, metabolism, and desired action

7. Combined pharmacotherapy is being used safely in children; same considerations in introducing multiple medicines apply to children as to adults

8. Antihistamines lower seizure threshold and cause delirium and worsening of tic disorders

9. Lithium is cleared rapidly by children, so they may require higher doses to stabilize a mood disorder

10. Valproate (Depakote) may be hepatotoxic in children under age 10

11. MAOIs are contraindicated in pediatric population due to dietary and other risks

12. Children both metabolize neuroleptics more rapidly and are more sensitive to their main effects

13. Stimulants are first line of treatment for attention deficit hyperactivity disorder (AD/HD) and this practice is generally continued through adolescence into adulthood

14. SSRIs are generally considered safe and effective for treatment of depression and some anxiety disorders in children

15. Buspirone (BuSpar) may be helpful in managing aggression and agitation in children with mental retardation or a pervasive development disorder (PDD) (Zimmerman, 1997)

- Medication Management For Adolescents

    1. Establishment of trust is essential because of developmental issues regarding control by authority

    2. More susceptible to extrapyramidal side effects

    3. Teens have poor fluid intake, which makes them susceptible to constipation, dry mouth, and urinary retention

    4. Vital signs need monitoring for potential hypotension

    5. Drowsiness may interfere with school

6. Abuse of medications include selling medications at school, especially antianxiety or sympathomimetic agents

7. Adolescent, family, and school professionals should understand indications, responses, interactions and compliance issues to facilitate proper adjustment of medication dosage

8. Adolescent, family, school and other psychiatric professionals must have reasonable expectations of medications

9. Monitor for potential overdose when patient is experiencing suicidal thoughts (Botz & Bidwell-Cerone, 1997)

Adolescent Behavioral Problems

- Violence

  1. Adolescent acting out behavior is rising; juvenile crime rate increased by 50% from 1985 to 1991

  2. Rate of victimization of teens is twice that of the general population.

  3. Girls 14 to 15 years of age have highest risk of any age group of being raped (Johnson, 1997)

  4. Violence by juveniles usually acted out on other juveniles; nearly one million juveniles between ages of 12 to 19 years of age are raped, robbed or assaulted . . . twice that of the general population

  5. Lethality of teenage violence is increasing; teenage violent death rate rose 13% between 1985 and 1991

  6. Teenage violent death rate is increasing; 12% to 31% of the general adolescent population have elevated depressive symptomatology placing them at risk for Major Depression

  7. Positive correlation between juvenile violent behavior and adult violent behavior

- Youth Gangs and Violence

  1. Antisocial behavior in adolescence positively associated with depression

  2. Conduct disorder associated with involvement with a delinquent peer group

3. Victims of teen violence are being killed rather than injured; (Johnson, 1997); increasingly, firearms are involved in adolescent homicide and suicide; teenage homicide rate has doubled since 1985

4. Gangs and cults—alienated adolescents who have not internalized social norms may align with deviant subcultures or gangs

   a. Gangs offer the adolescent the following:

      (1) Companionship

      (2) Loyalty

      (3) Identity

      (4) Status

   b. Cults

      (1) Specialized gangs organized around belief system expressed through ceremonies and rites

      (2) Usually led by charismatic authority figures who say they possess special powers

      (3) Leaders create atmosphere of awe to impress and recruit new members

      (4) Secrecy hides undesirable aspects of cult

      (5) Cohesiveness maintained by shared allegiance to belief system, rituals, and leader

      (6) Satanic cults offer adolescents a sense of power

      (7) Cults are antisocial because they reject prevailing social norms

      (8) Cults draw adolescents who are desperate, angry and alone by providing structure, mastery, control, and belonging (Haber, 1997)

- Runaways

   1. 500,000 to 2 million youngsters (mainly adolescents) run away from home each year and another 900,000 have no home (Mohr, 1998)

      a. Situational runaways—largest subgroup; circumstances include:

(1) Eldest daughters seeking relief from major household responsibilities (delegating family dynamics)

(2) Adolescents used as pawns in parental conflicts

(3) Parents trying to obstruct normal adolescent separation process (binding family dynamics)

(4) Reunion fantasy causing adolescents to run away as a ploy to pull parents together

b. Departure runaways—depressed and angry about treatment at home and hungry for affection and a sense of belonging; escape is a genuine survival tactic

c. Throwaways—youth who are asked to leave home (expelling family dynamics); usually endure lifestyles similar to departure runaways; approximately 200,000 to 600,000 have been thrown out, agree to leave, or are removed by authorities (Mohr, 1998)

2. Circumstances associated with departure runaways and throwaways include the following:

a. Parental criminal activity, violence, alcoholism, and addiction

b. Overall chaotic home environment

c. Physical, emotional, and sexual abuse and neglect

d. Conflicts over same-sex orientation

3. Population of children and adolescents with no social service support

a. Become homeless street people and often turn to prostitution, drug dealing, stealing and panhandling to survive; most cannot return home due to high degree of dysfunction

b. Vulnerable to exploitation; group at highest possible risk for rape, assault, homicide, depression, suicide, drug overdosing, pregnancies, poor nutrition, poor hygiene, sleep deprivation and STDs including HIV/AIDS and communicable diseases (Botz & Bidwell-Cerone, 1997; Haber, 1997; Mohr, 1998)

- Substance Abuse Disorders (SUD)

1. Prevalence rate among adolescents is 32%; higher among those at high risk for social impairment

2. Associated with mood, anxiety, and disruptive behavior disorders

3. Adolescent drug and alcohol abuse is major health problem and precedes later drug and alcohol dependency

4. Disrupts adolescent's ability to meet developmental tasks

5. Associated with:

   a. Accidents, suicides and psychiatric illness

   b. Dual diagnosis, especially depression, AD/HD, and conduct disorder

   c. Teenage pregnancy, infant morbidity and mortality, high risk sexual behavior and STD

      (1) Children of cocaine addicted mothers may experience difficulty in bonding; at risk for multiple problems, including low birth weight

      (2) Cocaine interferes with parental bonding and empathy

      (3) Infants born to alcohol dependent/alcohol addicted mothers are at risk for fetal alcohol syndrome; infants are difficult to soothe, are at high risk for later developmental abnormalities, disruptive behavior disorders and mental retardation

   d. Parental substance use

   e. Emotional distance between parent and adolescent and lack of involvement in adolescent's life

   f. Lack of supervision and discipline

   g. Low self-esteem, high population density, high crime (JAACAP, 1997g)

6. Developmental issues are often delayed, disrupted, or arrested when adolescents become substance abusers

7. Strong evidence to support a genetic or constitutional risk for SUD

8. Treatment programs use interventions similar to adult programs (12 Step programs, family involvement, reliance on group confrontation)

   a. Goal is to achieve abstinence

    b.   Address co-existing behavioral and psychiatric problems; family functioning, academic functioning and peer relations (JAACAP, 1997g)

    c.   Substance abuse is often a way of dealing with chronic stress and family dysfunction, so entire family must be targeted for intervention

CHILD MALTREATMENT

Incidence—1,012,000 children were victims of child abuse and neglect in 1994, a 27% increase over 1990; neglect = 45%, physical abuse = 25%, sexual abuse = 16%, psychological maltreatment = 6%, and "other" = 8%

Ages—twenty-seven percent of all victims were under 3 years, and another 20% were between 4 and 6 years of age (National Center of Child Abuse and Neglect (NCCAN), 1996)

Research agenda—needs to focus on case finding and prevention

Neglect—affects 1.2 million children by actual reports, probably impossible to estimate actual scope because neglect is easily overlooked

- Physical Neglect—most widely recognized and commonly identified form of neglect; includes failure to protect from harm or danger and provide for child's basic physical needs (shelter, food, clothing)

- Emotional Neglect—more difficult to document or substantiate, often beginning when children are too young to communicate or know they are not receiving appropriate care

    1.   Extreme form of neglect leads to nonorganic failure to thrive

    2.   American Humane Association describes emotional neglect as passive or passive/aggressive inattention to child's emotional needs, nurturing, or emotional well-being (Erickson & Egelund, 1996)

    3.   'Psychologically unavailable" parents overlook infants' cues and signals, especially cries and pleas for warmth and comfort

    4.   Has serious long term consequences for child; emotionally neglected children expect their needs will not be met, and do not even try to solicit care and warmth; they expect failure, therefore lack motivation

5. Neglectful parents:

    a. Lack an understanding of children's behavior and parent-child relationship

    b. Experience a great deal of stress

    c. Are socially isolated or unsupported

    d. Have a history of inadequate care themselves

6. Emotional availability of parents includes:

    a. Parental sensitivity

    b. Child responsiveness

    c. Parental nonintrusiveness

    d. Involvement of parent with child

- Medical Neglect

  1. Caregivers' failure to provide prescribed medical treatment for their children, e.g., immunizations, prescribed medication, recommended surgery

  2. May involve clash between parents' religious beliefs and recommendations of medical community

- Mental Health Neglect—caregivers' refusal to comply with recommended corrective or therapeutic procedures

- Educational Neglect—failure to comply with state regulations for school attendance (Erickson & Egelund, 1996)

Physical Abuse (Incidence and prevalence rates vary based on restrictiveness of definition)

- Child Characteristics Related To Abuse

  1. Early health problems increase risk

      a. Medical

      b. Intellectual

      c. Developmental aberrations

  2. Temperament/behavior

      a. Difficult temperament (impulsivity, crying)

      b. Conduct problems

      c. High activity

      d. Limited sociability

- Parental Characteristics Related To Abuse

  1. Heightened levels of distress or dysfunction

      a. Depression

      b. Physical symptoms

      c. Substance abuse

      d. Posttraumatic Stress Disorder (PTSD)

  2. Early physical punishment of parent

      a. Adults who experience or witness abuse during childhood are exposed to aversive models and use aggressive discipline with children

      b. Violence becomes transgenerational and multiplied; victims may reenact the trauma by identifying with the aggressor and acting out on others

      c. 30% of those abused as children abuse their own children.

  3. Personality disturbances

      a. Hostile personality

      b. Parental explosiveness

      c. Irritability and use of threats

  4. Cognitive style

      a. Negative cognitive attributional style—perceive children in negative light

      b. Belief in strict physical discipline

      c. Have high expectations of children in relation to age appropriate behaviors and cognitive skills

  5. Behavioral functioning

      a. Inconsistent child-rearing practices reflecting critical, hostile or aggressive management styles

      b. Poor problem solving ability; less attention-directing verbal and physical strategies, less mutual interaction in free play and problem solving situations

6. Biological factors—hyperarousal to stressful child as measured by autonomic arousal

7. Family system characteristics

   a. Coercive parent-child interactions

   b. Poor family relationships/family context of hostility

8. Experiences of abuse and violence are related to development of personality disorders, depressive, anxiety and dissociative disorders.

- Sexual Abuse

  1. Occurs between a child and adult, or older child; is defined as sexual contact or interaction for purpose of sexual stimulation/gratification of adult or older child (Monteleone, Glaze & Bly, 1994)

  2. Sexual acts range from least severe to most severe and intrusive

     a. Noncontact acts—making sexual comments to child, exposure, voyeurism, pornographic material viewing, inducing child to undress

     b. Sexual contact

        (1) Offender touching child's breasts, buttocks, genitals or asking child to touch his/her genitals

        (2) Frottage—rubbing genitals against victim's body or clothing for pleasure

        (3) Digital or object penetration

        (4) Oral sex—offender to child or child forced to perform on offender

        (5) Penile penetration—vaginal or anal

        (6) Intercourse with animals

  3. Circumstances of sexual abuse

     a. Dyadic

     b. Group sex

     c. Sex rings

     d. Sexual exploitation

      e. Child pornography

      f. Child prostitution

  4. Social conditions increasing risk of sexual abuse:

      a. Separated from both biological parents or runaway

      b. Raised in poverty

      c. Child handicapped

      d. Alcoholic family member

      e. Drug abusing family member

      f. Prostitution at home

      g. Transient adults living in home

      h. Mentally ill caretaker

      i. AIDS related disability of caretaker (Monteleone, Glaze, & Bey, 1994)

  5. Impact of sexual abuse on child

      a. Traumatic sexualization

      b. Stigmatization

      c. Betrayal

      d. Powerlessness

  6. Traumatic amnesia—may interfere with processing event and placing it in past memory (Whitfield, 1998)

- Ritual Abuse

  1. Abuse which occurs in a context linked to symbols or group activities with religious, magical or supernatural connotation; invocation of these symbols or activities, repeated over time, is used to frighten and intimidate children

  2. Intentional physical, sexual or psychological abuse of child by person responsible for child's welfare; such abuse is repeated and/or stylized; is typified by other acts, e.g., cruelty to animals, threats of harm to child, other persons and animals (Briere, 1996).

  3. Incidence difficult to determine due to problems in reporting, definition and categorization; professional skepticism; child's fear of reporting

4. Reports indicate a greater impact on victim than non-ritual abuse; ritually abused children demonstrate more symptoms on standardized assessments

5. Ritual abuse—receives a great deal of media attention, yet constitutes a very small proportion of the maltreatment (Briere, Berliner, Bulkley, Jenny & Reid, 1996)

Assessment of Child Maltreatment

- Conducted Within The Context Of The Environment
- Issues To Be Considered In Assessment

    1. Ethnicity and socioeconomic status

    2. Social desirability and reporting bias

    3. Professional roles may affect outcomes of assessment (interviewer bias, lack of training, leading questions)

    4. Use of standardized measures

    5. Multiaxial assessment

    6. Assessment information from children

        a. Behavioral report and /or observation

        b. Casual observations

        c. Mental status examination

        d. Projective assessments and drawings

        e. Projective storytelling/aperception tests

        f. Rorschach

        g. Cognitive assessments

        h. Bayley scales of infant development (BSID)

        i. Wechsler series of intelligence tests for children

        j. Kaufman assessment battery for children (K-ABC)

        k. Clinical Interviews

        l. Nondirective play sessions

        m. Structured psychiatric diagnostic interviews

    7. Assessment information from parents

      a.   The Child Behavior Checklist (CBCL)

      b.   The Vineland Adaptive Behavior scales (VABS)

8.   Family assessment

      a.   Standardized measures of family assessment

      b.   Clinical interviews

9.   Supplemental information

      a.   Teachers/school personnel

      b.   CBCL Teacher Report

      c.   Caseworkers

      d.   Foster parents/supplemental caretakers

10.   Assessment of risk of harm to self and/or others

      a.   Suicide

      b.   Self destructive behavior

      c.   Danger to others

      d.   Risk of revictimization

Maltreated Children and Therapy

- Reasons Most Children Are Brought To Therapy

    1.   Child is showing symptoms of abuse or neglect

    2.   Parents are concerned about how child is affected by abuse or neglect

- Child Factors That Affect Progress In Therapy

    1.   Willingness to participate in therapy

    2.   Ability to acknowledge experience of abuse or neglect

    3.   Capacity to use therapy

          a.   Genetic make-up

          b.   Level of functioning

          c.   Phase of development

          d.   Content and intensity of the event

     e. Accumulated life events and history of prior trauma

     f. Child needs reassurance to know that his /her needs will be addressed in therapy

- Essentials Components Of Successful Therapy

  1. Trust—physical and emotional

  2. Needs assessment

  3. History taking (essential)

  4. Family genogram (essential)

  5. Strong alliance with parent or caretaker

- Stages Of Therapy In Treating Sexual Assault (Hartman & Burgess, 1998)

  1. Management of defensive patterns

  2. Anchoring for safety

  3. Psychoeducation regarding complex trauma response

  4. Strengthen personal resources

  5. Surface trauma information

  6. Processing the trauma

  7. Future and transformation

- Assessment Of Sexual Abuse

  1. Specialized skill; should not be performed by professionals who have not been trained and supervised in this modality

  2. Recommended role of evaluator and therapist be kept separate (American Professional Society on the Abuse of Children [APSAC], 1997)

  3. Sexual acts are considered abusive when the following are present:

     a. Power differential

     b. Knowledge differential

     c. Gratification differential

  4. History is most difficult phase of evaluation and most important

5.   Both physical and behavioral assessment are necessary in establishing likelihood of abuse, however, majority of sexually abused children have no physical evidence

   a.   Child Sexual Behavior Inventory-3—valid instrument for assessing sexually abused children aged 2 to 12 (Friedrich, Berliner, Butler, Cohen, Damon, Shafram, 1996)

   b.   Sexualized behavior continues to be one of the most valid markers of sexual abuse in children (children who demonstrate sexual behavior)

      (1)   Sexual play

      (2)   Sexual talk

      (3)   Sexual actions, e.g., compulsive masturbation or attempts to engage others in sexual activity

      (4)   Touching other's genitals

      (5)   Asking others to touch them (Friedrich, et al., 1996)

- Sexual Abuse Treatment

   1.   Goals

      a.   Deal with effects of sexual abuse

      b.   Decrease risk for future abuse

   2.   Treatment issues for victim

      a.   Trust

      b.   Emotional reactions to sexual abuse

      c.   Responsibility for act

      d.   Altered sense of self

      e.   Anxiety and fear

      f.   Behavioral reactions to sexual abuse

         (1)   Sexualized behavior

         (2)   Aggression

         (3)   Runaway

         (4)   Self-harm

         (5)   Criminal activity

(6) Substance abuse

(7) Suicidal behavior

(8) Hyperactivity

(9) Sleep problems

(10) Eating problems

(11) Toileting problems

- Therapeutic questions

  1. What happened?

  2. Why did it happen?

  3. Why did you behave as you did then and since then?

  4. What will you do if something like this happens again?

- Modalities

  1. Group therapy

     a. Treatment of choice for sexual abuse except for patients who are too disturbed or disruptive

     b. Screen members

     c. Six to eight members; three to six with younger children

     d. Minimum of sixteen to twenty sessions

     e. Long term, open ended treatment helpful for adolescents

     f. Group should include several well socialized children (Friedrich, et al., 1996)

     g. Skills building for problem-solving (Bloomquist, 1996)

  2. Individual treatment (including play therapy)—also appropriate with an emphasis on alliance building

  3. Dyadic treatment—used to repair relationship between victim and nonoffending adult

  4. Family therapy—if reunification is in victim's best interest

  5. Use of multiple therapists indicated

     a. Range of services

     b. Shared responsibility for multiproblem families; one therapist can be overwhelmed with demands of highly needy families with multiple problems and multiple agency involvement

 c. Therapist support

 d. Co-therapy demonstrates a variety of roles to the patient

 e. Shared decision making (Faller, 1993)

6. Cognitive reactions to sexual abuse—child must be able to make sense of the abuse before it becomes suppressed, denied, or repressed and not resolved (Friedrich, et al., 1996)

7. Protection from future victimization

8. Pharmacotherapy to alleviate target symptoms, such as anxiety, depression or indications of posttraumatic stress

9. Therapy performed as part of a larger context in which safety, stability and support are provided (Friedrich, et al., 1996)

- Implications for Therapy With Ritual Abuse

 1. Higher incidence of PTSD

 2. Higher incidence of dissociative disorder

 3. Greater symptom severity

 4. Vicarious traumatization of the therapist because of greater impact on victim

Confidentiality

- Applies regardless of patient's age

- Information cannot be disclosed to outsiders without parental consent

- Decision to reveal information to parents is relative to child or adolescent's developmental age

 1. May be developmentally inappropriate to seek child's "consent" for disclosure to parents of information revealed during therapy

 2. May be developmentally and therapeutically appropriate to safeguard an adolescent's disclosures, even from parents

 3. Nurse should set ground rules for confidentiality during assessment/ evaluation

- If parent has abused or neglected a child, disclosure of confidential information to maltreating parent may be contraindicated regardless of the child's age

- Nurse should be familiar with legal concept of privilege

- Written records, notes, videotapes, drawings, and photographs may be subpoenaed

    1. Attorney issuing subpoena cannot require/force professional to produce records

    2. Subpoena does not override confidentiality requirement

    3. Patient should be consulted when subpoena for records is received

Legal issues in Child Abuse and Neglect

- First child abuse reporting laws enacted in 1963, following societal awareness of need for child protection

    1. C. Henry Kempe published the seminal article on Battered Child Syndrome in 1962.

    2. All professionals who work with children are mandated to report suspected abuse or neglect to designated child protection or law enforcement authorities.

        a. This includes both the generalist and specialist in psychiatric nursing

        b. Reporting laws override ethical duty to protect confidential information (Myers, 1992)

        c. Reporting requirement is triggered when there is evidence that would lead a competent professional to believe abuse or neglect is reasonably likely

        d. No requirement to prove abuse or neglect in order to file a report

        e. Professionals protected from retaliation for an unfounded or unsubstantiated report if report was made in good faith

        f. Misdemeanor charge for intentional failure to report

- Congress enacted Child Abuse Prevention and Treatment Act in 1974

    1. This established the National Center on Child Abuse and Neglect (NCCAN)

2. States must comply with Federal Guidelines to receive Federal funding, but have some choice how services are provided

- States have three kinds of laws (Pence & Wilson, 1992; Feller, 1992; Depanfilis & Salus, 1992)

    1. Reporting laws

        a. Define child abuse and neglect

        b. Specify conditions for state intervention in family life

        c. Encourage treatment approach rather than punitive

        d. Encourage coordination/cooperation among services

        e. Designate administrative structures for handling

    2. Juvenile and Family Court laws

        a. Emergency hearings—determine need for protection of alleged maltreated child

        b. Adjudicary hearings—determine if child has been maltreated

        c. Dispositional Hearings—determine action to be taken after adjudication

        d. Review hearings—review dispositions and determine need to continue placement for services and/or court intervention

    3. Criminal laws

        a. Define criminally punishable offenses

            (1) Law enforcement agencies investigate

            (2) Prosecutor decides if prosecution will occur

        b. Burden of proof beyond a reasonable doubt (stronger than in juvenile or family court)

        c. Defendants have full protection of 4th, 5th and 6th amendments (jury, cross examination, appointed counsel and speedy trial)

        d. Directed at deterring or rehabilitating defendant (probation or incarceration)

- Role(s) Of Clinical Nurse Specialist May Include:

    1. Evaluating children suspected of abuse

2. Providing therapy for abused children and for children experiencing legal proceedings related to abuse

3. Serving as expert witness in child abuse cases

4. Political action on behalf of children

5. Case management on behalf of children

- Nurses must be familiar with:

    1. Roles and responsibilities of various systems involved in child protection, including child protective services, police, and court system

    2. Emergency protective custody—all states provide mechanism to protect children in emergencies; police officers and in some states, child protective services' professionals and physicians have authority to take children into temporary protection custody; these laws have strict time limits

    3. Guidelines established for evaluation of children suspected of abuse (APSAC Guidelines, 1997)

    4. Laws in some states authorizing professionals to take pictures and x-rays without parental consent

- Expert Witness Testimony by CNS

    1. Before a person may testify as an expert witness, they must provide documentation of their expertise

        a. Educational accomplishments and licensure

        b. Specialized training, including board certifications, and continuing education

        c. Extent of experience with children or adolescents and direct clinical experience (% of practice time devoted to specified problem)

        d. Familiarity with relevant professional literature

        e. Membership in professional organizations

        f. Publications, presentations, teaching

        g. Honors, awards, professional recognition

    2. The form of expert testimony

        a. Opinion—expert witness permitted to offer professional opinions; expert must:

        (1)   Be reasonably confident of the opinion

        (2)   Employ appropriate methods of assessment and consider all relevant facts

        (3)   Understand pertinent clinical and scientific principles

        (5)   Be objective

        (6)   Provide rationale and information leading to the opinion

    b.   Answer to a hypothetical question

        (1)   Legal strategy whereby an attorney gives an extensive or lengthy, hypothetical statement and asks the expert to provide an answer to the hypothetical scenario

        (2)   Strategy generally falling out of favor

    c.   Expert testimony in the form of a dissertation

        (1)   Expert provides a lecture on a particular subject, e.g., the dynamics of a syndrome

        (2)   Testimony assists judge or jury to understand a phenomenon (Myers, 1992)

- Issues Regarding Child Testimony

    1.   Linked to interviewing of children

    2.   Interviews classified as investigative or therapeutic

    3.   Interviews conducted for purpose of treatment may be used in investigations

    4.   Goals for child investigative interviews include:

        a.   Minimizing trauma of the investigation

        b.   Maximizing information obtained

        c.   Minimizing contaminating effects of interview on the child's memory of the event

        d.   Maintaining integrity of the investigative process (Goodman & Bottoms, 1993)

    5.   Efforts underway to minimize gap between child's ability to testify and demands of legal system

- Sources Of Stress In Legal Proceedings Involving Children

  1. Long delays before trial which may:

     a. Create anxiety for victims

     b. Hamper therapeutic interventions.

     c. Affect child's memory (gives support to concept of videotaping early interviews)

  2. Lack of legal knowledge

     a. Preparation or orientation may help diminish child's anxiety

     b. Concept of "Court School" for child witnesses has been implemented; specialized training is available for child advocates to help orient children to courtroom procedures and stresses

  3. Intimidating courtroom environment

  4. Giving evidence in presence of accused

     a. Videotaped testimony and videolink can alleviate some stress

     b. Child's live testimony may have more impact on jury

     c. Possible prejudicing the defendant must be considered

  5. Being examined and cross-examined; difficulties for child include:

     a. Formality of interview procedures

     b. Unfamiliarity of language

     c. Challenging nature of cross-examination

     d. Time element in serious trials (Goodman & Bottoms, 1993)

- Forensic Nursing (Lynch & Burgess, 1998)

  1. CNS may serve as sexual assault nurse examiner (SANE) for children and adolescents

  2. CNS may have advanced training in collection of forensic evidence and classification of wounds

  3. CNS may review equivocal child death cases

  4. CNS may provide counseling for homicide victim's families

PSYCHOPATHOLOGY IN CHILDREN

Childhood Onset Schizophrenia (COS)

Early Onset Schizophrenia (EOS)

- Signs and symptoms
    1. Onset of psychotic symptoms before age 12 years (prepuberty) for COS; after for EOS; onset before age 6 years very rare
    2. Similarity of cognitive, neurologic, and linguistic deficits suggests the same disorder as adults, with greater severity and chronicity
    3. Same criteria used as for adults, but difficulties in applying criteria to children

- Differential Diagnosis
    1. Autism and other pervasive developmental disorders
    2. Neurological disorders
    3. Multidimensionally impaired (MDI)
        a. Mood lability and social ineptness present but not social withdrawal
        b. Most meet criteria for AD/HD
        c. Fleeting hallucinations
        d. Odd thinking, often in conjunction with language disorder
    4. Affective disorder—psychosis associated with bipolar disorder often misdiagnosed as schizophrenia
    5. Medical conditions and pharmacological agents (stimulants)
    6. Substance abuse
    7. Dissociative states
    8. Trauma related symptoms
    9. Associated with borderline personality disorder (Volkmar, 1996; (JAACAP), 1997f)
    10. Easier to diagnose in adolescents (EOS) than children (COS)
        a. Inability of preschool children to use rules of logic or notions

of reality makes it difficult to establish delusions or thought disorder

b. Focus on disorganized speech makes it difficult to evaluate a child with a language disorder

c. Hallucinations difficult to distinguish from sleep-related and other developmental phenomena

d. Need accurate information about premorbid functioning

- Nursing Diagnoses—same as adults
- Biological Origins

1. Neurodevelopmental models suppose a fixed lesion in interaction with a combination of genetic or nongenetic factors such as early viral CNS infection, autoimmune mechanisms or pregnancy/birth complication

2. Association of Asperger's with psychotic phenomena in children

3. Children with EOS may come from families with greater prevalence of disorder

4. Chromosomal abnormalities/prenatal insult

5. Eye-tracking abnormalities reported in adolescents at risk for schizophrenia; smooth pursuit abnormalities, or the inability to track a moving object with the eyes, specific for vulnerability to schizophrenia

6. Information processing deficits could underlie illogical thinking and loose associations

7. Position Emission Tomography (PET) evaluation shows striking right posterior parietal hypometabolism

- Mental Status Examination

1. Prodromal illness, exaggeration of that seen in adults

2. Motor clumsiness

3. Speech and language problems

4. Delay in language acquisition

5. Early diagnosis of disruptive or avoidant behaviors

6. Positive and negative symptoms

7. Auditory hallucinations most frequent, somatic and visual, less frequent

8. Higher baseline levels of thought disturbance

9. Loose associations and illogical thinking not typically seen in normal children after age 7

- Biochemical Approaches

    1. Similar medications used with both adults and children

    2. "Atypical" antipsychotics, such as risperidone and clozapine useful due to limited extrapyramidal side (EPS) effects; side effects of clozapine include agranulocytosis, and need close monitoring

    3. Comorbid depression may guide choice of agents in polypharmacy

    4. Since onset of therapeutic effect not apparent until some time after treatment started, rapid switching of agents is not helpful

    5. Stimulant use contraindicated due to capacity to induce psychotic symptoms (Volkmar, 1996)

- Psychotherapeutic Approaches

    1. Individual therapy based on:

        a. Developmental stage

        b. Degree of active thought disorder

        c. Ability to tolerate intimacy, and assessment of the degree of importance of the relationship to the child

        d. Encouragement of focus on reality of outside world

        e. Refocusing disordered thinking

        f. Setting limits on inappropriate behavior (Jongsma, Peterson & McInnis, 1996)

    2. Supportive therapy based on whether expression or suppression of affect is desired

    3. Expressive therapy

    4. Social skills training

    5. Special educational interventions

- Family Dynamics And Family Therapy

1. Parents often report children appeared normal at birth

2. Families experience profound sadness, guilt and self blame; older theories of "schizophrenogenic mothers" and cold, rejecting parents may still be held by some mental health professionals.

3. Parents may view self as victims of child's disorder

4. Lack of respite care and services places additional burdens on family

5. Family therapy with psychoeducational approaches foster clear communication

- Group interventions Enhance Socialization Skills

- Milieu Interventions

  1. Facilitation of child's highest level of functioning

  2. Facilitation of age appropriate skills

  3. Consistency and predictability essential

  4. Use isolation sparingly to facilitate child's integration into unit (Johnson, 1995)

  5. Staff needs education and help with child's uneven developmental presentation and variety in functioning

  6. Expectations must be realistic

- Community resources

  1. Support groups for parents

  2. National Association for the Mentally Ill (NAMI)

  3. Case management services to coordinate diverse services

  4. Federation of Families for Children's Mental Health

  5. Parents of Schizophrenics

- Nursing research agenda

  1. Outcome studies of treatment models that best facilitate patient functioning

  2. Impact of illness on siblings

PERVASIVE DEVELOPMENTAL DISORDERS (PDD)

Autistic Disorder (APA, 1994, p. 70)

- Signs and Symptoms

    1. Total of six items from a, b, and c, with at least two from a, and one each from b and c

        a. Qualitative impairment in social interaction as manifested by at least two of the following:

            (1) Marked impairment in use of multiple nonverbal behaviors such as eye-to-eye gaze, facial expression, body postures, and gestures to regulate social interaction

            (2) Failure to develop peer relationships appropriate to developmental level

            (3) Lack of spontaneous seeking to share enjoyment, interests or achievements with other people (e.g., by a lack of showing, bringing, or pointing out objeccts of interest)

            (4) Lack of social or emotional reciprocity

        b. Qualitative impairments in communication as manifested by at least one of the following

            (1) Delay in, or total lack of, the development of spoken language (not accompanied by an attempt to compensate through alternative modes of communication such as gesture or mime)

            (2) In individuals with adequate speech, marked impairment in the ability to initiate or sustain a conversation with others

            (3) Stereotyped and repetitive use of language or idiosyncratic language

            (4) Lack of varied spontaneous make-believe play or social imitative play appropriate to developmental level

        c. Restricted, repetitive patterns of behavior, interests and activities, as manifested by at least one of the following

(1) Encompassing preoccupation with one or more stereo-typed and restricted patterns of interest that is abnormal either in intensity or focus

(2) Apparently inflexible adherence to specific, nonfunctional routines or rituals

(3) Stereotyped and repetitive motor mannerisms (e.g., hand or finger flapping or twisting, or complex whole body movements)

(4) Persistent preoccupation with parts of objects

2. Delays or abnormal functioning in at least one of the following areas, with onset prior to age three

a. Social interaction

b. Language as used in social communication or

c. Symbolic or imaginative play

3. Disturbance not better accounted for by Rett's Disorder or Childhood Disintegrative Disorder

Note. From *Diagnostic and statistical manual of mental disorders* (4th ed.) (DSM-IV) (p. 70), by American Psychiatric Association, 1994, Washington, DC: American Psychiatric Press. Copyright 1994 by American Psychiatric Association. Reprinted with permission.

- Associated Features—the younger the child and more severe the impairment, the higher the number of associated features

1. Abnormal development of cognitive skills

2. Abnormal posture and motor behavior

3. Odd response to sensory input such as oblivion to pain or cold but hypersensitive to benign sounds, such as birds chirping; may have a fascination for some sensations of touch, such as velvet pillow

4. Abnormalities in eating, drinking or sleeping

5. Abnormalities of mood

6. Self-injurious behavior, such as head-banging, finger-biting, gouging skin

- Differential Diagnosis

    1. Mental retardation—even seriously impaired, can socialize and communicate in some way

    2. Schizophrenia rare in childhood

    3. Hearing impairments and specific developmental language and speech disorders

    4. Tic Disorders and Stereotypic Movement Disorder

    5. Other PDD

    6. Schizotypal or Schizoid Personality Disorder

Rett's Disorder

- Signs and Symptoms (APA, 1994, pp. 72-73)

    1. All of the following:

        a. Apparently normal prenatal and perinatal development

        b. Apparently normal psychomotor development through the first 5 months after birth

        c. Normal head circumference at birth

    2. Onset of all of the following after the period of normal development:

        a. Deceleration of head growth between ages of 5 and 48 months

        b. Loss of previously acquired purposeful hand skills between ages 5 and 30 months with the subsequent development of stereotyped hand movements (e.g., hand wringing or hand washing)

        c. Loss of social engagement early in the course (although often social interaction develops later)

        d. Appearance of poorly coordinated gait or trunk movements

        e. Severely impaired expressive and receptive language development with severe psychomotor retardation

            Note. From *Diagnostic and statistical manual of mental disorders* (4th ed.) (DSM-IV) (pp. 72-73), by American Psychiatric Association, 1994, Washington, DC: American Psychiatric

Press. Copyright 1994 by American Psychiatric Association. Reprinted with permission.

- Differential Diagnosis

    1. Autistic Disorder

    2. Childhood Disintegrative Disorder

    3. Mental Retardation

Childhood Disintegrative Disorder

- Signs and Symptoms (APA, 1994, pp. 74-75)

    1. Apparently normal development for at least the first two years after birth as manifested by the presence of age-appropriate verbal and non-verbal communication, social relationships, play and adaptive behavior

    2. Clinically significant loss of previously acquired skills (before age 10 years) in at least two of the following areas:

        a. Expressive or receptive language

        b. Social skills or adaptive behavior

        c. Bowel or bladder control

        d. Play

        e. Motor skills

    3. Abnormalities of functioning in at least two of the following areas:

        a. Qualitative impairment in social interaction (e.g., impairment in nonverbal behaviors, failure to develop peer relationships, lack of social or emotional reciprocity)

        b. Qualitative impairments in communication (e.g., delay in or lack of spoken language, inability to initiate or sustain a conversation, stereotyped and repetitive use of language, lack of varied make-believe play)

        c. Restricted, repetitive, and stereotyped patterns of behavior, interests, and activities, including stereotyped movement and mannerisms

> *Note.* From *Diagnostic and statistical manual of mental disorders* (4th ed.) (DSM-IV) (pp. 74-75), by American Psychiatric Association, 1994, Washington, DC: American Psychiatric Press. Copyright 1994 by American Psychiatric Association. Reprinted with permission.

- Differential Diagnosis—Another PDD or Schizophrenia

Asperger's Disorder

- Signs and Symptoms (APA, 1994, p. 77)

    1. Qualitative impairment in social interaction, as manifested by at least two of the following:

        a. Marked impairment in use of multiple nonverbal behaviors such as eye-to-eye gaze, facial expression, body postures, and gestures to regulate social interaction

        b. Failure to develop peer relationships appropriate to developmental level

        c. Lack of spontaneous seeking to share enjoyment, interests, or achievements with other people (e.g., by lack of showing, bringing or pointing out objects of interest to other people)

        d. Lack of social or emotional reciprocity

    2. Restricted, repetitive, and stereotyped patterns of behavior, interests, and activities as manifested by at least one of the following:

        a. Encompassing preoccupation with one or more stereotyped and restricted patterns of interest that is abnormal either in intensity or focus

        b. Apparently inflexible adherence to specific, nonfunctional routines or rituals

        c. Stereotyped and repetitive motor mannerisms (e.g., hand or finger flapping or twisting, or complex whole body movements)

        d. Persistent preoccupation with parts of objects

    3. Disturbance causes clinically significant impairment in social occupational or other important areas of functioning

    4. No clinically significant general delay in language (e.g., single words used by 2 years, communicative phrases used by age 3 years

5. No clinically significant delay in cognitive development of age appropriate self-help skills, adaptive behavior (other than in social interaction) and curiosity about the environment in childhood

6. Criteria not met for another PDD or Schizophrenia

Note. From *Diagnostic and statistical manual of mental disorders* (4th ed.) (DSM-IV) (p. 77), by American Psychiatric Association, 1994, Washington, DC: American Psychiatric Press. Copyright 1994 by American Psychiatric Association. Reprinted with permission.

Pervasive Developmental Disorder Not otherwise Specified (including Atypical Autism): Category used when there is a severe and pervasive impairment in the development of reciprocal social interaction, verbal and nonverbal communication skills, or when stereotyped behavior, interests and activities are present, but the criteria are not met for a specific PDD, Schizophrenia, Schizotypal Personalty Disorder, or Avoidant Personality Disorder.

ATTENTION-DEFICIT AND DISRUPTIVE BEHAVIOR DISORDERS: Behaviors that are disturbing to others and often socially disruptive. The behaviors are referred to as "externalizing" symptoms. They interfere with the child's social functioning and learning.

Attention-Deficit/Hyperactivity Disorder (AD/HD)

- Signs and Symptoms (APA, 1994, pp. 83-85)

  1. Either a or b

     a. Inattention—six or more of the following symptoms have persisted for at least six months to a degree that is maladaptive and inconsistent with developmental level:

        (1) Often fails to give close attention to details or makes careless mistakes in schoolwork, work or other activities

        (2) Often has difficulty sustaining attention in tasks or play activities

        (3) Often does not seem to listen when spoken to directly

        (4) Often does not follow through on instructions and fails to finish schoolwork, chores or duties in the workplace

(not due to oppositional behavior or failure to understand instructions)

(5)   Often has difficulties organizing tasks and activities

(6)   Often avoids, dislikes, or is reluctant to engage in tasks
that require sustained mental effort, e.g., schoolwork or
homework

(7)   Often loses things necessary for tasks or activities, e.g.,
toys, school assignments, pencils, books or tools

(8)   Often forgetful in daily activities

b.   Hyperactivity-Impulsivity—six (or more) of the following
symptoms have persisted for at least six months to a degree
that is maladaptive and inconsistent with developmental level:

(1)   Hyperactivity

(a)   Often fidgets with hands or feet or squirms in seat

(b)   Often leaves seat in classroom or in other situations in which remaining seated is expected

(c)   Often runs about or climbs excessively in situations in which it is inappropriate (in adolescents
or adults, may be limited to subjective feelings of
restlessness)

(d)   Often has difficulty playing or engaging in leisure
activities quietly

(e)   Often "on the go" or often acts as if "driven by a
motor"

(f)   Often talks excessively

(2)   Impulsivity

(a)   Often blurts out answers before questions have
been completed

(b)   Often has difficulty awaiting turn

(c)   Often interrupts or intrudes on others (e.g., butts
into conversations or games

2.   Some symptoms that cause impairment present before age seven

3. Some impairment from the symptoms present in two or more settings (e.g., school, home, work)

4. Must be clear evidence of clinically significant impairment in social, academic, or occupational functioning

5. Does not occur exclusively during the course of a Pervasive Developmental Disorder, Schizophrenia or other Psychotic disorder, and not better accounted for by Mood Disorder, Anxiety Disorder, Dissociative Disorder, or Personality Disorder.

  Note. From *Diagnostic and statistical manual of mental disorders* (4th ed.) (DSM-IV) (pp. 83-85), by American Psychiatric Association, 1994, Washington, DC: American Psychiatric Press. Copyright 1994 by American Psychiatric Association. Reprinted with permission.

- Associated Features

  1. Child may become alienated from peers due to inability to cooperate with others or follow game rules; excessive talking

  2. Child may engage in dangerous activities without considering consequences

  3. Symptoms may not be evidenced when child is in a highly structured, novel or one to one situation, or watching TV or playing video games.

  4. Age of onset before age seven (almost half before age four)

  5. Disorder often diagnosed at entry into school

  6. Low self-esteem, labile mood and temper tantrums

- Differential Diagnosis

  1. Considerations:

     a. Sometimes impossible to differentiate this diagnosis from response to a chaotic environment, including parenting problems

     b. Teacher reports somewhat more valid than family as the family may either normalize or be unaware what degree of compliance to expect from children at various ages.

  2. Rule out:

     a. Specific learning disabilities

  b. Acute situational reactions

  c. Adjustment disorders

  d. Conduct Disorder and Oppositional Defiant Disorder

  e. Mental retardation

  f. Pervasive developmental disorders

  g. Mood disorders, fear or anxiety

  h. Impaired vision or learning

  i. Seizures or sequelae of head trauma

  j. Acute or chronic medical illness

  k. Poor nutrition

  l. Insufficient sleep

  m. Various drugs which interfere with attention

    (1) Phenobarbital

    (2) Carbamazepine

    (3) Alcohol

    (4) Illicit drugs

    (5) Theophylline

  n. Early onset mania or bipolar illness (JAACAP, 1997c)

  o. Undifferentiated attention-deficit disorder—no impulsiveness or hyperactivity

 3. Utilize psychological evaluation and parent-teacher checklists:

  a. Achenbach's Child Behavior Checklist (CBCL)

  b. Teacher Report Form

  c. Barkley Home and School Situation questionnaire

  d. Conners Parent and Teacher rating scales

  e. Parent interviews including family history of ADD/ADHD, other disorders, family conflict

- Mental Status Examination

1. Observation in a free space situation, such as the playroom, is critical because the novelty of interview situation may encourage concentration

2. Age-appropriate overactivity is evaluated by quality of activity; AD/HD child has difficulty regulating his or her activity level to demands of the environment

3. Observe for symptoms of AD/HD oppositional behavior, aggressive behavior

- Nursing Diagnoses

    1. Coping, individual, ineffective

    2. Social interaction, impaired

    3. Self-concept, disturbance in self esteem

    4. Coping, ineffective family: compromised/disabling

- Genetic/Biological Origins/Biochemical Approaches

    1. May be sex-linked—more males than females

    2. Fathers may be alcoholic or have anti-social personality disorders

    3. Conduct disorder and specific developmental disorders more frequent in relatives

    4. Predisposing factors

        a. CNS abnormalities

        b. Disorganized, chaotic environments

        c. Noradrenergic, dopaminergic and serotonergic abnormalities

        d. Family history of AD/HD

    5. Diagnostic studies—hyper/hypothyroid may be contributing factor

    6. Psychopharmacology—between 70 and 80% of children with AD/HD respond to medication

        a. Methylphenidate hydrochloride (Ritalin) is prescribed most frequently

            (1) Divided doses, up to 1 mg/kg

            (2) Side effects—reduced appetite and insomnia

            (3) Growth retardation noted in some studies

           (4)   Risk of misuse of stimulants increased in adolescents

      b.   Pemoline and dextroamphetamine sulfate also used

      c.   Bupropion—contraindicated in children/adolescents with seizure disorders

- Intrapersonal Origins/Psychotherapeutic Interventions

  1. Retarded ego development

  2. Low self-esteem

  3. Play therapy—structured, one to one with frequent reinforcement and incentives for evidence of self control, "point system" and other behavioral interventions for positive reinforcement

  4. Careful environmental control—tasks and chores broken down into short, manageable components; homework done in short periods with opportunities for breaks

  5. Convey unconditional positive regard as these children often have low self-esteem and respond to positive reinforcement

  6. Avoid teasing

  7. Assist with organization and planning

  8. Approach child with firmness, consistency and limit-setting as well as patience

- Family Dynamics/Family Therapy

  1. Dysfunctional family system

  2. Sociopathic, alcoholic, conduct disordered relatives

  3. Chaotic environment—promote consistency and schedules

  4. Family therapy and parenting classes; teach negotiation, problem solving and contingency contracting

  5. Bibliotherapy for parents

     (1)   Barkley, R. A. (1995). *Taking charge of ADHD*. NY: Guilford.

     (2)   Hallowell, E., & Ratey, J. (1994). *Driven to distraction*. NY: Pantheon.

.

(3) Kelly, K., & Ramundo, P. (1996). *You mean I'm not lazy, stupid or crazy?* NY: Fireside Books.

7. Behavioral reinforcement from family therapist

8. 'Time out" vs. physical punishment

9. Offer diversions, such as tapes and stories to counteract the AD/HD child's constant chatter

- Group Approaches/Therapy/Self-Help

  1. Promote and encourage parent support group

  2. Parenting Classes

  3. Parents need information on structuring and planning the child's milieu at home (see Milieu interventions below)

  4. Skills building for anger management, decreasing impulsivity and rules compliance (Bloomquist, 1996)

- Milieu interventions

  1. Children with a primary diagnosis of AD/HD usually do not meet criteria for hospitalization unless they have other diagnoses such as Major Depression and Posttraumatic Stress Disorder

  2. Limit-setting

  3. Point system

  4. Behavioral charts and schedules

  5. Decrease external stimuli

  6. Provide for large muscle activity to discharge motor activity

  7. Limit setting on disruptive behavior

  8. Clear explanation of expectations

  9. Encourage positive peer activities

  10. Multidisciplinary coordination involving child's teachers

  11. Provide opportunities and incentives for success

  12. Academic skills training

  13. Social skills training and problem-solving

  14. Therapeutic recreation

- Community resources

  1. Support groups such as Attention Deficit Disorder Association (ADDA), Attention Deficit Information Network (AD-IN), and Children with ADD (CHADD)

  2. Parenting classes—Systematic Training for Effective Parenting (STEP) and Parent Effectiveness Training (PET) classes

Conduct Disorder (CD)

- Signs and Symptoms (APA, 1994, pp. 90-91)—a persistent pattern of behavior which causes clinically significant impairment in social, academic or occupational functioning and in which the basic rights of others or major age-appropriate societal norms and rules are violated as manifested by the presence of three or more of the following criteria in the past 12 months, with at least one criterion present in the past 6 months

  1. Aggression to people and animals

     a. Often bullies, threatens, or intimidates others

     b. Often initiates physical fights

     c. Has used a weapon that can cause serious physical harm to others (e.g., a bat, brick, broken bottle, knife, gun)

     d. Has been physically cruel to people

     e. Has been physically cruel to animals

     f. Has stolen while confronting a victim (e.g., mugging, purse snatching, extortion, armed robbery

     g. Has forced someone into sexual activity

  2. Destruction of Property

     a. Has deliberately engaged in fire setting with the intention of causing serious damage

     b. Has deliberately destroyed others' property (other than by fire setting)

  3. Deceitfulness or Theft

     a. Has broken into someone else's house, building or car

     b. Often lies to obtain goods or favors or to avoid obligations (i.e., "cons" others)

     c. Has stolen items of nontrivial value without confronting a victim (e.g., shoplifting, but without breaking and entering; forgery)

  4. Serious violation of rules

     a. Often stays out at night despite parental prohibitions, beginning before age 13

     b. Has run away from home overnight while living in parental or parental surrogate home (or once without returning for a lengthy period)

     c. Is often truant from school, beginning before age 13 years

       Note. From *Diagnostic and statistical manual of mental disorders* (4th ed.) (DSM-IV) (pp. 90-91), by American Psychiatric Association, 1994, Washington, DC: American Psychiatric Press. Copyright 1994 by American Psychiatric Association. Reprinted with permission.

- Associated with:
  1. Early use of tobacco, alcohol, nonprescribed drugs
  2. Lack of empathy, guilt or remorse; often blames others.
  3. Low self esteem covered by bravado with low frustration tolerance, irritability, and recklessness are common
  4. Poor academic achievement
  5. Other conditions including anxiety and depression; specific developmental disorder; AD/HD is a common co-morbid finding
  6. Adolescent chemical dependency has a high degree of co-morbidity
  7. Adult Axis II disorder of Antisocial Personality may be given by age 18

- Differential diagnosis
  1. Not diagnosed by single acts of antisocial behavior, but by persistent and repetitive pattern
  2. Different from oppositional defiant disorder in that the rights of others are violated as well as major age appropriate social norms
  3. Bipolar disorder usually represents brief manic episodes
  4. AD/HD

   5. Substance abuse

   6. PTSD

   7. BPD

   8. Adjustment disorder

   9. Narissistic personality disorder

  10. Schizophrenia (JAACAP, 1997e)

- Mental Status Examination (common findings in Conduct Disorder)

  1. May present as angry or superficially friendly; self-centered, lacks empathy or concern for others

  2. Major defenses include denial, projection; blames or implicates others

  3. Poor insight

  4. May attempt to bully examiner and behave in coercive or threatening ways

- Nursing Diagnoses

  1. Coping, ineffective, individual

  2. Violence, potential for, self directed or directed toward others

  3. Anxiety

  4. Adjustment, impaired

  5. Self-concept, disturbance in: body image self-esteem, role performance; personal identity

  6. Coping, ineffective family: compromised/disabling

  7. Social interaction, impaired

- Genetic/Biological Origins/Biochemical Approaches

  1. Common in children with antisocial and alcoholic parents

  2. Associated conditions, such as AD/HD, depression or posttraumatic stress disorder may be treated pharmacologically

  3. Drug screens to identify drug use and abuse

- Intrapersonal Origins/Psychotherapeutic Interventions

  1. Fixed in separation-individuation phase

2. Retarded ego development; id driven

3. Child maltreatment and associated parental substance abuse and psychiatric illness

4. Poverty, psychosocial toxicity, lack of supportive community structure (JAACAP, 1997e)

5. Psychotherapy (the earlier the intervention occurs, the better the outcome)

   a. Security and trust provide climate for growth

   b. Self-esteem enhanced by behavioral change and increased autonomy

   c. Understand dynamics of anger to establish locus of control; skills building in anger management (Bloomquist, 1996)

   d. Recognize and express feelings to eliminate dysfunctional defenses

   e. Provide for processing grief and loss

   f. Computer-assisted self evaluation and provision of alternatives helpful due to massive use of denial to cover vulnerability

- Family Dynamics/Family Therapy

   1. Multiple moves or schools

   2. Inconsistent management; harsh discipline; poor parenting

   3. History of parental rejection

   4. Shifting of parent figures

   5. Paternal absence, alcoholism and parental mental illness

   6. Large family size

   7. Early institutional living

   8. Association with delinquent sub-group

   9. Isolates self in family

   10. Court involvement/Child Protective Services; often known to multiple agencies

   11. Family therapy aimed at intervening in dysfunctional dynamics and training in new approaches

      a. Work with strengths

      b. Train parents to be consistent and decrease both overly permissive and overly harsh responses

      c. Foster self-responsibility, differentiation of self and decrease blaming communication

      d. Allow for expression of grief and tenderness

      e. Multiple family therapy approaches may be beneficial

      f. Family stress management

- Group approaches

  1. Allow for confrontation

  2. Test new ways of relating, including practicing empathy

  3. Model effective coping

  4. Form healthy relationships with non-CD peers; promote appropriate peer network

  5. Utilize exercises designed to deal with feelings, facilitate trust and develop healthy coping skills

  6. Psychosocial skills-building

  7. Refer to Alateen or Children of Alcoholics (COA) group

  8. Chemical dependency assessment and referral to appropriate 12 Step program or adolescent intensive outpatient program

  9. Anger management

  10. Alternatives to sexual promiscuity; sex education program (Jongsma, et al., 1996)

- Milieu Interventions

  1. Crisis shelters when indicated, residential treatment or group homes

  2. Provide for physical safety of patient and others

  3. Promote regulation of impulse control

  4. Promote positive problem-solving abilities

  5. Promote healthy expression of anger, such as providing safe place, e.g., gymnasiums etc

6. Provide structured mechanisms for learning trust, such as Ropes Program, Escape to Reality, etc.

7. Disseminate accurate information about staff changes, turnover, etc. as changes may reawaken old abandonment issues

8. Job and independent living skills training

9. Primary nursing promotes bonding with adult

- Community resources

    1. Appropriate 12 step Program

    2. Big Brother, Big Sister programs

    3. CASA (Court Appointed Special Advocates)

    4. Promote sports, fitness activities.

    5. Outward Bound therapeutic programs; Boot camps

    6. Parents Involved Network

    7. Federation of Families for Children's Mental Health

    8. Case management is essential due to multiple agency involvement and family tendency to seek help only in times of crisis.

    9. Coordination with school and appropriate other community systems, such as juvenile probation and parole

Oppositional-Defiant Disorder

- Signs and Symptoms (APA, 1994, pp. 93-94)

    1. A pattern of negativistic, hostile and defiant behavior lasting at least 6 months during which four (or more) of the following are present

        a. Often loses temper

        b. Often argues with adults

        c. Often actively defies or refuses to comply with adults' request or rules

        d. Often deliberately annoys people

        e. Often blames others for his or her mistakes or misbehavior

        f. Often touchy or easily annoyed by others

        g. Often angry and resentful

      h.   Often spiteful or vindictive

2. Disturbance in behavior causes clinically significant impairment in social, academic or occupational functioning

3. Behaviors do not occur exclusively during the course of a Psychotic or Mood Disorder.

4. Criteria are not met for Conduct Disorder and if the individual is age 18 years or older, criteria are not met for Antisocial Personality Disorder

    Note. From *Diagnostic and statistical manual of mental disorders* (4th ed.) (DSM-IV) (pp. 93-94), by American Psychiatric Association, 1994, Washington, DC: American Psychiatric Press. Copyright 1994 by American Psychiatric Association. Reprinted with permission.

- Differential Diagnosis
    1. Diagnosis only made if behavior is more common than that of other children of the same age; usually defiance is only seen with adults and peers the child knows well, and is justified by the child
    2. Conduct Disorder
    3. Passive Aggressive Personality Disorder
    4. Chemical dependency
    5. AD/HD

- Mental Status Examination
    1. Few signs of disorder are seen on mental status examination
    2. When confronted with behavior, client often utilizes projection and blames others
    3. Associated features include labile mood, bad temper and low frustration tolerance
    4. History, including teacher reports, essential

- Nursing Diagnoses
    1. Coping, ineffective, individual
    2. Violence, potential for, self directed or directed toward others
    3. Anxiety

4. Adjustment, impaired

5. Self-concept, disturbance in: body image, self-esteem, role performance; personal identity

6. Coping, ineffective family: compromised/disabling

7. Social interaction, impaired

- Genetic/Biological Origins/Biochemical approaches

    1. No information on familial pattern

    2. Age at onset by eight years, no later than early adolescence

    3. Medication for associated AD/HD

    4. Antidepressants for associated depression

        a. SSRI

        b. Bupropion

        c. Imipramine (Tofranil)—may be utilized with children over 12; FDA guidelines for ECG changes must be followed

        d. Lithium carbonate—augmentation of other medicine; may help decrease aggression

- Intrapersonal Origins/Psychotherapeutic Approaches

    1. May be related to physical or sexual abuse, or both

    2. Play therapy to encourage awareness of feelings, facilitate disclosure of issues, learn new ways of effective coping

        a. Board games

        b. Talking, Feeling, Doing Game

        c. The Ungame

        d. Therapeutic stories

        e. Role playing

    3. Art therapy—drawing, modeling, clay, sand tray to process unconscious issues

    4. Promote self-esteem and self-worth

    5. Skill building in interpersonal relationships, anger management, increasing compliance and effective problem-solving (Bloomquist, 1996)

6. Social skills training

- Family Dynamics/Family Therapy

    1. Utilize family therapy to promote healthy family interaction and decrease tendency to pathologize child

    2. Support parental hierarchy

    3. Explore alternate ways of coping, especially assisting parents to avoid playing into oppositional tendencies

- Group Approaches/Group Therapy

    1. Encourage verbalization of feelings and develop positive social support mechanisms

    2. Learn alternate ways of coping

    3. Psychodrama encourages trying out new behaviors

    4. Provide positive reinforcement

    5. Social skills groups

    6. Promote positive peer relationships

- Milieu Approaches

    1. Children with this diagnosis are rarely admitted to inpatient settings, although they may have a dual diagnosis with a major mental health problem such as depression or bipolar disorder

    2. Environmental activities and group process are necessary, as well as those mentioned under Conduct Disorder

- Community resources

    1. Parenting classes, such as STEP and PET

    2. Sports and team activities

    3. Wilderness and Outward Bound type programs

    4. Camps, YMCA, YWCA programs

    5. Big Brother, Big Sister

    6. Review resources in Conduct Disorder

PERSONALITY DISORDERS

Although personality disorders are not generally included in the disorders of infancy, childhood and adolescence, the presentation, defenses and symptomatology of these disorders are presaged by the childhood disruptive behavior disorders. According to DSM IV, APA, 1994 one may see the following personality disorders or the initial signs in older children or adolescents:

I. Antisocial

II. Avoidant

III. Borderline

- Signs and Symptoms—see Behavioral Syndromes and Disorders of Adult Personality chapter
- Biological/Intrapersonal Origins of Personality Disorders
    1. Faulty ego functioning may be related to developmental arrests in childhood as well as genetic predisposition and trauma; see Behavioral Syndromes and Disorders of Adult Personality chapter
    2. Primitive defenses of personality disorders triggered by experiences of poor parenting, family dysfunction, and inadequate caretaking
    3. Children reared in this environment have low self-esteem, lack trust and have poor social skills
    4. Early trauma, including physical abuse and sexual abuse
- Family Dynamics
    1. Parents lack empathy and affection; often rejecting and chaos ridden
    2. Family substance abuse, mental illness, abuse and violence
    3. Review family and environmental dynamics for Conduct Disorder

MOOD DISORDERS IN CHILDREN AND ADOLESCENTS

Depression: Prevalence of depression is extremely low up until age 9, but rises sharply from ages 9 to 19, especially in females (Lewisohn, Clarke, Seeley & Rhode, 1994)

- Signs and Symptoms

1. Same diagnostic criteria are utilized for children and adolescents as for adults

2. The criteria for weight change or appetite disturbance in children is failure to achieve expected gain, or greater than 5% loss of body weight in 1 month

3. Declining academic performance

4. Isolation and refusal to communicate

- Comorbidity with other diagnoses include:

    1. Conduct Disorders and Oppositional Defiant Disorder

    2. School phobias

    3. Learning problems

    4. Attention Deficit Disorders

    5. Chemical dependency

    6. Anxiety disorders

    7. Specific developmental disorders

    8. Chronic illness

    9. Grief and loss/bereavement

- Familial Patterns—experiences of abuse and violence, runaways, family chemical dependency and having one or both parents with a mood disorder increases the risk

- Suicide

    1. Adolescent depression is positively associated with suicidal behavior

    2. Suicide rising among adolescents with mood disorders

    3. Suicide attempts in children younger than age 12 relatively rare (Johnson, 1997)

    4. Suicide attempts rise sharply at age 13 to 14 years

    5. Third leading cause of death for youth age 15 to 24 years

        a. Highest rates occur in white males

        b. Next highest nonwhite males

    6. Risk factors for suicide

    a.   Affective illness—depression or mania

    b.   Parental divorce

    c.   Use of firearms

    d.   Antisocial or aggressive behavior

    e.   Family history of suicidal behavior

7. Signs of suicide

    a.   Change in grades

    b.   Giving away possessions

    c.   Decreased interest in after school activities

    d.   Few friends

    e.   Breakup with girlfriend or boyfriend

    f.   Pressure by family to stop dating one person

    g.   Wearing black

    h.   Listening to morose or violent music

    i.   Drug and/or alcohol use

    j.   Discussing suicide

    k.   Self-mutilation (Botz & Bidwell-Cerone, 1997)

8. Cluster suicides may be preceded by exposure to fictional suicide in media, completed suicide in a school system and friendship with someone who has completed suicide.

9. Reducing suicide contagion

    a.   Avoid simplistic explanations for suicide

    b.   Do not engage in repetitive discussion of the recent suicide event

    c.   Do not provide graphic descriptions of suicide

    d.   Do not glorify suicide or persons who commit it

    e.   Focus on deceased's nonsuicide characteristics (Botz & Bidwell Cerone, 1997)

10. Nursing interventions include:

    a.   Monitoring potential for self-harm

b. Focusing on the motivations of the suicidal youngster

c. Coordinating the support system

d. Working with school based crisis teams

e. Reinforce patient's open expression of underlying feelings

- Medication management includes the use of SSRIs—sertraline, fluoxetine, fluvoxamine, and paroxetine, as well as tricyclics and atypical antidepressants, e.g., bupropion, mirtazapine

    1. Tricyclic antidepressant (TCA) seizures occur more frequently in children than in adults

    2. Rapid clearance may mean that therapeutic response takes longer in children than in adults

Bipolar Disorders (often not diagnosed or misdiagnosed in children and adolescents)

- Signs and Symptoms

    1. Adolescents—resemble the adult course of illness; 20% of all cases present prior to age 19 (JAACAP, 1997d)

    2. Children younger than age 9 more likely to present with irritability and affective lability (Johnson, 1995)

    3. Older children present with labile moods, paranoia, grandiose delusions and other psychotic symptoms

    4. Severe behavioral deterioration

    5. Psychological testing may be utilized in diagnostic evaluation

        a. Children's Depression Inventory (CDI)

        b. School-Age Depression Listed Inventory (SADLI)

        c. Bellevue Index of Depression (BID)

        d. Children's Depression Rating Scale—Revised

        e. Mania Rating Scale

- Differential diagnosis

    1. Drugs e.g., corticosteroids, sympathomimetics, isoniazid, antidepressants, stimulants

2. Abusive substances, e.g., amphetamines, cocaine, inhalants, phencyclidine (JAACAP, 1997d)

3. Endocrine disorders, such as hyperthyroidism

4. Neurologic conditions, such as head trauma, temporal lobe seizures, tumors, HIV, multiple sclerosis

5. Infections—Encephalitis, influenza, syphilis

6. The following psychiatric conditions

   a. Childhood disruptive disorders

   b. PTSD

   c. Substance abuse

   d. Schizophrenia

   e. Schizoaffective disorder

   f. Borderline personality disorder

   g. Agitated depression

- Mental Status Examination—presentation similar to adults

  1. Adolescents may have psychotic symptoms

  2. Markedly labile and erratic symptoms

  3. Severe behavioral deterioration

- Nursing Diagnoses

  1. Same as for adult bipolar disorders

  2. Alterations in parenting

- Genetic/Biologic Origins

  1. Affects both sexes equally

  2. Males more affected in early onset cases

- Biochemical approaches

  1. Medication management addresses manic or mixed symptoms, depressive symptoms and prevention of relapses (JAACAP, 1997d)

  2. Lithium

     a. Renal clearance of lithium higher in children than in adults;

children and adolescents may require higher dosages to achieve therapeutic blood levels (Antai-Otong, 1995)

b. Complete physical examinations and baseline laboratory studies must be done prior to initiating drugs

c. Children and adolescents often tolerate Lithium better than adults

d. Dosage ranges from 600 mg daily for a weight of 15 to 25 kg given in divided doses to 1500 mg per day for a weight range of 50 to 60 kg given in divided doses

3. Anticonvulsant mood stabilizers

a. Carbamazepine (Tegretol) is given in doses of 15 to 30 mg/kg/day

b. Valproic acid (Depakene) given in non-response to Lithium or Tegretol—dose is 25 to 60 mg/kg/day, with a blood level of 50 to 120 mEq/L

c. Benzodiazepines possible adjunct for acute mania

d. Neuroleptics

e. Antimania agents

f. ECT (JAACAP, 1997d)

- Intrapersonal Origins/Psychotherapeutic Interventions

1. Mania runs in families—bipolar parents may exercise inadequate parenting techniques

2. Cohort effect indicates increased incidence of bipolar illness in individuals born after 1940

3. Hospitalization often indicated

4. Age specific psychotherapy/play therapy

- Family Dynamics/Family Therapy

1. Psychoeducational approaches essential

2. Support and empathy

3. Biological origins of this disorder must be taken into account (therapist may be dealing with several bipolar persons in family)

- Group approaches

1. Play group

2. Self-esteem group

3. 'Time out" provided to protect other group members

4. Address associated psychological problems

5. Anger management

- Milieu Interventions

  1. Same as adults, but modified for developmental level

  2. Must provide safe environment for other patients

FEEDING AND EATING DISORDERS OF INFANCY OR EARLY CHILDHOOD

Pica

- Signs and Symptoms (APA, 1994, p. 96)

  1. Persistent eating of non-nutritive substances for a period of at least one month (such as dirt, plaster, hair, bugs, and/ or pebbles)

  2. The eating of non-nutritive substances is inappropriate to the developmental level

  3. The eating behavior is not part of a cultural practice.

  4. If the eating behavior occurs exclusively during the course of another mental disorder (e.g., Mental Retardation, PDD, Schizophrenia), it is sufficiently severe to warrant independent clinical attention

     Note. From *Diagnostic and statistical manual of mental disorders* (4th ed.) (DSM-IV) (p. 96), by American Psychiatric Association, 1994, Washington, DC: American Psychiatric Press. Copyright 1994 by American Psychiatric Association. Reprinted with permission.

- Community resources

  1. Public health nurses

  2. Well-child clinics

  3. Lead poisoning prevention programs

  4. Social services

Rumination Disorder of Infancy

Partially digested food is brought up into the mouth without nausea, retching, disgust. The food is ejected, or chewed and reswallowed. The condition is potentially fatal. There may be weight loss or failure to gain weight.

- Signs and Symptoms (APA, 1994, p. 98)

  1. Repeated regurgitation and rechewing of food for a period of at least 1 month following a period of normal functioning

  2. The behavior is not due to an associated gastrointestinal or other medical condition (e.g., esophageal reflux)

  3. The behavior does not occur exclusively during the course of Anorexia Nervosa or Bulimia Nervosa—if the symptoms occur exclusively during the course of Mental Retardation or PDD they are sufficiently severe to warrant independent clinical attention

     Note. From *Diagnostic and statistical manual of mental disorders* (4th ed.) (DSM-IV) (p. 98), by American Psychiatric Association, 1994, Washington, DC: American Psychiatric Press. Copyright 1994 by American Psychiatric Association. Reprinted with permission.

- Differential Diagnosis

  1. Congenital anomalies (e.g., pyloric stenosis)

  2. GI infections

- Nursing Diagnoses

  1. Altered nutrition, less than body requirements

  2. Ineffective family coping

  3. Altered family process

- Genetic/Biological Origins—no information; spontaneous remissions are common

- Family Dynamics/Family Therapy

  1. Parents may become alienated from the infant due to their frustration and his/her failure to respond

  2. Noxious odor of the regurgitate may cause parent to avoid holding the infant

3. Health teaching regarding nature of illness and suggestions for coping are essential

- Community resources—Public health nursing

Anorexia and Bulimia

Eating disorders are a great risk for adolescents. Anorexia has a mortality rate of 10 to 15%. Hallmarks of these disorders are secretiveness, denial of the problem, and resistance to therapy or any treatment that will lead to weight gain (Mohr, 1998; Hartman & Burgess, 1998).

- Signs and Symptoms

    1. Classic DSM-IV criteria may not be applicable.

    2. Begins in late school age (10 to 12); Onset most common between 12 to 18 years of age.

    3. Child does not have to lose the percentage of weight applicable for an adult with an eating disorder

        a. Prepubertal children have lower percentage of body fat and thin children may become unhealthy quickly

        b. Boys and girls present with childhood anorexia

        c. Affects 1 in 200 adolescent females

- Intrapersonal Origins/Psychotherapeutic Interventions

    1. Adolescent anorexia

        a. Consider issues relative to puberty

        b. Separation dynamics and increased independence from family

        c. Increased autonomy in problem solving

        d. Peer pressure, including sexuality

            (1) Difficulty with interpersonal intimacy and closeness

            (2) May have a history of sexual trauma

    2. Adolescent bulimia

        a. Generally not common in children; begins between age 13 to 18

        b. Initiation into process of major life choices

3. Treatment of anorexia and bulimia

    a. Close coordination with medical care

        (1) Establish minimum daily caloric intake

        (2) Food journal

        (3) Monitor vomiting, binging, exercise and laxative abuse

    b. Implemented within the context of the adolescent's developmental, social, and academic needs

    c. Individual

    d. Group

    e. Family therapy—major component; need to understand dynamics of the family as a system (Antai-Otong, 1995)

    f. Bibliotherapy

OTHER DISORDERS OF INFANCY CHILDHOOD OR ADOLESCENCE

Separation Anxiety Disorder

- Signs and Symptoms (APA, 1994, p. 113)

1. Developmentally inappropriate and excessive anxiety concerning separation from home or from those to whom the individual is attached, as evidenced by three (or more) of the following:

    a. Recurrent excessive distress when separation from home or major attachment figures occurs or is anticipated

    b. Persistent and excessive worry about losing or possible harm befalling, major attachment figures

    c. Persistent and excessive worry that an untoward event will lead to separation from a major attachment figure (e.g., getting lost or being kidnapped)

    d. Persistent reluctance or refusal to go to school or elsewhere because of fear of separation

    e. Persistently and excessively fearful or reluctant to be alone or without major attachment figures at home or without significant adults in other settings

    f.   Persistent reluctance or refusal to go to sleep without being near a major attachment figure or to sleep away from home

    g.   Repeated nightmares involving theme of separation

    h.   Repeated complaints of physical symptoms (such as headaches, stomachaches, nausea, or vomiting) when separation from major attachment figures occurs or is anticipated

2.   The duration of disturbance is at least 4 weeks

3.   The onset is before age 18 years

4.   The disturbance causes clinically significant distress or impairment in social, academic (occupational), or other important areas of functioning.

    Note. From *Diagnostic and statistical manual of mental disorders* (4th ed.) (DSM-IV) (p. 113), by American Psychiatric Association, 1994, Washington, DC: American Psychiatric Press. Copyright 1994 by American Psychiatric Association. Reprinted with permission.

- Differential diagnosis

  1.   Somatic complaints

  2.   Developmentally appropriate separation anxiety

  3.   Overanxious disorder

  4.   Panic disorder with agoraphobia

  5.   PDD or Schizophrenia

- Mental Status Examination

  1.   May refuse to separate from parent

  2.   May cling or cry and fuss if parent tries to leave; if separates, checks frequently in spite of reassurances and knowledge that parent is close by

- Nursing Diagnoses

  1.   Anxiety—mild, moderate, severe

  2.   Coping, ineffective individual

  3.   Powerlessness

  4.   Self-esteem, situational, low

  5.   Social interaction, impaired

6. Social isolation

7. Fear

- Genetic/Biological Origins/Biochemical Approaches

    1. Specific developmental disorders involving language and speech may predispose to this condition

    2. Mothers with anxiety disorders more common in this population according to some studies

    3. More common in females than males

- Interpersonal Origins/Psychotherapeutic Interventions

    1. Moderate to catastrophic stressor as defined on Axis IV

    2. More research needed on genetic vs. environmental transmission

    3. Brief, symptom focused therapy approaches:

        a. Psychodrama

        b. Art work

        c. Play therapy utilizing role play, doll house, sand box, puppets to explore anxieties, fears and worries

        d. Therapeutic games, storytelling to expand awareness

        e. Emphasis on symptom reduction, empowerment, mastery and control

        f. Goal is to decrease symptoms quickly to enhance functioning, avoid permanent dysfunction

        g. Relaxation training may be helpful—diversion, deep breathing; muscle relaxation (Jongsma et al., 1996)

- Family Dynamics/Family Therapy

    1. Decrease anxiety and rigidity in parental system

    2. Decrease conflict and increase problem-solving

    3. Clarify communication

    4. Increase individual autonomy and decrease fusion

    5. Take focus off child as symptom-bearer

    6. Educate parents re: developmentally normal anxiety

7. Educate parents to decrease their own anxiety and over-protection

- Group Approaches

    1. Self-esteem group

    2. Play therapy group

    3. Theraplay

    4. Organized and informal play/sports opportunities

- Milieu Interventions

    1. Highly unusual to admit these children to an inpatient setting; treated as outpatients

    2. Organization and predictability helpful, while gradually fostering child's independence and self-reliance

- Community Resources

    1. Educational programs for parents

    2. Church and sports activities

Selective Mutism (Elective Mutism)

- Signs and Symptoms (APA, 1994, p. 115)

    1. Consistent failure to speak in specific social situations (in which there is an expectation for speaking, e.g., at school) despite speaking in other situations.

    2. Disturbance interferes with educational or occupational achievement or with social communication.

    3. The duration of the disturbance is at least 1 month (not limited to the first month at school)

    4. The failure to speak is not due to lack of knowledge of, or comfort with the spoken language required in social situation

    5. The disturbance is not better accounted for by a communication disorder (e.g., stuttering) and does not occur exclusively during the course of a PDD, Schizophrenia or other Psychotic disorder

        Note. From *Diagnostic and statistical manual of mental disorders* (4th ed.) (DSM-IV) (p. 115), by American Psychiatric Association, 1994, Washington, DC: American Psychiatric Press. Copyright 1994 by American Psychiatric Association. Reprinted with permission.

- Differential Diagnosis

  1. Severe or Profound Mental Retardation, Pervasive Developmental Disorder, Developmental Expressive Language Disorder

  2. Children of families who have recently emigrated to a country of a different language

  3. Organic factors/medical problems

- Mental Status Examination

  1. Attempts to engage the patient in conversation are futile, although the presence of adequate receptive language is apparent

  2. May communicate by gestures, nodding or shaking head, or by short monotone utterances

- Nursing Diagnosis

  1. Impaired communication

  2. Altered Socialization

  3. Altered Family Process

  4. Ineffective individual coping

  5. Parental role conflict

- Biological Origins/Biochemical Approaches

  1. May be related to neorobiological precursor of anxiety disorder

  2. Fluoxetine has been shown to decrease anxiety and mutism (JAA-CAP, 1997b)

- Intrapersonal Origin/Psychotherapeutic Interventions

  1. Associated with shyness and other oppositional behavioral problems

  2. Case histories report symptoms developed following reprimand for verbalization

  3. Challenging to treat since these patients don't talk to therapist and often passively refuse nonverbal communication

  4. Psychoanalysis reportedly is beneficial

  5. Behavior therapy may be beneficial

  6. Resolve core conflict contributing to mutism so patient speaks consistently in all social situations

- Family Dynamics/Family Therapy
    1. Maternal overprotection
    2. Major personality or psychiatric conflict or a combination of both
    3. Families seen as vulnerable to a hostile world
    4. Symptom is seen as an expression of family conflict
    5. Silence used as manipulation
    6. Increased rate of psychiatrically ill/abnormal family dynamics
    7. Family therapy and school counseling essential
        a. Confront family denial so parents cooperate with treatment plan
        b. Assist in developing realistic expectations
        c. Teach effective communication skills to family
        d. Utilize parent-training models to enhance child and family coping (Elder, 1997)
- Group Approaches—not indicated
- Milieu Intervention—provide reinforcement for verbal responses
- Community Resources
    1. Parenting classes
    2. Socialization and sports activities

Reactive Attachment Disorder of Infancy or Early Childhood

- Signs and Symptoms (APA, 1994, p. 118)
    1. Markedly disturbed and developmentally inappropriate social relatedness in most contexts, beginning before age 5 years, as evidenced by either a or b
        a. Inhibited Type—persistent failure to initiate or respond in a developmentally appropriate fashion to most social interactions, as manifested by excessively inhibited, hypervigilant, or highly ambivalent and contradictory responses (e.g., the child may respond to caregivers with a mixture of approach, avoidance, and resistance to comforting, or may exhibit frozen watchfulness)

  b. Disinhibited Type—diffuse attachments as manifested by indiscriminate sociability with marked inability to exhibit appropriate selective attachments (e.g., excessive familiarity with relative strangers or lack of selectivity in choice of attachment figures)

2. Disturbance in criteria 1 is not accounted for solely by developmental delay (as in Mental Retardation) and does not meet criteria for PDD

3. Pathogenic care, as evidenced by at least one of the following:

  a. Persistent disregard of the child's basic emotional needs for comfort, stimulation, and affection, (harsh punishment or consistent neglect by caregiver)

  b. Persistent disregard of child's basic physical needs (nutrition, housing, freedom from physical danger including sexual abuse)

  c. Repeated changes of primary caregiver that prevent formation of stable attachments (e.g., frequent changes in foster care)

4. Presumption that the care in 3 is responsible for the disturbed behavior in 1.

  Note. From *Diagnostic and statistical manual of mental disorders* (4th ed.) (DSM-IV) (p. 118), by American Psychiatric Association, 1994, Washington, DC: American Psychiatric Press. Copyright 1994 by American Psychiatric Association. Reprinted with permission.

- Differential Diagnosis

  1. Mental Retardation or Pervasive Developmental Disorder, such as Autistic Disorder

  2. Children with severe neurological abnormalities, including deafness, blindness, profound multisensory defects, major central nervous system disease, or severe chronic physical illness

- Mental Status Examination

  1. Lack of developmentally appropriate social responsiveness

  2. Apathy and lack of interest in environment

  3. Child may stare, have weak cry and poor muscle tone, as well as low motility

4. Home visit often required to investigate neglect or abuse, as caregiver reports not reliable

- Nursing Diagnosis
    1. Altered role performance, parenting
    2. Altered family processes
    3. Altered comfort
    4. Ineffective family coping (disabled)
    5. Potential for injury
    6. Altered communication
    7. Unilateral neglect
    8. Altered growth and development

- Intrapersonal Origins/Psychotherapeutic Approaches—response to neglect/provision of adequate caretaking

- Family Dynamics
    1. Parents—severe character pathology
    2. Severe depression, isolation, and lack of support systems
    3. Lack of bonding in first weeks of life
    4. Transgenerational pattern of dysfunctional parenting, abuse, neglect, and mental illness
    5. Overwhelming psychosocial stresses in parents with emotional deficits

- Family Therapy
    1. Engage relevant family members in treatment
    2. Identify family stresses
    3. Assess family resources
    4. Assess and intervene in dysfunctional conflicts affecting child's well-being
    5. Supervise care
    6. Recommend out-of-home placement if necessary

- Milieu Approaches

    1. Does not meet criteria for psychiatric hospitalization

    2. Patient may be placed in infant home or pediatric unit to treat other conditions while awaiting placement; cuddling and stimulation essential; staff may model appropriate behavior for parents

- Community Resources

    1. Community mental health parent support groups

    2. Parenting classes

    3. Public health nursing

    4. Pediatric/family centered outpatient program

    5. Child protective services

    6. Child abuse prevention services

    7. Multidisciplinary team approach—case management and coordination of care essential

Stereotypic Movement (Formerly Stereotypy/Habit) Disorder

- Signs and Symptoms (APA, 1994, p. 121)

    1. Repetitive, seemingly driven and nonfunctional motor behavior (e.g., hand-shaking or waving, body-rocking, head-banging, mouthing of objects, self-biting, picking at skin or bodily orifices, hitting own body)

    2. The behavior markedly interferes with normal activities or results in self-inflicted bodily injury that requires medical treatment (or would result in an injury if preventive measures were not used). Specify "With Self-injurious behavior"

    3. If Mental Retardation is present, the stereotypic or self-injurious behavior is of sufficient severity to become a focus of treatment.

    4. The behavior is not better accounted for by a compulsion (as in Obsessive Compulsive Disorder), a tic (as in Tic Disorder), a stereotypy that is part of a PDD or hair pulling (as in Trichotillomania).

    5. The behavior is not due to the direct physiological effects of a substance or a general medical condition.

    6. The behavior persists for 4 weeks or longer.

    Note. From *Diagnostic and statistical manual of mental disorders*

(4th ed.) (DSM-IV) (p. 121), by American Psychiatric Association, 1994, Washington, DC: American Psychiatric Press. Copyright 1994 by American Psychiatric Association. Reprinted with permission.

- Differential Diagnosis

  1. Normal rocking and thumb-sucking are common in normal infants and young children.

  2. Pervasive Developmental Disorder, Tic Disorder and Obsessive Compulsive Disorder

- Mental Status Examination—behavior appears compulsive and involuntary

- Nursing Diagnosis

  1. Physical mobility, impaired

  2. Potential for injury

- Biological Origins

  1. Common in mental retardation

  2. Associated with congenital deafness and blindness

  3. Associated with degenerative and CNS disorders

  4. Temporal-lobe epilepsy and severe schizophrenia

  5. May be induced by certain psychoactive substances such as amphetamine, in which case the diagnosis of Psychoactive Substance-Induced Organic Mental Disorder should also be made

- Biochemical Treatment

  1. Haloperidol 0.5 to 16 mg/day; side effects include sedation, headache, extrapyramidal symptoms, tardive dyskinesia, neuroleptic malignant syndrome, orthostatic hypotension, photosensitivity, anorexia, constipation, paralytic ileus, impaired liver function, hypersalivation, agranulocytosis, anemia, leukopenia, cough reflex suppression, laryngeal edema, brochospasm, diaphoresis

  2. Lithium carbonate (Lithium) 600 to 2100 mg in 2 to 3 divided doses; keep blood levels to 0.4 to 1.2 mEq/L; adverse reactions include vomiting, headache, tremor, weight gain

  3. Opiate antagonists are presently under study

- Family Dynamics/Family Therapy: Provide family support and information re: management and pharmacology

CHILDHOOD AND ADOLESCENT ANXIETY DISORDERS

Powerlessness, increased dependency, impaired self-esteem and poor social skills are common manifestations of anxiety disorders in children. Child and adolescent anxiety disorders are on a continuum with, and may become adult anxiety disorders. Retrospective studies of adults with anxiety disorders indicated that 65% had two or more anxiety disorders as children. Insecurely or ambivalently attached infants develop more anxiety diagnoses in childhood and adolescence. Behavioral inhibition is a risk factor in the development of anxiety disorders in young children. Anxiety disorders in children do not appear in isolation. They are part of an array of other symptoms and traits.

Social Phobia (see Anxiety and Stress Related Disorders chapter)— avoidant behaviors in children and adolescents are manifested as persistent or extremely constricted social interaction with unfamiliar people. There is fear of acting in a humiliating or embarrassing manner.

- Signs and Symptoms (Additional criteria for children APA, 1994, pp. 416-417)

  1. Must be evidence of capacity for age-appropriate social relationships with familiar people and the anxiety must occur in peer settings, not just in interactions with adults

  2. Anxiety may be expressed by crying, tantrums, freezing, or shrinking from social situations with unfamiliar people.

  3. Children may not realize that fear is excessive or unreasonable as adults may.

  4. In individuals under age 18 years, the duration is at least 6 months.

     Note. From *Diagnostic and statistical manual of mental disorders* (4th ed.) (DSM-IV) (pp. 416-417), by American Psychiatric Association, 1994, Washington, DC: American Psychiatric Press. Copyright 1994 by American Psychiatric Association. Reprinted with permission.

- Differential Diagnosis for Anxiety Disorders

  1. Physical conditions

      a. Hypoglycemic episode

      b. Hyperthyroidism

      c. Cardiac arrythmias

      d. Caffeinism

      e. Pheochromocytoma

      f. Seizure disorders

      g. Migraine

      h. CNS disorders

  2. Medication reactions

      a. Antihistamines

      b. Anti-asthmatics

      c. Sympathomimetics

      d. Antipsychotics

      e. Non-prescription drugs, e.g., diet pills, cold medicine (JAA-CAP, 1997b)

  3. Mood disorders

  4. AD/HD

  5. Adjustment disorder

  6. Substance use disorder

- Etiology

  1. Modeling of shy aloof behaviors by primary caregivers

  2. Child abuse

  3. Early traumatic childhood losses

  4. Chronic medical problems

  5. Impaired social skills

- If continues into adulthood, becomes avoidant personality disorder

Generalized Anxiety Disorder (Includes Overanxious Disorder of childhood) (see Anxiety and Stress Related Disorders chapter)

- Children with this disorder are extremely sensitive

- Overanxious behavior is exaggerated during times of stress
- Overly concerned about social performance and competency

Obsessive-Compulsive Disorder

- Thought to be rare in children until recently
- Symptoms in children include obsessive thoughts, rituals, such as washing, checking and repeatedly rewriting letters or numbers until perfect
- Adults realize the behaviors are unreasonable; children may not

Panic Disorder: Uncommon before the prepubertal period; peak age of onset is 15 to 19 years of age

Posttraumatic Stress Disorder (see Anxiety and Stress Related Disorders chapter)

- Signs and Symptoms

  1. Repetitive play in which themes or aspects of trauma are expressed and re-experienced

  2. Sexualized play indicative of sexual knowledge greater than would be expected of a child's developmental age; may be an indicator of suspected abuse

  3. Loss of recently acquired developmental skills or language skills is often a way the avoidant criteria are expressed

     Note. From *Diagnostic and statistical manual of mental disorders* (4th ed.) (DSM-IV) (p. 428), by American Psychiatric Association, 1994, Washington, DC: American Psychiatric Press. Copyright 1994 by American Psychiatric Association. Reprinted with permission.

Treatment measures for Children and Adolescents with Anxiety Disorders: Should be an adjunct to behavioral and/or psychotherapeutic interventions

- Biochemical approaches

  1. SSRI

  2. Fluvoxamine

3. Trycyclic antidepressants (imipramine, clomipramine)—use customary TCA protocol including baseline vital signs, ECG and serum levels

4. Benzodiazepines (used on short term basis)

   a. Clonazepam—behavioral inhibition can be a side effect

   b. Alprazolam

5. Beta blockers—block physiological symptoms of anxiety

6. Buspirone (Bernstein, Borchadt, & Perwein, 1996; JAACAP, 1997b)

7. Other medications such as antispasmodics and antihistamines

- Psychotherapeutic Goals

  1. Overcome fear of threat

  2. Differentiate and understand various feelings

  3. Elevate self-esteem and feelings of security

  4. Understand the link between feelings, thoughts and behaviors

  5. Understand that arousal is a symptom of fear

  6. Enhance problem solving skills

  7. Gain a sense of mastery

  8. Develop adaptive coping skills

  9. Resolve core conflicts

  10. Eliminate anxiety

- Psychotherapy

  1. Systematic desensitization

  2. Exposure and response prevention

  3. Cognitive behavioral therapy

- Family Therapy: Psychoeducation for parents to help reinforce healthy parenting skills

  1. Support child's increasing autonomy and competence

  2. Modify family functioning

TIC DISORDERS

Tics are defined as sudden, rapid, recurrent, nonrhythmic, motor movements, vocalization, repetitive movements, gestures or utterances that mimic some aspect of normal behavior. Tics cannot be controlled, but can be suppressed for varying lengths of time. They are worsened by stress and diminished during sleep.

Simple Motor Tics: Eye blinking, facial grimacing

Simple Vocal Tics: Coughing, throat clearing, sniffing, snorting, barking

Complex Motor Tics: Facial gestures, grooming behaviors, touching

Complex Vocal Tics

- Repeating words and phrases out of context
- Coprolalia—use of socially unacceptable words
- Palilalia—repeating one's own sounds or words
- Echolalia—repeating the last heard sound or word
- Echokinesis—repeating someone else's movements

Tourette's Disorder

- Signs and Symptoms (APA, 1994, pp. 100-103)

  1. Both multiple motor and one or more vocal tics have been present at some time during the illness, although not necessarily concurrently.

  2. Tics occur many times a day (usually in bouts) nearly every day or intermittently throughout a period of more than 1 year, and during this period there is never a tic-free period of more than 3 consecutive months.

  3. The disturbance causes marked distress or significant impairment in social, occupational, or other important areas of functioning.

  4. The onset is before 18 years.

  5. The disturbance is not due to the direct physiological effects of a substance (e.g., stimulants) or a general medical condition (e.g., Huntington's disease or postviral encephalitis).

Note. From *Diagnostic and statistical manual of mental disorders* (4th ed.) (DSM-IV) (pp. 100-103), by American Psychiatric Association, 1994, Washington, DC: American Psychiatric Press. Copyright 1994 by American Psychiatric Association. Reprinted with permission.

- Associated with ADHD and OCD in clinical populations
- Differential Diagnosis
  1. Abnormal motor movements associated with neurologic disorders
  2. Organic mental disorders
  3. Schizophrenia
- Mental Status Examination
  1. The definitive manifestations of these disorders may be present on assessment, or the caretaker may describe the salient features
  2. There may be associated anxiety due to social situation embarrassment
  3. Depressed mood is common
- Nursing Diagnosis
  1. Impaired social interaction due to communication barriers
  2. Impaired verbal communication
  3. Powerlessness
  4. Anxiety related to unexpected manifestation of tics
  5. Ineffective individual coping related to anxiety
  6. Chronic low self-esteem
  7. Altered sensory/perception—kinesthetic
- Genetic/Biological Origins
  1. Age-dependent expression of symptoms
  2. Familial patterns reported for all cases of tic disorders—more common in first degree biological relatives of people with Tourette's
  3. OCD more common in first degree biological relatives of those with Tourette's than those with other tic disorders
  4. At least three times more common in males than females

     5.   Controversy over association with:

        a.   Exposure to phenothiazines

        b.   Head trauma

        c.   Administration of CNS stimulants

        d.   Intrauterine environment

           (1)   Maternal life stress

           (2)   Complications of pregnancy

           (3)   First trimester nausea

     6.   EEG abnormalities in 50%

- Biochemical Approaches

     1.   Haloperidol (Haldol) effective in chronic tic disorders and Tourette's

        a.   Children over 12 years

           (1)   Initial dose—1 to 15 mg in divided doses, with gradual increase to 100 mg to bring symptoms under control

           (2)   Maintenance dose—9 mg daily

        b.   Children under 12 years

           (1)   Initial dose—0.5 to 1.5 mg daily; dosage increased by 0.5 mg increments

           (2)   Maintenance dose—1.5 mg daily

        c.   Side effects

           (1)   Similar to piperazine phenothiazines

              (a)   Low incidence of sedation and autonomic effects

              (b)   High incidence of extrapyramidal reactions

           (2)   Food and Drug Agency Pregnancy Category C

     2.   Pimozide (Orap)—strongly antidopaminergic like haloperidol (Haldol)

     3.   Clonidine (Catapres)

        a.   Not as effective as Orap or Haldol

        b.   No tardive dyskinesthesia risk

- Intrapersonal Origins/Psychotherapeutic Interventions

  1. Behavioral therapy effective in symptom modulation

  2. Symptoms may be exacerbated by stress; autogenic relaxation and stress management may help the patient to self-regulate

  3. Massed practice—behavioral technique where patient practices intentionally, the undesired behavior

  4. Acceptance by therapist is a key in treatment

- Family Dynamics/Family Therapy

  1. Parents need guidance in understanding biological determinants of this disorder and in recognizing compulsive nature of behavior

  2. Punishment may reinforce symptom

  3. Efforts to help child overcome socialization problems should be emphasized

- Group approaches

  1. May benefit from inclusion in a diverse group with opportunity to receive support from other members

  2. Self-help is an important aspect of care and support groups are available in larger cities

- Milieu

  1. Rarely admitted to inpatient unit unless associated with depression or AD/HD

  2. Provide opportunity to process feelings of differentness in the milieu as an extension of normal adolescent growth and development

- Community resources

  1. Gilles de la Tourette Foundation

Chronic Motor or Vocal Tic Disorder

- Signs and Symptoms (APA, 1994, p. 104)

  1. Single or multiple motor or vocal tics (i.e., sudden rapid, recurrent, nonrhythmic, stereotyped motor movements or vocalizations), but not both, have been present at some time during the illness.

  2. The tics occur many times a day nearly every day or intermittently throughout a period of more than 1 year, and during this period

there was never a tic-free period of more than 3 consecutive months.

3. The disturbance causes marked distress or significant impairment in social, occupational, or other important areas of functioning.

4. The onset is before age 18 years.

5. The disturbance is not due to the direct physiological effects of a substance (e.g., stimulants) or a general medical condition (e.g., Huntington's disease or post-viral encephalitis.

6. Criteria have not been met for Tourette's Disorder.

Note. From *Diagnostic and statistical manual of mental disorders* (4th ed.) (DSM-IV) (p. 104), by American Psychiatric Association, 1994, Washington, DC: American Psychiatric Press. Copyright 1994 by American Psychiatric Association. Reprinted with permission.

Transient Tic Disorder

- Signs and Symptoms (APA, 1994, p. 105)

1. Single or multiple motor and/or vocal tics (i.e., sudden, rapid, recurrent, nonrhythmic, stereotyped motor movements or vocalizations

2. The tics occur many times a day, nearly every day for at least 4 weeks, but for no longer than 12 consecutive months.

3. The disturbance causes marked distress or significant impairment in social, occupational, or other important areas of functioning.

4. The onset is before age 18 years.

5. The disturbance is not due to the direct physiological effects of a substance (e.g., stimulants) or a general medical condition (e.g., Huntington's disease or postviral encephalitis).

6. Criteria have never been met for Tourette's Disorder or Chronic Motor or Vocal Tic Disorder.

7. Specify if single episode or recurrent

Note. From *Diagnostic and statistical manual of mental disorders* (4th ed.) (DSM-IV) (p. 105), by American Psychiatric Association, 1994, Washington, DC: American Psychiatric Press. Copyright 1994 by American Psychiatric Association. Reprinted with permission.

Tic Disorder Not Otherwise Specified: Tics that do not meet criteria for a specific Tic disorder

- Differential Diagnosis for all Tic Disorders except Tourette's

    1. Other movement disturbances

    2. Neurological conditions

    3. Medication reaction

- Biochemical Approaches—medication only used in very severe cases of Chronic Motor or Vocal Tic Disorder

ELIMINATION DISORDERS

Enuresis

- Signs and Symptoms (APA, 1994, pp. 109-110)

    1. Repeated voiding of urine into bed or clothes (whether involuntary or intentional).

    2. The behavior is clinically significant as manifested by either frequency of twice a week for at least 3 consecutive months or the presence of clinically significant distress or impairment in social, academic (occupational), or other important areas of functioning

    3. Chronological age is at least 5 years (or equivalent developmental level).

    4. The behavior is not due exclusively to the direct physiological effect of a substance (e.g., a diuretic) or a general medical condition (e.g., diabetes, spina bifida, a seizure disorder).

    5. Specify nocturnal only, diurnal only or nocturnal and diurnal

        Note. From *Diagnostic and statistical manual of mental disorders* (4th ed.) (DSM-IV) (pp. 109-110), by American Psychiatric Association, 1994, Washington, DC: American Psychiatric Press. Copyright 1994 by American Psychiatric Association. Reprinted with permission.

- Differential Diagnosis

    1. Medical conditions

    2. Urinary tract infection

    3. Anxiety disorders, e.g., phobias related to toileting

- Mental Status
    1. Child may have low self-esteem due to caretaker rejection or social ostracism by peers
    2. Incidence of associated major mental illness is greater among those with Functional Enuresis than in the general population
- Associated Conditions
    1. Functional Encopresis, Sleepwalking Disorder, Sleep Terror
    2. Associated with other behavioral disorders and psychopathology, however, associated disorders may stem from enuresis
- Nursing Diagnosis: Urinary incontinence, functional
- Biological Origins/Biochemical Approaches
    1. Low functional bladder volume
    2. More males than females
    3. 75% have first-degree biological relative with disorder
    4. Imipramine
        a. 1.5 mg/kg/day to no more than 5 mg/kg/day
        b. Side effects include:
            (1) Dry mouth
            (2) Constipation
            (3) Tachycardia
            (4) Drowsiness
            (5) Postural hypotension
            (6) Cardiac conduction slowing
        c. ECG monitoring essential with baseline
- Intrapersonal Origins/Psychotherapeutic Interventions
    1. Secondary enuretics have same rate of emotional or behavioral problems as primary enuretics
    2. Psychotherapy alone is not effective treatment, but may be helpful with associated psychiatric conditions

3. Hypnotherapy may be effective, although duration of recovery has not been substantiated

4. Behavioral techniques (Conditioning)

    a. Mowrer apparatus (bell and pad awakens child when he wets and works by a combination of Pavlovian conditioning, avoidance learning, and placebo effect

    b. Intermittent reinforcement and overlearning reduce relapse

    c. Retention control training

    d. Training rapid awakening

    e. Reinforcement for daytime micturition

    f. Avoiding negative social consequences

    g. Encourage active participation

    h. Encourage patient responsibility

    i. Challenge/confront non-compliance (Jongsma et al., 1996)

Encopresis

- Signs and Symptoms (APA, 1994, p. 107)

    1. Repeated passage of feces into inappropriate places (e.g., clothing or floor) whether involuntary or intentional.

    2. At least one such event a month for at least 3 months.

    3. Chronological age is at least 4 years (or equivalent developmental level).

    4. The behavior is not due exclusively to the direct physiological effects of a substance (e.g., laxatives) or a general medical condition except through a mechanism involving constipation.

    5. Specify with or without constipation and overflow incontinence.

    Note. From *Diagnostic and statistical manual of mental disorders* (4th ed.) (DSM-IV) (p. 107), by American Psychiatric Association, 1994, Washington, DC: American Psychiatric Press. Copyright 1994 by American Psychiatric Association. Reprinted with permission.

- Nursing Diagnoses

    1. Altered elimination, bowel

2. Bowel incontinence

- Genetic/Biological Origins/Biochemical Approaches

    1. 15% of fathers of encopretics were encopretic

    2. Ratio of male to female encopretics ranges from 66% to 88% of samples

    3. Common with mental retardation but poorly defined

    4. Inadequate physiological functioning of defecation

- Intrapersonal Origins/Psychotherapeutic Interventions

    1. Social learning theory attributes disordered learning or insufficient learning

    2. Secondary encopresis involves learned avoidant behavior, reinforced by delay of painful defecation

    3. Psychogenic theories formulated by Freud—compliance vs. opposition in "anal period"

    4. Treatment determined by thorough assessment

        a. Toilet training needed if appropriate training has not taken place

        b. Positive behavioral reinforcement of appropriate toileting behavior

        c. Secondary encopresis related to more serious psychopathology—need to treat high levels of anxiety, anger or depression

        d. If encopresis in response to severe environmental stress, modifying stressor brings relief

- Family Therapy for Enuriesis and Encopresis

    1. Orient family counseling to supporting behavioral techniques

    2. Treat family psychopathology if present; some theorists postulate issues of paternal distance and maternal anxiety, as well as parental absence

    3. Support and management alternatives lessens parental pressure on child, enabling learning to take place; parental management training (PMT) can be effective

    4. Explore rigidity in toilet training

5. Confront and challenge hostile and critical behavior

6. Interrupt cycle of hostile dependent angry interactions

7. Identify and defuse secondary gains (Jongsma, et al., 1996)

- Milieu Interventions: Behavioral techniques as outlined should be incorporated in care plan

- Community resources: Parenting classes

COMMUNICATION DISORDERS

Expressive Language Disorder

- Signs and Symptoms (APA, 1994, p. 58)

  1. Scores obtained from standardized individually administered measures of expressive language development are substantially below those obtained from standardized measures of both nonverbal intellectual capacity and receptive language development. Disturbance may manifest clinically by symptoms that include having a remarkably limited vocabulary, making errors in tense, or having difficulty recalling words or producing sentences with developmentally appropriate length or complexity.

  2. The difficulties interfere with academic or occupational achievement or with social communication.

  3. Criteria are not met for Mixed Receptive-Expressive Language Disorder or a Pervasive Develpmental Disorder.

  4. If Mental Retardation, a speech-motor or sensory deficit, or environmental deprivation is present, the language difficulties are in excess or those usually associated with these problems. (Code on Axis III)

     Note. From *Diagnostic and statistical manual of mental disorders* (4th ed.) (DSM-IV) (p. 58), by American Psychiatric Association, 1994, Washington, DC: American Psychiatric Press. Copyright 1994 by American Psychiatric Association. Reprinted with permission.

Mixed Receptive-Expressive Language Disorder

- Signs and Symptoms (APA, 1994, p. 60-61): The scores obtained from a battery of standardized individually administered measures of both receptive and expressive language development are substantially below those obtained from standardized measures of nonverbal intellectual capacity. Symptoms include those for Expressive Language Disorder as well as difficulty understanding words, sentences, or specific types of words, such as spatial terms.

Note. From *Diagnostic and statistical manual of mental disorders* (4th ed.) (DSM-IV) (pp. 60-61), by American Psychiatric Association, 1994, Washington, DC: American Psychiatric Press. Copyright 1994 by American Psychiatric Association. Reprinted with permission.

Phonological Disorder

- Signs and Symptoms

  1. Failure to use developmentally expected speech sounds that are appropriate for age and dialect (e.g., errors in sound production, use, representation, or organization such as, but not limited to, substitutions of one sound for another [use of /t/ for target /k/ sound] or omissions of sounds such as final consonants

  2. The difficulties in speech sound production interfere with academic or occupational achievement or with social communication.

  3. If Mental Retardation, a speech-motor or sensory deficit, or environmental deprivation is present, the speech difficulties are in excess of those usually associated with these problems. (Code on Axis III)

     Note. From *Diagnostic and statistical manual of mental disorders* (4th ed.) (DSM-IV) (p. 63), by American Psychiatric Association, 1994, Washington, DC: American Psychiatric Press. Copyright 1994 by American Psychiatric Association. Reprinted with permission.

Stuttering

- Signs and Symptoms (APA, 1994, p. 65)

  1. Disturbance in the normal fluency and time patterning of speech (inappropriate for the individual's age), characterized by frequent occurrences of one or more of the following

     a. Sound and syllable repetitions

     b. Sound prolongations

     c. Interjections

     d. Broken words (e.g., pauses within a word)

e.   Audible or silent blocking (filled or unfilled pauses in speech)

f.   Circumlocutions (word substitutions to avoid problematic words)

g.   Words produced with excess of physical tension

h.   Monosyllabic whole-word repetitions (e.g., "I-I-I see him")

2.   The disturbance in fluency interferes with academic or occupational achievement or with social communication.

3.   If a speech-motor or sensory deficit is present, the speech difficulties are in excess of those usually associated with these problems. (Code on Axis III)

Note. From *Diagnostic and statistical manual of mental disorders* (4th ed.) (DSM-IV) (p. 65), by American Psychiatric Association, 1994, Washington, DC: American Psychiatric Press. Copyright 1994 by American Psychiatric Association. Reprinted with permission.

Communication Disorders Not Otherwise Specified (APA, 1994, p. 65)

- Do not meet criteria for specific Communication Disorder
- Example: A voice disorder (abnormality of vocal pitch, loudness, quality, tone or resonance)

Note. From *Diagnostic and statistical manual of mental disorders* (4th ed.) (DSM-IV) (p. 65), by American Psychiatric Association, 1994, Washington, DC: American Psychiatric Press. Copyright 1994 by American Psychiatric Association. Reprinted with permission.

The Following Refers to all Communication Disorders

- Differential Diagnosis for Communication Disorders
  1.   Hearing impairment or other sensory deficit
  2.   Speech-motor deficit
  3.   Normal dysfluencies that occur in young children
  4.   Severe environmental deprivation (for Phonological Disorder and Expressive Language Disorder)
  5.   Neurological deficit
  6.   Mental retardation with learning disabilities

7. Autistic disorder (for Expressive Language Disorder)

8. Mental retardation (for Expressive Language Disorder)

9. Acquired aphasia due to general medical condition (for Expressive Language Disorder)

10. Spastic dysphonia

11. Anxiety disorder

- Mental Status Variations

    1. Often causes the speaker great anxiety and fearfulness of speaking

    2. Speech rate may be altered

    3. Motor movements frequently accompany stuttering such as eye blinks, tics, tremors of the face and head, fist clenching

    4. Severity of symptoms may increase under pressure to communicate, such as during interview

- Nursing Diagnoses

    1. Impaired verbal communication

    2. Anxiety

- Genetic/Biological Origins

    1. Familial pattern noted in Communication Disorders

    2. Stuttering—research supports genetic evidence for origin of stuttering

        a. Male to female ratio is three to one

        b. Fifty percent of first degree biological relatives affected

    3. May have generalized neurological soft signs

    4. No factors have been shown to be clearly associated with recovery

    5. Approximately 80% recover before age 16

    6. Females more commonly recover than males

- Psychotherapeutic and Behavioral Interventions

    1. Therapy should focus on overcoming associated anxiety and frustration

2. Relaxation training, positive self-talk and stress management may help provide a sense of mastery and self-control

3. Teach self-control strategies

- Family Therapy

    1. Family may help raise child's self esteem

    2. Assist parents to understand and be empathetic with patient

    3. Contributory family dysfunctional patterns addressed; confront interactions that maintain dysfunction

    4. Challenge denial surrounding deficit in order to support actual interventions

    5. Promote realistic expectations, e.g., filling in pauses (Jongsma et al., 1996)

- Group Approaches: Overcome low self-esteem and impairment of social functioning

- Community Resources

    1. Speech and hearing therapy—usually not covered by third party payers.

    2. School systems may have special education services

LEARNING DISORDERS

There is a great deal of controversy over the inclusion of these as mental disorders. Often there is no sign of psychopathology. Detection and treatment takes place within the school system. May be associated with other Axis I disorders.

Reading Disorder (APA, 1994, p. 50)

- Reading achievement, as measured by individually administered standardized tests of reading accuracy or comprehension, is substantially below that expected given the person's chronological age, measured intelligence and age-apppropriate education.

- The disturbance significantly intereferes with academic achievement or activities of daily living that require reading skills.

- If a sensory deficit is present, the reading difficulties are in excess of those usually associated with it.

Mathematics Disorder (APA, 1994, p. 51)

- Mathematical ability, as measured by individually administered standardized tests, is substantially below that expected, given the person's chronological age, measured intelligence, and age-appropriate education.

- The disturbance significantly interferes with academic achievement or activities of daily living that require mathematical ability.

- If a sensory deficit is present, the difficulties in mathematical abiliby are in excess of those usually associated with it.

Disorder of Written Expression (APA, 1994, p. 53)

- Writing skills, as measured by an individually administered standardized tests (or functional assessments of writing skills), are substantially below those expected given the person's chronological age, measured intelligence, and age-appropriate education.

- The disturbance significantly interferes with academic achievement or activities of daily living that require the composition of written texts (e.g., writing grammatically correct sentences and organized paragraphs

- If a sensory deficit is present, the learning difficulties are in excess of those usually associated with it.

Learning Disorder not otherwise specified (APA, 1994, p. 53)

- Disorders in learning that do not meet criteria for any specific learning disorder.

- Might include problems in all three areas (reading, mathematics, written expression)

- Problems significantly interfere with academic achievement even though performance on tests measuring each individual skill is not substantially below that expected given the person's chronological age, measured intelligence, and age-appropriate education

  Note. From *Diagnostic and statistical manual of mental disorders* (4th ed.) (DSM-IV) (pp. 50-53), by American Psychiatric Association, 1994, Washington, DC: American Psychiatric Press. Copyright 1994 by American Psychiatric Association. Reprinted with permission.

MOTOR SKILLS DISORDER

Developmental Coordination Disorder

- Signs and Symptoms (APA, 1994)

    1. Performance in daily activities that require motor coordination is substantially below that expected given the person's chronological age and measured intelligence. This may be manifested by marked delays in achieving motor milestones (e.g., walking, crawling, sitting) dropping things, "clumsiness," poor performance in sports or poor handwriting.

    2. The disturbance significantly interferes with academic achievement or activities of daily living.

    3. Not due to a general medical condition (e.g., cerebral palsy, hemiplegia, or muscular dystrophy) and does not meet criteria for PDD

- Differential Diagnosis

    1. Mental retardation

    2. Neurological disorders

    3. Pervasive Developmental Disorders

    4. AD/HD

    5. Elective mutism

    6. Inadequate schooling

    7. Impaired vision or hearing

    8. PTSD induced regression and loss of recently acquired skills

- Mental Status Variations

    1. Determined by history, observation

    2. Teacher report/checklists essential

- Nursing Diagnoses

    1. Growth and development, altered

    2. Ineffective individual coping

    3. Self-concept, disturbance in

    4. Communication, impaired, verbal

5. Knowledge deficit or Learning need (specify)

- Genetic/Biological Origins/Biochemical Approaches

  1. Perinatal injury of various kinds

  2. No information on sex ratio for the arithmetic and coordination disorders; the others are from two to four times more common in males than females

  3. Prevalence rate is 2 to 10% of population

  4. Some show history in first-degree biologic relatives

  5. No evidence that medication directly benefits children with these disorders; may be used for associated conditions

- Individual Psychotherapy

  1. May be helpful with issues of low self-esteem and school failure

  3. Collaboration with school guidance counselor and school counseling may be helpful

- Family Dynamics/Family Therapy: Families may need assistance in parent management strategies and psychoeducational approaches may be in order

- Group approaches: May be helpful in self-esteem issues and to help overcome feelings of differentness

- Community resources: Educational intervention depends upon degree of impairment

  1. National Learning Disabilities Association

  2. Federation for Children with Special Needs

MENTAL RETARDATION (MR)

Mild Mental Retardation—IQ level 50 to 55 to approximately 70

- Can develop social and communication skills
- Acquisition of academic skills to sixth grade level
- Acquire skills for minimum self-support
- Can live in the community
- May need guidance and support during stress

Moderate Mental Retardation—IQ level 35 to 40 to 50 to 55

- 10% of the population with MR
- Can talk and communicate
- Can profit from vocational training, but unlikely to progress beyond second grade level
- May have difficulties with social conventions
- Can live in supervised group homes
- Need supervision and guidance under stress

Severe Mental Retardation—IQ level 20 to 25 to 35 to 40

- 3% to 4% of people with MR
- Little or no communicative speech during pre-school, may learn speech during school-age years
- Can be taught limited hygiene skills
- Can "sight-read" some survival words, as "EXIT" 'STOP' 'MEN" 'WOMEN'
- May perform simple tasks under close supervision
- May live in the community in group homes or with families, in the absence of an associated handicap

Profound Mental Retardation—IQ level below 20 or 25

- 1% to 2% of people with MR
- Minimal capacity for sensorimotor functioning
- Motor development, self care and communication skills may improve if appropriate training provided
- May live in group homes, intermediate care facilities or with families
- Need day programs or sheltered workshop

Mental Retardation Severity Unspecified: Strong presumption of mental retardation but person's intelligence is untestable by standard tests

- Signs and symptoms for Mental Retardation (APA, 1994, pp. 41-42)

1. Significantly subaverage intellectual functioning—I.Q. of 70 or below on an individually administered IQ test (for infants, a clinical judgment of significantly subaverage intellectual functioning).

2. Concurrent deficits or impairments in present adaptive functioning (i.e., the person's effectiveness in meeting the standards expected for his or her age by his or her cultural group) in at least two of the following areas: communication, self-care, home-living, social/interpersonal skills, use of community resources, self-direction, functional academic skills, work, leisure, health, and safety.

3. The onset is before age 18 years

> *Note.* From *Diagnostic and statistical manual of mental disorders* (4th ed.) (DSM-IV) (pp. 41-42), by American Psychiatric Association, 1994, Washington, DC: American Psychiatric Press. Copyright 1994 by American Psychiatric Association. Reprinted with permission.

- Associated Disorders

  1. The more severe the retardation, the greater the likelihood of other abnormalities in one or more systems

  2. In Down syndrome, social skills are much higher than could be expected for the level of retardation

  3. Prevalence of mental disorders at least three or four times higher than in the general population

  4. Common associated disorders

     a. Pervasive Developmental Disorders

     b. AD/HD

     c. Stereotypic Movement Disorder

- Mental status variations—needs to be adjusted to level of retardation

  1. Passivity

  2. Dependency

  3. Low self-esteem

  4. Low frustration tolerance

  5. Aggressiveness

  6. Poor impulse control

    7. Stereotyped self-stimulating and self-injurious behavior

- Nursing diagnoses

    1. Impaired verbal communication

    2. Aggression

    3. Impaired social interaction

    4. Altered growth and development

    5. Self care deficit(s)

    6. Self concept disturbance

    7. Powerlessness

- Genetic/Biologic Origins/Biochemical Approaches

    1. Hereditary factors in 5% of cases

    2. Inborn metabolism errors (Tay-Sachs disease; phenylketonuria)

    3. Single gene abnormalities (Tuberous sclerosis)

    4. Chromosomal aberrations (translocation Down syndrome, Fragile X syndrome)

    5. Early alterations of embryonic development (30%)

        a. Maternal alcohol consumption causing prenatal damage due to toxins

        b. Pregnancy and perinatal problems (10%)

        c. Fetal malnutrition, prematurity or hypoxia

        d. Maternal trauma—pregnant women are at higher risk for injury due to family violence than non-pregnant women

    6. Physical disorders acquired in childhood

- Biochemical approaches are Diagnostic and Symptom Specific

    1. Concomitant mental disorder must be specifically treated, as antidepressants for depression, or stimulants for AD/HD

    2. Agitation, aggression, and tantrums may respond to antipsychotics; high dosage, low potency drugs more cognitively dulling than low dosage, high potency drugs

    3. Aggressive or self-abusive behaviors may be controlled with Lithium

    4. Tantrums and aggression may be controlled with carbamazepine and propanolol

       a. Carbamazepine (Tegretol)

         (1) 10 mg/kg/day to 20 to 30 mg/kg/day

         (2) Therapeutic blood level 4 to 12 μg/mL

         (3) Side effects include drowsiness, nausea, vertigo, psychosis

         (4) Monitor CBC and LFTs for blood dyscrasias and hepatotoxicity

       b. Propanolol

         (1) Has a wide dosage range

         (2) Side effects include dizziness, fatigue, insomnia, depression, nausea, diarrhea, bronchospasm

- Intrapersonal Origins/Psychotherapeutic Interventions

    1. Psychosocial deprivation, lack of stimulation, and complications of other mental disorders

    2. Behavior modification specific for acting-out

    3. Supportive treatment that raises self-esteem may be helpful for the higher functioning patient

- Family Dynamics/Family Therapy

    1. Dysfunctional family processes, such as abusive and chemically dependent families

    2. Families who undernurture and understimulate

    3. Therapy geared to correcting dysfunctional processes without pathologizing family; promote rewarding, praising

    4. Deficits of mentally retarded child create severe stress for family; pattern of overprotection and overcompensation may develop

    5. Families need both respite care and help in focusing on the child's strengths as well as realistic expectations

    6. Psychoeducational approaches to engender family cooperation with programs

- Group Approaches

1. Traditional, insight-oriented group not indicated

2. Behavior modification, educational group may be helpful

3. Multiple family group therapy decreases family's sense of isolation, stress, and provides a forum for sharing effective management strategies

4. Socialization groups useful

5. Skills building

- Milieu Interventions

   1. Mental retardation, per se, is no longer generally considered criteria for admission to a psychiatric inpatient setting

   2. Day care settings or sheltered workshops provide milieu

   3. Community meetings helpful in group home, day care settings or workshop setting

   4. Designed to address specific problematic behaviors

   5. Aggressive behaviors are in response to over-whelming lack of power experienced by these children

   6. Child needs help in coping with teasing, and protection from harm by others

- Community resources

   1. Numerous resources in larger metropolitan areas

   2. Rural areas have extremely limited resources

   3. Steady decline in services in last twenty years

   4. Retarded adults with supervision are reliable and effective workers for routine tasks

   5. Federation for Children with Special Needs

   6. National Information Center for Handicapped Children and Youth

Questions
Select the best answer

1. Estimates of children and adolescents experiencing a mental disorder in the United States are:

   a. 10 million
   b. 7.5 million
   c. 250,000
   d. 2.5 million

2. Psychiatric disorders among children and adolescents are:

   a. Decreasing
   b. Stable
   c. Probably increasing
   d. Difficult to assess

3. Since the 1960s, the suicide rate for youngsters age 15 to 19 has:

   a. Declined
   b. Doubled
   c. Stayed the same
   d. Tripled

4. Children of immigrants who experience a lack of acculturation may be at greater risk for;

   a. PTSD
   b. PDD
   c. Mental retardation
   d. Depression

5. Risk factors are those which increase the likelihood of developing an emotional mental disorder. Which of the following risk factors increases the intensity of all other risk factors?

   a. Physical and sexual abuse
   b. Adolescent parents
   c. Divorce, parental conflict, and family instability
   d. Poverty

6. Biological or genetic factors that negatively impact a child's mental health include:

a. Personality characteristics
b. Low birth weight
c. Problem solving ability
d. Normal intellectual development

7. Life in a blended family may increase the risk of developing inadequate coping skills due to:

   a. Child support issues
   b. Step-siblings replacing peers
   c. Visitation schedules disrupting family routines
   d. Economic pressures for all parents to work

8. Children in foster care are at very high risk for developing psychiatric disorders. One reason for this may be due to:

   a. Cutbacks in funding
   b. Poorly selected foster families
   c. Lack of turnover in placement
   d. Lack of permanency preventing development of significant interpersonal relationships

9. A major factor in lack of access to health care for children in the United States is the lack of health insurance and:

   a. Inadequate numbers of prepared mental health professionals to provide needed services
   b. Poor follow through by foster parents
   c. Inadequate primary prevention by school nurses
   d. Poor psychiatric skills among primary care providers

10. Teens are victimized at a rate that is_____ that of the general population.

    a. Twice
    b. Three times
    c. Four times
    d. Five times

11. Which group has the highest risk of being raped?

    a. Girls 16-18
    b. Boys 11-14
    c. Boys 6-8
    d. Girls 14-15

12. Violence by juveniles is most often inflicted on which population?

    a. Other juveniles
    b. Younger children
    c. Middle Aged adults
    d. Elderly people

13. Cults are attractive to alienated adolescents who have not internalized social norms. Cults are usually led by:

    a. Adults who provide substitute parenting to the adolescent
    b. Same sexed peers with organizational skills
    c. Charismatic authority figures who claim to possess certain powers
    d. Peers who have dabbled in Satanism

14. Runaways are a population of children and adolescents who are at high risk for emotional and physical health problems. Family forces which contribute to runaway behavior include delegating dynamics. Which of the following is an example of delegating dynamics?

    a. Preventing the adolescent from after school activities
    b. Telling the adolescent to move out when he finishes high school
    c. A single father using the adolescent girl as a maternal figure for the younger siblings
    d. Physical abuse of the adolescent

15. A 15 year old girl's parents divorced and proceeded to continue to argue with each other around issues of child support and visitation. The girl was interrogated about life at each parent's home by the other, and the mother prevented visitation when the child support check was late. In addition, the mother became angry when the youngster came back from visitation and reported having a good time. The girl ran away and stayed with different friends for 10 days. This is an example of which type of runaway?

    a. Departure
    b. Situational
    c. Throwaway
    d. Emotional survival

16. Harry, age 16, ran away from home because his parents were both abusive alcoholics. There was little structure or predictability in the home environment, with people often moving in or out. Harry became a "street person'. Harry is at high risk for:

a. Victimization and exploitation
b. Having a reunion fantasy
c. Developing a gender identity disorder
d. Having difficulty with time management

17. Amy, age 19, is addicted to crack cocaine and becomes pregnant. She continues drug use while pregnant. A serious problem that may occur due to her addiction is low birth weight. Another serious problem may be:

a. Pervasive developmental disorder
b. Failure to thrive
c. Failure to bond
d. High utilization of health services

18. Adolescent substance abuse affects what percentage of the adolescent population?

a. 12%
b. 46%
c. 24%
d. 32%

19. Substance abuse is potentially more serious among adolescents because:

a. They are difficult to manage at home
b. There are few 12 Step programs for youngsters
c. There is an interference with developmental issues
d. It perpetuates substance abuse throughout the generations

20. The incidence of child abuse and neglect has:

a. Increased 27% between 1990 and 1994
b. Declined 27% between 1990 and 1994
c. Stabilized between 1990 and 1994
d. Been impossible to properly evaluate

21. A three year old boy regularly arrives at the day care center inappropriately dressed for cold weather. He appears undernourished and is often dirty. This may be an example of:

a. Medical neglect
b. Emotional neglect
c. Physical neglect
d. Passive inattention

22. The type of neglect which is difficult to document or substantiate is:

    a. Medical neglect
    b. Emotional neglect
    c. Physical neglect
    d. Educational neglect

23. Suzanne is a three year old who was born prematurely and spent the first several months of her life in the hospital. When she was sent home, she was on a cardiac monitor. Suzanne was slow to walk, talk, and toilet train. What is her risk for experiencing abuse?

    a. Less than most children, as her parents will want to protect her
    b. No different from any other child, as children do not bring on abusive behavior
    c. Slightly higher than other children
    d. Higher than other children due to the fact that early health and medical problems increase risk of abuse

24. Jeffrey is a six year old who has AD/HD and difficulty attending to social cues. He is always on the go and is noted to have behavior problems in school. What, if any, is Jeffrey's risk of being abused?

    a. No different from other children
    b. Greater than others
    c. Less than others
    d. Impossible to predict

25. Donna Barry, a single mother, brings her daughter Lorraine, age 7, in for a evaluation of "behavior problems". Ms. Barry speaks about Lorraine in negative terms. She acknowledges that Lorraine does not present a problem at school, and says she spanks Lorraine if her room is not cleaned to Ms. Barry's satisfaction. Lorraine appears to be anxious and somewhat depressed. An appropriate intervention would be:

    a. Counseling aimed at teaching Ms. Barry effective management skills
    b. Reporting Ms. Barry for child abuse.
    c. Referring Lorraine for medication management
    d. Asking Lorraine's teacher to report any unusual bruising

26. Assessment of child sexual abuse requires specialized skills and training. It is important that the interviewer use age appropriate language, provide a safe environment, and avoid leading questions. An example of a leading question is:

a. What happened after you went to bed?
b. Where did you touch him?
c. He put his fingers in your bottom, didn't he?
d. Tell me what happened next.

27. Most children who have been maltreated are in therapy because they are showing symptoms of being abused or neglected and:

    a. Social services requires treatment of the child
    b. Therapy enables the child to be a better witness
    c. Therapy may be used to gather information to prosecute the perpetrator
    d. The parents are concerned about how the child is affected by the abuse or neglect

28. Cynthia is a five year old kindergarten child who was digitally penetrated by her babysitter's teenage son. She is usually eager to come to her therapist's office and has been able to describe what happened to her. Other factors that may impact on her progress in treatment include:

    a. The perpetrator's apology to Cynthia
    b. The babysitter's apology to Cynthia
    c. The therapist's alliance with the parent
    d. Cynthia's mother's abuse history

29. A primary focus in the beginning of therapy with abused children includes establishing trust and rapport and:

    a. Integrating the child's thoughts about herself
    b. Helping the child to take risks
    c. Reliving or reexperiencing the abuse
    d. Determining the child's coping style

30. Helping the child to develop ways to cope effectively with symptoms, accessing abuse memories, sensations, thoughts and feelings is a focus of which stage of therapy?

    a. Assessment
    b. Beginning
    c. Middle
    d. Termination

31. Sexual acts are abusive clinically when there is a differential between the victim and the offender in terms of power, knowledge and:

    a. Gratification
    b. Intellect
    c. Socioeconomic level
    d. Gender

32. In assessing sexual abuse, current recommendations regarding the role of evaluator and therapist are that they should be:

    a. Kept separate
    b. Integrated
    c. Done in different agencies
    d. Aimed at keeping the child's story consistent for court purposes

33. Danny is a six year old boy who reported to his teacher that his stepfather often fondles him and forces him to suck his penis. A physical examination reveals no evidence of sexual abuse. Which of the following statements is true?

    a. Most sexually abused children show physical signs of abuse
    b. Most sexually abused children are molested by persons outside the home
    c. The majority of children who are sexually abused have no physical evidence of abuse
    d. It is probable that someone coached Danny to say negative information about the stepfather.

34. Conditions that increase the likelihood of a child being sexually abused are life apart from both biological parents, poverty, mental illness of a caretaker and:

    a. Having a grandparent in prison
    b. Academic failure
    c. Attention deficit hyperactivity disorder
    d. Alcoholic family member

35. The clinical nurse specialist has developed specialized skills in the treatment of sexually abused children. The intervention regarded as the treatment of choice for sexually traumatized children is:

    a. Conjoint family therapy
    b. Solution focused therapy
    c. Analytical play therapy
    d. Group therapy

36. Advantages of co-therapists in working with sexually abused children include:

    a. Greater protection from further victimization

b. Greater consensus on validation of the abuse
c. Protection from further victimization
d. Shared responsibility for multiproblem families

37. Common target symptoms related to child sexual abuse that may be alleviated by pharmacotherapy include anxiety, depression and

a. Poor school performance
b. Regressed behavior
c. Soiling
d. Posttraumatic symptoms

38. Ritual abuse is defined as the intentional physical, sexual or psychological abuse of a child when the abuse is repeated and stylized and typified by acts such as cruelty to animals, threats of harm to the child, other people or animals. Which of the following is true of ritual abuse?

a. The impact on the victim is greater than in other forms of abuse and the children are more symptomatic as assessed by standardized instruments.
b. There is less impact on the victim than in other forms of abuse because of a greater tendency on the part of the victim to dissociate.
c. The ritually abused child's parents have a greater sense of control than when their children are victimized in non-ritualized ways.
d. This type of abuse is well documented and thoroughly researched.

39. The clinical nurse specialist working with children must be aware of the laws regarding reporting child abuse. Which of the following provides a guideline for the nurse?

a. All abuse must be thoroughly investigated by the CNS before it is reported.
b. The reporting requirement does not require proving abuse before reporting.
c. There is generally a felony charge for intentional failure to report.
d. The reporting laws do not override the ethical duty to protect confidential information.

40. Who decides whether or not the clinical nurse specialist is qualified as an expert witness?

a. The nurse
b. The nurse's peers
c. The attorney issuing a subpoena

d. The judge

41. Professionals who qualify as expert witnesses are permitted to offer opinions about which they are confident. In arriving at an opinion, it must be demonstrated that the expert considered all relevant facts, employed appropriate methods of assessment and:

    a. Is advocating for the patient
    b. Has a doctoral degree
    c. Interviewed all parties in a dispute
    d. Demonstrates objectivity

42. Interviews of children may be therapeutic or investigative. It is important in conducting investigative interviews that the interviewer:

    a. Makes sure that sufficient evidence is gathered for a prosecution in spite of the impact on the child of repeated interviews
    b. Minimizes the investigative trauma for the victim
    c. Is qualified as an expert witness
    d. Reports all details of the child's disclosures to the child's therapist.

43. Sources of stress for children experiencing legal proceedings include:

    a. The constitutional right for the offender to have a speedy trial
    b. Lack of familiarity with the courtroom environment
    c. Going to "court school'
    d. Rapid changes in development

44. The major stressor for children who testify in trials of accused abusers is:

    a. Unfamiliarity with legal terminology
    b. The judge's black robes
    c. Confronting the accused
    d. Lack of memory for the events over time

45. States must comply with Federal child abuse and neglect guidelines to receive Federal funds, yet have autonomy in deciding how services are provided to abused and neglected children. The types of laws which are relevant to reporting, intervention and prevention of child abuse include reporting laws, criminal laws and:

    a. Affirmative action laws
    b. Sexual harassment statutes
    c. Anti-pornography statutes

d. Juvenile and family court laws

46. Rationale for parents "rooming in" with a sick child are theories of:

   a. Ego development
   b. Attachment
   c. Psychodynamic development
   d. Communication

47. Marylou is a four-year-old hospitalized with a severe upper respiratory infection. Her mother notes that she has begun wetting the bed after being dry for the last two years. She expresses her concern to the consultation liaison nurse clinical specialist. In helping the mother to understand this change in her daughter's behavior, the nurse should teach the mother about which of the following:

   a. Learning strategies for relaxing
   b. Understanding concepts of regression in illness
   c. Promoting family functioning
   d. Retraining toileting

48. Children hospitalized with chronic illnesses need opportunities for stress management, play and related activities, promoting family functioning and:

   a. Learning and academic activities
   b. Learning ways to express hostility by abreaction
   c. Family therapy
   d. Continuing relations with their outpatient therapist

49. Childhood onset schizophrenia is defined as an onset of psychotic symptoms at approximately which age?

   a. Before age 16
   b. By age 8
   c. Between 4 and 10
   d. before age 12

50. Childhood onset schizophrenia is considered:

   a. The same disorder as adult schizophrenia
   b. A different disorder from adult schizophrenia
   c. A pervasive developmental disorder
   d. Related primarily to poor prenatal nutrition

51. Differential diagnosis of childhood onset schizophrenia needs to take into consideration that symptoms may yield the possibility of neurological disorders, affective disorders, and:

    a. Trauma related symptoms
    b. Reactive attachment disorder
    c. Developmental learning disorder
    d. Anxiety disorder NOS

52. Brain scans of children with childhood onset schizophrenia show:

    a. Left posterior parietal hypometabolism
    b. Right posterior parietal hypometabolism
    c. Left anterior temporal hypermetabolism
    d. Right anterior temporal hypermetabolism

53. Children with schizophrenia show loose associations and illogical thinking. This type of thought disturbance is:

    a. Typically seen in normal children between ages 5-11.
    b. Unusual before age 6 in normal subjects
    c. Not typically seen in normal children after age 7
    d. Not responsive to medication management.

54. Treatment of childhood schizophrenia involves the use of medications that are similar to adult medication. Care should be exercised in the use of which medications which may cause psychotic symptoms?

    a. Minor tranquilizers
    b. SSRIs
    c. Stimulants
    d. Antiparasitical agents

55. An appropriate intervention for the schizophrenic child on an inpatient unit would be:

    a. Tailoring rules and expectations to his or her level of functioning
    b. Using isolation to protect the other children from anxiety about the schizophrenic child's odd behavior
    c. Facilitation of age appropriate skills through having the same rules for everyone
    d. Having high expectations to promote development of skills

56. The community mental health case manager in child and adolescent psychiatric

nursing may be called upon to coordinate care for the schizophrenic child. This may include arranging for hospitalization if indicated, involving the families with NAMI, referring to a child study team and:

    a. Providing direct services
    b. Prescribing medication to a stressed parent
    c. Arranging for respite care
    d. Providing inpatient services.

57. Four year old Nicholas screams when he is held, does not go to a caretaker when hurt, plays in isolation with the same object for long periods of time, has numerous rituals, and cannot tolerate the sound of computer keys clicking. A possible diagnosis to screen for would be:

    a. Attention deficit hyperactivity disorder
    b. Oppositional defiant disorder
    c. Reactive attachment disorder
    d. Pervasive developmental disorder

58. Andy, age 2, had a history of normal development for the first six months of life as well as apparently normal prenatal and perinatal development. After six months, his head growth slowed down, he began to wring his hands constantly, showed a decline in social engagement, had a poorly coordinated gait, and showed impaired expressive language and psychomotor retardation. The most likely diagnosis would be:

    a. Mild mental retardation
    b. Childhood disintegrative disorder
    c. Rett's disorder
    d. Autistic disorder

59. Adult personality disorders may be presaged by which of the following child and adolescent disorders?

    a. Reactive attachment disorder
    b. Dysthymia
    c. School phobia
    d. Oppositional defiant disorder

60. Which of the following of the personality disorders may be diagnosed in older children or adolescents?

    a. Narcissistic
    b. Borderline

    c. Schizotypal

    d. Phobic

61. Depression is unusual up until the age of:

    a. 10

    b. 13

    c. 7

    d. 9

62. Change in weight or appetite disturbance are vegetative signs of depression. This criteria is modified in children to include failure to achieve expected gain or:

    a. Greater than 5% loss of body weight in one month

    b. Greater than 10% loss of body weight in one month

    c. Loss of 5 pounds in three months

    d. Weight gain of 5% in 6 weeks

63. Depression in children is comorbid with many other disorders, including:

    a. Childhood onset schizophrenia

    b. Childhood disintegrative disorder

    c. Anxiety disorders

    d. Rumination disorder of infancy

64. The risk of a child having a mood disorder increases with which of the following:

    a. Family chemical dependency

    b. Divorce of the child's parents

    c. Change in schools

    d. Obesity

65. Suicide among adolescents increases markedly at which age?

    a. 15-17

    b. 13-14

    c. 15-24

    d. 17-20

66. The highest suicide rates occur in:

    a. Black males

b. Black females
c. White males
d. White females

67. Two youngsters in a small school successfully complete suicide. The clinical nurse specialist is invited to do a crisis debriefing for the school personnel. It is important to help the staff to avoid simplistic explanations for the suicide and:

   a. Avoid graphic descriptions of the suicides
   b. Glorify the deceased
   c. Focus on the deceased's nonsuicide characteristics
   d. Pretend as if nothing had happened

68. Bipolar children and adolescents usually require dosing that is:

   a. Lower than adults
   b. Divided in smaller doses
   c. The same as adults
   d. Higher than adults

69. Bipolar youngsters are often a diagnostic challenge. Children less than 9 who are manic are usually:

   a. Extremely aggressive
   b. Difficult to soothe
   c. Good team players
   d. Irritable with emotional lability

70. Which of the following conditions may present in a similar way to bipolar illness in children?

   a. Neurological conditions, such as head trauma
   b. Munchausen's syndrome by Proxy
   c. Chromosomal abnormalities
   d. Hepatitis

71. The age of onset for anorectic youngsters is most commonly between:

   a. 10-14
   b. 12-18
   c. 14-19
   d. 9-12

72. What is important for the nurse to keep in mind when evaluating a child who has lost weight due to anorexia?

    a. The same percentage of body weight lost applies to children and adults
    b. 3% weight loss in children is diagnostically certain for anorexia
    c. Anorectic children do not lose weight if attention is not focused on them
    d. Children do not have to lose the percentage of weight applicable for an adult with an eating disorder.

73. Stephen, age 7, throws up his breakfast every morning before school. The least likely disorder is:

    a. Separation anxiety disorder
    b. School phobia
    c. Bulimia
    d. Anxiety disorder not otherwise specified

74. Which of the following is essential to include in developing a plan of care for an adolescent with an eating disorder?

    a. Art therapy to uncover childhood trauma
    b. Music therapy
    c. Psychodynamic approaches to ascertain the underlying motivations for difficulties with food
    d. Family therapy to modify dysfunctional patterns which maintain the disorder

75. The peak age of onset of Panic Disorder is:

    a. 10-12
    b. 15-19
    c. 14-16
    d. 10-15

76. Play therapy in which the child tells a story and a therapist also tells a story in reciprocal fashion is a technique that enables a child to express his or her:

    a. Ways of behaving
    b. Cultural norms
    c. Unconscious feelings
    d. Autonomy

77. Marcie is a nine year old girl with severe attention deficit hyperactivity disorder. Her parents have developed a chart which tracks Marcie's ability to manage and succeed at her various responsibilities and activities. This technique is part of which type of therapy used with children?

    a. Cognitive therapy
    b. Family therapy
    c. Behavior therapy
    d. Solution focused therapy

78. Which of the following is a strong predictor of positive outcomes for a child who has an DSM IV diagnosis?

    a. Intellectual abilities
    b. Positive peer relationships
    c. Parental involvement in therapy
    d. Absence of chemical dependency issues in Family of origin

79. Many children and adolescent inpatient settings are based on which of the following models:

    a. Family systems model
    b. Community mental health model
    c. Medical model
    d. Strategic and solution focused model

80. 'Time out" is a way for a child to reflect upon his or her behavior and regain control. Time in "time out" is generally determined by which of the following:

    a. Two minutes for each day on the unit
    b. One minute for each year of development
    c. Level of care
    d. Staffing adequacy

81. Joshua, a new boy on the unit, runs up to the nurses' station and crosses over a line meant to keep the children at some distance from the staff. This is the first time you have seen him do this. Which would be the most appropriate response?

    a. Smiling at him because it is important to help him feel welcome
    b. Ignoring the behavior
    c. Saying "Josh, remember the unit rules we reviewed earlier today? No running and no crossing the line. The rules are posted in the dining room if you aren't sure'

    d. 'Stop running. If you do that again, you'll have to go to time out in your room.'

82. Which of the following is not a medication considerations for children?

    a. Children differ in response to a medication's main and side effects
    b. When medicating children, start slow, titrate carefully, use the lowest effective dose
    c. Children may metabolize and eliminate medications more rapidly
    d. Antihistamines are safe over the counter medications which have no effect on psychotropic medications.

83. Kevin is a 12 year old boy recently diagnosed with bipolar disorder. In planning medication management for Kevin it is important to remember:

    a. Children, adolescents and adults require the same dosing range
    b. Lithium is hepatotoxic to children
    c. Lithium is cleared rapidly by children, so they may need higher doses to stabilize a mood disorder
    d. Lithium is only used for augmentation in children

84. The clinical nurse specialist is discussing medication management with a 16 year old adolescent. It is important to remember that adolescents are often resistant to complying with medication due to:

    a. Resistance to perceived control by authority
    b. The success of anti-drug education
    c. Side effects
    d. A resurgence of interest in "natural medicines'

85. Adolescents may abuse medications by giving or selling them to their friends. Which medications are likely to be abused this way?

    a. Major tranquilizers
    b. Antianxiety agents
    c. MAO inhibitors
    d. SSRIs

86. Skills training as a therapeutic intervention has as its goal:

    a. Career preparation
    b. Arts and crafts therapy
    c. Competence in mastering developmental tasks
    d. Activities of daily living training

87. Which of the following interventions encourages the child to express feelings or reenact loss or trauma?

    a. Structured play
    b. Supportive therapy
    c. Behavioral play
    d. Mutual story tellling

88. The child psychiatric nurse clinical specialist provides a sand tray with small figures and objects to encourage a child to tell a story by setting up a scene. This is known as:

    a. Structured play therapy
    b. Nondirective play therapy
    c. Solution focused play therapy
    d. Stress management

89. One of the most serious outcomes of substance abuse disorders (SUD) among adolescents is which of the following:

    a. Lack of social mobility
    b. Interruption of developmental tasks
    c. Poor social skills training
    d. Conflict with parents

90. Adolescent substance abuse would be more likely in which of the following families?

    a. Rural farming family
    b. Emotionally detached parents with lack of involvement in youth's life
    c. Dual career parents
    d. Parents who are not involved with community issues

91. Seven year old Danielle was sexually assaulted by the babysitter's adolescent son. She has no memory of the event, and has been diagnosed as having traumatic amnesia. Which of the following is a probable outcome of the experience of amnesia?

    a. Traumatic amnesia interferes with the processing of the event and placing it in past memory
    b. The child is protected from the effects of the abuse
    c. She will likely recall the event when she is ready
    d. She will recall the event in traumatic dreams

92. Conditions to be ruled out in establishing a diagnosis of Attention Deficit Hyperactivity Disorder would include:

    a. Seizures or sequelae of head trauma
    b. Posttraumatic stress disorder
    c. Hypersomnia
    d. Selective mutism

93. Which of the following is contraindicted for the treatment of Attention Deficit Disorder if there is a coexisting seizure disorder?

    a. Tricyclic antidepressants
    b. SSRIs
    c. Mirtazapine
    d. Bupropion

94. Benzodiazepines may be used on a short term basis for children with anxiety disorders. A side effect of clonazepam is:

    a. Behavior inhibition and shyness
    b. Behavior disinhibition
    c. Cardiotoxicity
    d. Excessive clinginess

95. Which of the following is NOT TRUE of adolescents with an eating disorder?

    a. The adolescent is a high risk patient
    b. Adolescents with eating disorders tend to be extremely secretive about their illness
    c. The mortality rate is 10 to 15%
    d. They are extremely compliant with treatment

96. The latest consensus regarding selective mutism is that:

    a. It is a form of social phobia
    b. Medicine is ineffective in the treatment of this condition
    c. These patients have highly controlling parents
    d. Most of these children have associated hearing problems

Answers

1. b	32. a	64. a
2. c	33. c	65. b
3. d	34. d	66. c
4. d	35. d	67. a
5. d	36. d	68. d
6. b	37. d	69. d
7. c	38. a	70. a
8. d	39. b	71. b
9. a	40. d	72. d
10. a	41. d	73. c
11. d	42. b	74. d
12. a	43. b	75. b
13. c	44. c	76. c
14. c	45. d	77. c
15. b	46. b	78. c
16. a	47. b	79. a
17. c	48. a	80. b
18. d	49. d	81. c
19. c	50. a	82. d
20. a	51. a	83. c
21. c	52. b	84. a
22. b	53. c	85. b
23. d	54. c	86. c
24. b	55. a	87. d
25. a	56. c	88. a
26. c	57. d	89. b
27. d	58. c	90. b
28. c	59. d	91. a
29. d	60. b	92. a
30. c	61. d	93. d
31. a	62. a	94. a
	63. c	95. d
		96. a

BIBLIOGRAPHY

American Nurses' Association. (1994). *Statement on Psychiatric and Mental Health Nursing Clinical Nursing Practice and Standards of Psychiatric-Mental Health Nursing Practice.* Washington, DC: Author.

American Professional Society on the Abuse of Children. (1997). *Guidelines for psychosocial evaluation of suspected sexual abuse in children.* Chicago: APSAC.

American Psychiatric Association. (1994). *Diagnostic and statistical manual of mental disorders (4th ed.).* Washington, DC: author.

Antai-Otong, D. (Ed.). (1995). *Psychiatric nursing:Biological and behavioral concepts.* Philadelphia: W. B. Saunders.

Assessment and treatment of children and adolescents with anxiety disorders. (1997b). *Journal of the American Academy of Child & Adolescent Psychiatry,* 36(10), Supplement, 69s-84s.

Assessment and treatment of children, adolescents and adults with Attention-deficit/hyperactivity disorder. (1997c). *Journal of the American Academy of Child & Adolescent Psychiatry,* 36(10), Supplement, 85s-121s.

Assessment and treatment of children and adolescents with bipolar disorder. (1997d). *Journal of the American Academy of Child & Adolescent Psychiatry,* 36(10), Supplement, 157s-176s.

Assessment and treatment of children and adolescents with conduct disorder. (1997e). *Journal of the American Academy of Child & Adolescent Psychiatry,* 36(10), Supplement, 122s-139s.

Assessment and treatment of children and adolescents with schizophrenia. (1997f). *Journal of the American Academy of Child & Adolescent Psychiatry.* 36(10), Supplement, 177s-193s.

Assessment and treatment of children and adolescents with substance use disorders. (1997g). *Journal of the American Academy of Child & Adolescent Psychiatry.* 36(10), 140s-156s.

Bernstein, G. A., Borchardt, C. M., & Perwein, A. (1996). Anxiety disorders in children and adolescents: A review of the past 10 years. *Journal of the American Academy of Child and Adolescent Psychiatry,* 35(9), 1110-1119.

Biederman, J., Faraone, S. V., Milberger, S., Jettonl, J. G., Chen, L., Mick, E., Greene, R. W., & Russell, R. L.(1996). Is childhood oppositional defiant disorder a precursor to adolescent conduct disorder? *Journal of the American Academy of Child and Adolescent Psychiatry,* 35(9), 1193-1204.

Bloomquist, M. (1996). *Skills training for children with behavior disorders.* New York: Guilford Press.

Botz, J. R., & Bidwell-Cerone, S. (1997). Adolescents. In J. Haber, J. Krainovich-Miller, B. Leach McMahon, P. Price-Hoskins. *Comprehensive psychiatric nursing* (5th ed. pp. 739-760). St. Louis: Mosby Year Book.

Briere, J., Berliner, L., Bulkley, J., Jenny, C. l., & Reid, T. (1996). *The APSAC handbook on child maltreatment.* Thousand Oaks: Sage Publications.

Brodeur, A. E., & Monteleone, J. A. (1994). *Child Maltreatment: A clinical guide and reference.* St. Louis: G. W. Medical Publishing.

Cantwell, D. P. (1996). Attention deficit disorder: A review of the past 10 years. *Journal of the American Academy of Child and Adolescent Psychiatry, 35*(8), 978-987.

DePanfilis, D., & Salus, M. (1992). *A coordinated response to child abuse and neglect.* Washington, DC: National Center on Child Abuse and Neglect.

DeVane, C. L., & Sallee, F. R. (1996). Serotonin selective reuptake inhibitors in child and adolescent psychopharmacology: A review of published experience. *Journal of Clinical Psychiatry, 57*(20), 55-66.

Elder, J. H. (1997). Defining parent training for practice and research. *Journal of the American Psychiatric Nurses Association, 3*(4), 103-110.

Erickson, M. E., & Egelund, B. (1996). Child neglect. In J. Briere, L. Berliner, J. A. Bulkley, C. Jenny, & T. Reid, (Eds.). *The APSAC handbook on child maltreatment* (pp. 4-20). Thousand Oaks, CA: Sage Publications.

Faller, K. C. (1993). *Child sexual abuse: Intervention and treatment issues.* Washington, DC: National Center on Child Abuse and Neglect.

Feller, J. (1992). *Working with the courts in child protection.* Washington, DC: National Center on Child Abuse and Neglect.

Friedrich, W. Berliner, L., Butler, J., Cohen, J., Damon, L., & Shafram, C. (1996). Child Sexual Behavior: An Update with the CSBI-3. *The APSAC Advisor,* (9)4, 13-14.

Gaudin, J. (1993). *Child neglect: A guide for intervention.* Washington, DC: National Center on Child Abuse and Neglect.

Goodman, G., & Bottoms, B. L. (Eds.). (1993). *Child victims, child witnesses.* New York: The Guilford Press.

Haber, J., Krainovich-Miller, B., Leach McMahon, A., & Price-Hoskins, P. (1997). *Comprehensive psychiatric nursing* (5th ed.). St. Louis: Mosby Year Book.

Hartman, C. R., & Burgess, A. W. (1998). Treatment of complex sexual assault. In A. W. Burgess (Ed.), *Advanced practice psychiatric nursing* (pp. 397-418). Stamford, CT: Appleton & Lange.

Hovey, J. D., & King, C. (1996). Acculturative stress, depression and suicidal ideation among immigrant and second generation latino adolescents. *Journal of the American Academy of Child and Adolescent Psychiatry, 35*(9), 1183-1192.

Hendren, R. L. (1996). Management of psychosis in adolescents suffering from schizophrenia and bipolar disorder. *Essential Psychopharmacology,* (1), 38-53.

Johnson, B. S. (1997). *Psychiatric mental health nursing* (4th ed.). Philadelphia: J. B. Lippincott.

Johnson, B. S.(1995). *Child, adolescent & family psychiatric nursing*. Philadelphia: J. B. Lippincott.

Jongsma, A., Peterson, L. M., & McInnis, W. P. (1996). *The child and adolescent psychotherapy treatment planner*. New York: Wiley & Sons.

Kendler, K. S. (1996). Parenting: A genetic-epidemiologic perspective. *American Journal of Psychiatry, 153*(1), 11-20.

Kingston, L., & Prior, M. (1995). The development of patterns of stable, transient, and school-age onset aggressive behavior in young children. *Journal of the American Academy of Child and Adolescent Psychiatry, 34*(3), 348-358.

Krauss, J. (1993). *Health care reform: Essential mental health services*. Washington, DC: American Nurses Publishing.

Leaf, P. J., Alegria, M., Cohen, P., Goodman, S.H., Horwitz, S. M., Hoven, C. W., Narrow, W. E., Vaden-Kiernan, M., & Regier, D. A. (1996). Mental health service use in the community and schools: Results from the four-community MECA study. *Journal of the American Academy of Child and Adolescent Psychiatry, 35*(7), 889-897.

Lewisohn, P. M., Clarke, G. N., Seeley, J. R. & Rohde, P. (1994). Major depression in community adolescents: Age at onset, episode duration, and time to recurrence. *Journal of the American Academy of Child and Adolescent Psychiatry. 33*(6), 809-818.

Lynch, V. A., & Burgess, A. W. (1998). Forensic nursing. In A. W. Burgess, (Ed.), *Advanced practice psychiatric nursing (pp. 473-490). Stamford, CT: Appleton & Lange.*

McKenna, K. M., Gordon, C. T., & Rapoport, J. L. (1994). Childhood-onset schizophrenia. *Journal of the American Academy of Child and Adolescent Psychiatry, 33*(6), 771-781.

Monteleone, J. A., Glaze, S., & Bly, K. M. (1994). Sexual abuse: An overview. In A. E. Brodeur & J. A. Monteleone (Eds.), *Child maltreatmentL A clinical guide and reference* (pp. 113-131). St. Louis: G. W. Medical Publishing.

Mohr, W. (1998). Issues in the care of adolescent clients. In A. W. Burgess (Ed.), *Advanced practice psychiatric nursing* (pp. 285-302). Stamford, Ct.: Appleton & Lange.

Myers, J. E. B. (1992). *Legal issues in child abuse and neglect.* Newbury Park: Sage Publications.

Nakane, Y., & Rapoport, J. L. (1995). Childhood onset schizophrenia. *Current Approaches to Psychoses, 4*(10), 1-5.

National Center of Child Abuse and Neglect (1996). *Study findings: National study of the incidence and severity of child abuse and neglect.* Washington, DC: Department of Health and Human Services.

Pence, D., & Wilson, C. (1992). *The role of law enforcement in the response to child abuse and neglect.* Washington, DC: National Center on Child Abuse and Neglect.

Pilowsky, D. J., & Kates, W. G. (1996). Foster children in acute crisis: Assessing critical aspects of attachment. *Journal of the American Academy of Child and Adolescent Psychiatry. 35*(8), 1095-1097.

Psychiatric assessment of children and adolescents. (1997a). *Journal of the American Academy of Child & Adolescent Psychiatry, 36*(10), Supplement, 4s-20s.

Risley-Curtiss, C. (1996). The health status and care of children in out-of-home care. *APSAC Advisor, 9*(4), 1-7.

Rosen, S. L. (1998). Working with children in foster care. In A. W. Burgess (Ed.), *Advanced practice psychiatric nursing* (pp. 371-396). Stamford, CT: Appleton & Lange.

Scahill, L., & Lynch, K. (1994). Tricyclic antidepressants: Cardiac effects and clinical implications. *Journal of Child and Adolescent Psychiatric Nursing, 7*(1), 37-39.

Stowell, J. (1994). Evaluating the adolescent substance abuser. *Directions in Rehabilitation Counseling, 5*(2), 2-12.

Urquiza, A. J., & Winn, C. (1995). *Treatment for abused and neglected children: Infancy to age 18.* Washington, D.C. National Center on Child Abuse and Neglect.

Volkmar, F. R., (1996). Childhood and adolescent psychosis: A review of the past 10 years. *Journal of the American Academy of Child and Adolescent Psychosis. 35(7)*, 843-851.

Walsh, E., & Randell, B. P. (1995). Seclusion and restraint:What we need to know. *Journal of Child and Adolescent Psychiatric Nursing, 8(1)*, 28-40.

Weller, E. B., & Weller, R. A. (1991). Mood disorders. In M. Lewis (Ed.), *Child and adolescent psychiatry: A comprehensive textbook (pp. 646-663). Baltimore, MD: Williams & Wilkins.*

Whitfield, C. L. (1998). Trauma and memory. In A. W. Burgess (Ed.), *Advanced practice psychiatric nursing* (pp. 171-186). Stamford, CT: Appleton & Lange.

Zimmerman, M. L., (1997). Infants and children. In J. Haber, J. Krainovich-Miller, B. Leach Mc Mahon, P. Price-Hoskins. *Comprehensive psychiatric nursing.* (5th ed., pp. 715-738). St Louis: Mosby Year Book.

The Larger Mental Health Environment

Janice V. R. Belcher

Mental Health Care Delivery System

- The number and variations of psychiatric-mental health delivery care settings have greatly increased since the 1970s.

- In the United States, the major focus has been in treatment of mental disorders, not the prevention of mental disorders.

- Types of settings

  1. Acute care inpatient settings, either psychiatric units in general hospitals or in psychiatric hospitals.

     a. Often psychiatric units specialized in adults, children, adolescent, alcohol, substance abuse and/or geriatrics.

     b. In recent years, changing reimbursement of inpatient stays has resulted in shorter psychiatric lengths of stays.

     c. From this decline in hospitalization days, many psychiatric units offer an array of services including partial hospitalization, outpatient and home care

     d. Today, most patients that are admitted to the hospital are in crisis with the treatment goal of stabilization.

     e. Inpatient treatment is focused on preventing harm to oneself or others and the need for multidisciplinary assessment and stabilization.

  2. Public mental hospital settings

     a. Deinstitutionalization, which began in 1970s, has reduced the census of the public mental hospitals established by state governments.

     b. Over the last 30 years, public mental hospital census has declined over 75% while the number of admissions have doubled.

     c. Public mental hospitals have seen an increase in admission rates of younger, violent patients.

     d. The goals of deinstitutionalization are:

        (1) To save clients from debilitating effects of lengthy, restrictive periods of hospitalization.

        (2) To return the client to home and community as soon as possible after hospitalization.

(3) To maintain the client in the community for as long as possible.

e. In general, the public mental hospital patient population decreased by returning the patients to their families, transferring them to nursing homes and by shifting them into the community where unfortunately some became homeless street people because community support did not work.

3. Ambulatory settings

a. Community Mental Health Centers (CMHC)

(1) The CMHC Act passed by Congress in 1963 supported mental health centers and deinstitutionalization in all fifty states.

(2) This legislation represented a shift from the focus of the mentally ill in public mental hospitals to flexible, community care.

(3) A principle in the development of CMHC was that people with mental illness have a right to treatment in the least restrictive environment.

(4) In 1965, the five essential services for a federally funded CMHC were inpatient services, outpatient services, partial hospitalization, and consultation and education.

(5) The legislation provided federal funding to local communities for construction and staffing of CMHC, with the understanding that funding would eventually shift to state and local resources.

(6) In 1975, seven other essential services were added including children's services, geriatric services, aftercare, state hospital pre-screening, drug abuse treatment, alcohol abuse treatment, and transitional housing.

(7) After deinstitutionalization, the patients were discharged from public mental health hospitals to a CMHC system so that the CMHC staff could provide adequate follow-up.

(8) CMHC experienced the following problems working with discharged public mental health hospital patients:

(a) Many discharged patients found it difficult to adjust to independent community living because patients needed a slow, gradual introduction to independent living.

(b) Patients had difficulty keeping appointments and complying with medication schedules.

(c) Many patients became involved in a revolving door syndrome or had many, short hospital admissions.

(9) CMHC are successful in working with chronic patients by using crisis intervention, extensive community outreach programs, supportive living arrangements, and work programs.

(10) Psychiatric emergency crisis/walk-in programs are centralized community mental health programs that offer face-to-face evaluations of patients 24 hours a day.

(a) 57% of these programs are community-based and some are located in conjunction with a general hospital emergency department (Geller, Fisher, & McDermeit, 1995).

(b) Emergency services were originally targeted for suicide prevention and outpatient treatment of acute psychosis.

(c) Since waiting times for treatment at CMHC can be long, crisis programs provide care for the acutely decompensated chronically mental ill patient living in the community (Hillard, 1994).

(11) Psychiatric emergency services have continued to evolve in the community over the last 10 years as most urban settings have centralized emergency services in one or a few sites.

(a) Most rural areas are coordinating networks of emergency services at a limited number of sites, usually in a general hospital.

(b) Many emergency services have expanded roles so that patients can stay for several days.

(c) Some programs offer community outreach programs whereby staff go into the community to work with patients.

(d) Many emergency services start long term medication regimes such as anti-depressants.

(12) The current state of mobile crisis services by a 50 state survey (Geller et al, 1995):

(a) Seventy-three percent of the states had mobile emergency services and provided services in private homes, hospital emergency rooms, residential programs, shelters, correctional facilities, bus and train stations, and general hospital medical units.

(b) Mobile crisis units were reported to provide for patients and families: earlier interventions, improved access to care, support for families, minimizing patient's trauma.

4. Partial Hospitalization Programs (PHP) are ambulatory treatment programs that include the major, diagnostic, medical, psychiatric, and prevocational treatment modalities designed for patient with serious mental disorders who require coordinated, intensive, and multidisciplinary treatment not provided in the usual outpatient setting. (Rosie, Azim, Piper, & Joyce, 1995).

a. The four functions of partial hospitalization include:

(1) Treatment of acutely ill patients who would be inpatients

(2) Rehabilitation of patients who are in transition from acute inpatient to outpatient care

(3) Intensive treatment of patients who do not require inpatient care but who may benefit from more intensive care than it is possible to provide on an outpatient basis

(4) Long-term maintenance of chronic psychiatric patients

b. For maximum treatment effectiveness, partial hospitals should match the functional level of patients with treatment intensity.

(a) An intensive group-oriented psychotherapy program may lead to deterioration of acutely ill patients.

        (b)   If low functioning patients are treated with patients needing intensive group-oriented psychotherapy, the intensity of the program may be diluted.

5. Other Community Settings

    a. There are many emerging psychiatric nurse roles including case managers, psychiatric home health nurses, psychiatric community outreach nurses, psychiatric nurses who practice in vocational and rehabilitation centers and psychiatric nurses who work in a variety of collaborative practice settings.

    b. A psychiatric nurse who is a case manager can work with patients, families, and groups over the continuum of care, for example from an inpatient setting to community-based care such as an outpatient clinic or home.

    c. According to Easterling, Avie, Wesley & Chimner (1995), case management is a clinical system that focuses on the accountability of an identified individual or group by:

        (1) Coordinating patient or group patient care across an illness episode or continuum of care (for example, clinic to hospital to home)

        (2) Ensuring and facilitating achievement of quality and clinical cost outcomes

        (3) Negotiating, obtaining, and coordinating services and resources needed by patients/families

        (4) Intervening at key points for individual patients (for example, using critical pathways)

        (5) Addressing and resolving patient patterns that cause poor quality-cost outcomes within collaborative teams

        (6) Creating opportunities and systems of health care to enhance patient outcomes

    d. A community mental health nurse who works in therapy with individuals, families or group should be Masters prepared.

    e. Community mental health nurses assist patients with a range of psychological problems and are concerned with the patient's stress, coping and adaptation.

f. Community mental health nurses assist individuals and families to anticipate the course of events in the mental health care system.

g. Psychiatric mental health nursing in home health

   (1) In recent years, there has been an increased need for psychiatric nurses in the home.

   (2) A criteria for providing home health is usually that the patients are homebound or their illnesses result in them not being able to leave their home.

   (3) Three groups of common homebound patients include:

       (a) People living alone especially the elderly

       (b) People with medical illnesses especially chronic illnesses

       (c) Chronically mentally ill people

   (4) The psychiatric nurse may provide:

       (a) Direct care giving, such as assisting a depressed patient to perform his/her activities of daily living

       (b) Counseling, such as assisting a depressed patient to modify negative thinking

       (c) Education, such as teaching a depressed patient about his/her antidepressant medication side effects

       (d) Referral, such as scheduling an appointment when the patient needs medication adjustment

       (e) Health promotion for patients and family, such as guiding the families in preparing balanced nutritional meals.

5. Outpatient Private practice

   a. Since the 1960s, psychiatric nurses have engaged in private practice, especially clinical specialists who hold ANA Certification in Advanced Practice (Peplau, 1990).

   b. Nurses can practice solo or with other health care professionals

   c. Nurses' private practice can include a variety of functions including individual and family assessment; individual, group, and family psychotherapy; and prescribing psychotropic medication.

   d. In general, barriers to Certified Psychiatric Clinical Nurse Specialists include difficulty in obtaining third party reimbursement, limited autonomy in organized practice settings and low salaries (Merwin, Fox & Bell, 1996).

   e. The following are important considerations in working in private practice. The private practitioner:

     (1) Has the client as the primary obligation

     (2) Determines who the client will be

     (3) Determines the techniques to be used in service to this client

     (4) Determines practice professionally, not bureaucratically

     (5) Receives a payment directly from or in behalf of the client

     (6) Is educated in a graduate program

     (7) Is sufficiently experienced as an Advanced Practice Nurse

     (8) Adheres to Advanced Practice Nursing values, standards, and ethics and is professionally responsible

     (9) Is licensed and certified where applicable to engage in private practice

   f. Disadvantages of private practice:

     (1) Economic uncertainties of private practice and possible financial difficulties

     (2) Professional isolation, loneliness, and lack of advancement

     (3) Malpractice suits

(4) Total responsibility for professional accountability and professional competence

g. Establishing a viable private practice

(1) Evaluate whether solo or group practice is desirable

(2) Create a financial management system

(3) Obtain malpractice and office liability insurance

(4) Establish criteria for hiring employees and using consultants

(5) Ensure that private practice is geographically accessible

(6) Successful marketing strategies include specialization and courteous attention to referrals

Managed Care—An Internal Force of Change Within the Mental Health Delivery System

- Managed care is a health care strategy designed to achieve the positive outcomes that can result from adopting price competition while controlling for unfavorable effects.

- For competitive low prices, there must be a variety of health care providers such as hospitals, physicians, Health Maintenance Organizations (HMOs).

- For competitive low prices, health care providers must keep their costs low for example, use cost containment strategies.

- Along with low prices, health care providers must provide a quality service.

- Health care changes as the result of managed care.

1. Change of provider incentives, change from fee for service reimbursemant to capitation

a. Fee for service reimbursement is the traditional method of paying health care providers where providers determined what health care services the patient needs, and the insurer passively paid for each service received by the patient according to the reasonable charge in a given geographical area.

b. Capitation is a preset amount of money allocated to provide set services for a population over a stated period of time, regardless of service used. Typically, an employer or third party payor will contract with a behavioral managed care company or a provider organization to provide comprehensive mental health care for a lump sum payment. The managed care company and/or the provider organization then decides what care the patient needs.

    c.   In capitation, the managed care company and/or the provider organization incurs more risks if health care costs for a group of people exceed the capitated payment.

2. Need for standards to evaluate quality clinical practice and patient outcomes.

3. Need to evaluate changing clinical practice patterns such as declining psychiatric length of stay and effect on patient outcomes.

4. Need to improve linkages among inpatient and outpatient providers.

- Organizational changes needed in managed care

    1.   Understanding of fee for service versus capitation reimbursement

    2.   Promotion of team-based care or creating a seamless organization

    3.   Aggressive promotion of self-care

    4.   Case management for high cost, high use members

    5.   Continuous improvement emphasis

- Impact of managed care on hospital nurses (Buerhaus, 1994)

    1.   Decreasing hospital wages since the hospital obtains lump sum (capitation) and may incur more risk

    2.   Decreasing patient length of stay which results in more staff lay-offs, buyouts, retirement, and termination

    3.   Down-sizing of hospitals including contracting (outsourcing) some services

    4.   Tracking specific patient hospital and nursing costs resulting in more administrative tasks

    5.   Substituting of lower skill workers for higher skill workers to lower labor costs

- Ethical dilemmas in managed care

1. Early patient discharge because of financial incentives

2. Providers limiting and denying patient treatments and options because of financial incentives which may result in denial of care.

3. Providers monitoring and controlling patient treatments and resources

- Impact of managed care on Advanced Practice Nurses (Buerhaus, 1994)

  1. Substituting Advanced Practice Nurses for physicians

  2. Increasing demand by capitation plans for Advanced Practice Nurses who provide cost effective care

  3. Professional conflicts among different providers who provide similar services

  4. Increasing responsibility of Advanced Practice Nurses to lower costs and monitor patients' resource consumption

- **Types of Health Care Insurance Plans**

  1. Health Maintenance Organizations (HMO) are organizations that receive money from consumers in exchange for a promise to provide all health care required during a defined period of time. Consumers have restricted choice of health care providers, no cost for services beyond insurance payment, restricted choice to hospitals, reduced cost to employers who buy the insurance. (Cleverley, 1997).

  2. Preferred Provider Organizations (PPO) are programs which contract with health care providers to provide health care services to consumers usually at a discounted rate. Consumers have some restricted choice by using contracted health care providers, copay for services, access to contracted hospitals, some reduced cost to employers who buy the insurance (Cleverley, 1997).

  3. Traditional fee for service insurance plan—consumers have freedom of choice of health care providers, usually pay a deductible and 20% of outpatient charges, unlimited access to choice of hospitals, employers usually pay a higher cost but employees have freedom of choice.

  4. Combinations and variations of HMOs, PPOs and traditional fee for service.

External Forces Interacting with the Mental Health System

- Social issues
  1. Role behavior
     a. Stereotyping behavior is useful in examining roles such as men and women, nurse and physician, and female patient and male therapist, male patient and female therapists.
     b. In general, there are distinct beliefs about the characteristics of men and women.
        (1) Male characteristics reflect competence such as competitiveness, independence, and objectivity.
        (2) Females are perceived as being opposite of these characteristics and are dependent, noncompetitive, and subjective.
        (3) Men are perceived as being blunt and unable to express feelings.
        (4) Women are seen as having tact, are aware of other's feelings, and are able to express their feelings.
        (5) These sex role stereotypes can impact many areas of a person's life including:
            (a) A person's self esteem and prescribed role in society
            (b) The nurse-client therapeutic relationship
            (c) Nursing roles with other health care disciplines
  2. Power
     a. Defined as the potential of an individual or a group to influence the behavior of another
     b. Types of power (Marquis & Huston, 1994)
        (1) Legitimate power—power gained by a title or official position
        (2) Expert power—power gained through knowledge expertise
        (3) Reward power—power obtained by the ability to grant favors, or to reward others with what they value

(4) Coercive power—power obtained on fear of punishment

(5) Referent power—power obtained by an individual because of an association with others

c. Strategies for acquiring and using power in communities and organizations (Marquis & Huston, 1994)

(1) Present a powerful image and assume authority in your interactions

(2) Learn to speak the community's or organization's language

(3) Acquaint yourself with who is powerful and network

(4) Seek experts' advice and build a knowledge base

(5) Increase visibility and use the politicians' priorities to speak your needs

(6) Empower others by sharing knowledge and increasing team building

- Health care policy and political issues

    1. According to Health System Review (1996), current health care legislative issues include concerns about:

        a. Health care coverage for the uninsured and other vulnerable populations such as children, women, and the chronically ill

        b. Restricting managed care and hospital consolidation

        c. Creating or expanding Medicaid coverage to include managed care and/or case management programs on state levels

        d. Using provider report cards which measure various quality and cost aspects of patient care, for ranking different hospitals or health care providers (e.g., average length of stay in hospital)

    2. Mental health care policy and political issues

        a. The care of people with mental health disorders is challenged by their vulnerability and lack of voice in the political process.

        b. Key past mental health legislation

            (1) In 1935, the Social Security Act influenced mental health care because of the shift from state to the federal government in the care of ill people.

(2) In 1955, the Mental Health Study Act created the Joint Commission on Mental Illness and Health that recommended shift of patient populations from state hospital systems to community mental health systems.

(3) In 1963, the Community Mental Health Centers Act created community mental health centers and led to deinstitutionalization. Federal funds were to match state funds in creating CMHC.

(4) In 1975, the Developmental Disabilities Act focused on the rights and treatment of people with developmental disabilities and provided a foundation for individuals with mental disorders.

(5) In 1977, the President's Commission on Mental Health supported community mental health centers, protection of human rights, and insurance for mentally ill people.

(6) In 1986, the Protection and Advocacy for Mentally Ill Individuals Act provided advocacy programs for mentally ill people.

(7) In 1990, the Americans with Disabilities Act promoted employment opportunities and prohibited discrimination for all people with disabilities including mental disorders.

(8) In 1998, the Mental Health Parity Act of 1996, prohibited lifetime or annual limitations on mental health coverage for certain insured employees.

c. According to Health System Review (1996), the best method for mental health insurance coverage such as HMO, PPO or traditional fee for service model is being debated by state and federal legislators in the mental health care arena

d. National health care agenda, under the Public Health Service, Healthy People 2000 (U.S. Department and Health and Human Services, 1990) creates a national focus on promoting health and preventing disease. The following are areas related to mental health and mental disorders:

      (1)   Reducing suicide, especially among children and adolescents and in jails

      (2)   Reducing mental disorders among adults

      (3)   Reducing adverse affects from stress

      (4)   Increasing community supports for people with mental disorders

      (5)   Increasing treatment for people with depressive disorders

      (6)   Increasing access to care for people with personal and emotional problems

      (7)   Increasing mental functioning assessment for both children and adults by primary care providers

   e. Strategies for psychiatric-mental health nurses to serve as change agents for addressing mental health issues:

      (1)   Write and verbalize concerns and solutions to legislative bodies and the media.

      (2)   Seek membership on community committees that recommend or formulate policy.

      (3)   Be familiar with the legislative process, obtaining copies of bills and making presentations at local, state, and federal hearings.

3.   The impact of financial issues on health care (McCloskey & Grace, 1994)

   a. The U. S. finances health care by both public and private monies.

   b. With the passage of Medicare and Medicaid legislation in 1965, the federal government embarked upon a significant subsidy to health care greatly increasing access to care.

   c. The public-sector share of health care costs is expected to grow from its current 40.6% to 42.5% by 2000.

   d. It has been estimated that the number of persons with serious and persistent mental health care problems range from 1.7 to 2.4 million. Hollingsworth & Sweeney (1997) estimated that

> Wisconsin's average annual expenditure per patient with serious mental illness was $14,000 in 1994 dollars.

4. Reimbursement for Advanced Practice Nursing

    a. Types of reimbursements (McCloskey & Grace, 1994)

        (1) Fee-for-service reimbursement. Current trends throughout the country indicate that probably less than 20% of mental health care will be delivered through the traditional fee-for-service model.

        (2) Capitation. Mental health capitation refers to paying a set amount of money for mental health services for a defined group of people.

        (3) Medicare reimburses health care for the elderly and some disabilities by this federal program. Hospitals are now reimbursed a flat amount based (Diagnostic Related Group) upon the patient's medical diagnosis, age, surgical procedure, and comorbidity (existence of other medical conditions). Home care, including psychiatric home care, is reimbursed under Medicare.

        (4) Medicaid is a federally assisted and state-administered program for the indigent.

        (5) Reimbursement for clinical nurse specialists

            (a) ANA House of Delegates has adopted resolutions supporting direct reimbursement for nursing services by both public payers (Medicaid, Medicare, the Civilian Health and Medical Program of the Uniformed Services (CHAMPUS), and the Federal Health Benefits Program and private payers (insurance companies and health care service contractors such as Blue Cross/Blue Shield).

            (b) Medicare Part B reimburses clinical nurse specialists regardless of geographic area if services are within the scope of practice of the CNS.

            (c) Medicaid reimburses clinical nurse specialists at state's discretion. Advanced practice nurses are reimbursed in twenty eight states.

    (d)   CHAMPUS reimburses certified psychiatric clinical nurses specialists.

    (e)   FEHB (Federal Employee Health Benefit Program) reimburses clinical nurse specialists.

(6)   Contract Payment and Services

    (a)   Nurses can develop contracts to provide specific services independently for patient subgroups being served by HMOs or other health care providers.

    (b)   Many times, these providers are interested in the cost of the service and who can legally and safely provide that service.

    (c)   Service contracting is a matter of defining a required service for a group of clients that is difficult to provide with existing staff.

    (d)   Reasons promoting contractual liaisons (Marshall, 1994) include defining a particular population, increasing profitability for selected health care professionals and lowering cost for third-party payers and facilities.

(7)   Strategies for Advanced Practice Nurses to obtain third-party reimbursement (Streff, 1994)

    (a)   Networking by the leadership and membership of nursing organizations with elected officials and administrators of major corporations who have investment in cost effective health care.

    (b)   Networking with national insurance corporations.

    (c)   Assessing political climate and preparing to submit and resubmit bills for reimbursement.

    (d)   Maintaining political vigilance by providing bill sponsors and supporters with a clearly stated fact sheet, a definition of scope of practice, a cost analysis, and a projection of the impact of the bill.

    (e)   Persistent lobbying for the bill by continued networking with legislators, nursing associations, health care providers and community groups.

    (8) Billing for private practice (Billings, 1993)

      (a) Not all clients have or want to work with insurance, some will pay for services themselves

      (b) Give new clients a handout so the financial arrangement will be clear

      (c) Before the first visit, have the client check with their insurance to see what services are covered or whether visit needs to be preauthorized

      (d) On the first visit, use an initial data form to obtain all necessary information such as date of birth, social security number and insurance information

      (e) If the client is filing for his/her own reimbursement, provide the necessary information

      (f) If the client requests your assistance, approach the insurer with the assumption that you will be reimbursed

      (g) If need be, apply to become an authorized provider

      (h) One way to increase referrals is to develop a relationship with the referral source

    (9) Questions that assist in determining private practice charges:

      (a) How much do other Advanced Practice Nurses providing a similar service in the area charge?

      (b) How much do other similar helping professionals in the area charge?

      (c) What is your level of experience and education?

      (d) What do third-party payers say are ''reasonable and customary charges'' for professionals in your area?

      (e) What is the most attractive rate for the clientele that you hope to attract?

    (10) Private practice in managed care (Godschalx, 1996)

(a) To take advantage of capitation, nurses must broaden their ideas of evaluation and treatment.

(b) In fee for service reimbursement, the nurse must evaluate the client to obtain a diagnosis and to match the client to available services. Reimbursement is based upon the diagnosis.

(c) In capitation, reimbursement is not based on diagnosis so that a variety of treatment approaches can be tried.

Leadership and Management

- Leadership Theory and Roles

  1. Leadership is the process of influencing others toward goal setting.

  2. Gardner identifies the tasks of leaders as being: envisioning goals, affirming values, motivating, managing, achieving workable unity, explaining, serving as a symbol, representing the group, and renewing their energy (Swansburg, 1996).

  3. Early leadership studies focused on identifying leadership traits in individuals such as intelligence, personality and abilities.

  4. Studies of leadership styles in the 1930s by Lewin and colleagues examined the decision-making styles of leaders:

     a. Autocratic—leaders make decisions alone

     b. Democratic—leaders involve followers in the decision-making process.

     c. Laissez-faire—leaders are permissive and allow followers to have complete autonomy.

  5. Hersey and Blanchard Life-Cycle of Situational Leadership (Swansburg, 1996)

     a. Assumes that the type of leadership depends on the situation

     b. The three main factors to consider in the leadership process are: the leader, the situation, and level of maturity (readiness) of the followers

     c. As a follower becomes more mature, the follower needs less structure (task structure) and more focus on building relationships in the group (relationship behavior).

    d. Leadership strategies vary depending on the follower and include:

        (1) Telling—for followers who are immature and need high task structure and low relationship behavior; leaders provide specific instructions and closely supervise performance

        (2) Selling—for followers who are a little less immature and need high task structure and high relationship behavior; leaders explain decisions and provide opportunity for clarification

        (3) Participating—for followers who are more mature and need low task structure and high relationship behavior; leaders share ideas and facilitate decision making

        (4) Delegating—for followers who are mature and need low task structure and low relationship behavior; leaders turn over responsibility for decisions and implementation

- Management Theory and Roles

  Classical management theory describes the functions of management as planning, directing, organizing and evaluating.

  1. Planning

     a. Using epidemiology for planning priorities

         (1) Epidemiology is the study of disease in human populations.

         (2) Epidemiologists are concerned with patterns of disease such as communicable, congenital and chronic illnesses within a population.

         (3) Epidemiology focuses on characterizing health outcomes in terms of what, who, where, when, and why. For example, what is the disease? Who is affected by the disease? When do disease related events occur? Why did the disease related events occur?

         (4) Epidemiological research has shown a positive relationship between physical and psychiatric disorders and that the strength of this relationship varies among different populations.

(5) Epidemiological findings assist researchers and funding agencies to establish priorities to guide future research.

(6) Epidemiology has been useful in examining mental illness caused by poisoning, chemicals, drug usage, nutritional deficiencies, biological agents and electrolyte imbalances (Stuart & Sundeen, 1996).

(7) The following epidemiological triangle is useful to explain the presence or absence of illness:

   (a) Host or population characteristics in the occurrence, nonoccurrence, or prognosis of an illness. Includes factors such as age, gender, marital status, ethnicity, race, religion, national origin, genetics, life-style behaviors.

   (b) Agent or cause. Includes infectious agents (bacteria, viruses, fungi, parasites), physical agents (radiation, heat, cold, machinery), or chemical agents (heavy metals, toxic chemicals, pesticides).

   (c) Environment or surroundings. Includes factors such as population density, education, occupation, income, housing, social support, rainfall, habitat, levels of stress, satisfaction, noise, resources, access to care and temperature.

(8) The identification of risk factors is important for planning for populations most likely to suffer illness or injury.

   (a) Psychosocial risk factors include developmental or situational events that occur at a certain time that can create a vulnerable point for an individual. An example is suicide. Adolescents have a high suicide rate.

   (b) Workers who lose their jobs are especially vulnerable to depression, illness, and family conflicts.

b. Incorporating community assessment into planning

   (1) Community needs assessment includes assessing social indicators or examining community characteristics such as income, race, population density, and crime.

     (2) More information on the community needs can be obtained from key informants in the community or people who work in the community such as clergy, social service and health care providers.

     (3) Community forums can provide community members an opportunity to express their needs. Important in community assessment is viewing the community as a partner so that interventions can be community-focused.

     (4) One community assessment wheel (Anderson & McFarlane, 1995) assesses the areas of physical environment, education, safety and transportation, health and social services, communication, economics, politics and government, and recreation.

     (5) The systems model focuses on developing a comprehensive system of care and coordinating mental health services. Interventions include creating community support services, service coordination and case management. (Worley, 1996)

c. Planning community interventions

     (1) Primary prevention is an intervention to reduce the incidence of disease by promoting and preventing disease processes.

     (2) Secondary prevention is an intervention such as depression screening that detects disease in early stages.

     (3) Tertiary prevention is an intervention that attempts to reduce the severity of a clinically apparent disease.

d. Planning children's health issues

     (1) Children compose one third of our population.

     (2) Major health problems include injuries and acute illness.

     (3) Behavioral problems include eating disorders, attentional problems, substance abuse, conduct disorders and delinquency, sleep disorders, and school maladaptation.

     (4) A child's coping mechanisms are influenced by the individual development level, temperament, previous stress

experiences, role models, and support of parents and peers.

    (5)   Healthy People 2000 (National Health Promotion and Disease Prevention Objectives, by Public Health Service, 1991) supports programs for decreasing smoking, reducing gun violence, and promoting playground safety.

e.   Planning women's health

    (1)   Programs need to focus on women's psychosocial and physiological well-being

    (2)   Women are more likely to suffer from major depression and phobias. (Jones & Trabeaux, 1996)

        (a)   Women have twice the rate of depression than men even when income level, education and occupation are controlled.

        (b)   Women 18-44 years have the highest rates of depression.

        (c)   Factors that contribute to depression in women include unhappy intimate relationships, history of sexual and physical abuse, reproductive events, multiple roles, ethnic minority status, low self esteem, poverty and unemployment

    (3)   Three major causes of mortality in women are heart disease, cancer, and cerebrovascular disease.

f.   Planning men's health

    (1)   Men are physiologically more vulnerable evidenced by more male infants deaths and shorter predicted lifespan. Many reasons account for this difference including genetics, risk-taking behaviors, and ignoring warning signals.

    (2)   Males have more significant death rates in AIDS, suicides, homicides, and accidents.

    (3)   Male suicide rate is four times higher than females and the eighth leading cause of death overall.

          (a)   The highest suicide risk group is men aged 15 to 44.

          (b)   Men are more likely to make a serious attempt to kill themselves rather than use it as a cry for help.

          (c)   Suicide risk factors for men include unmarried, unemployed, previous attempt, positive family history and suffering from terminal illness or other medical condition.

    (4)   Alcohol disorders remain high for men—chronic liver disease and cirrhosis are health diseases affecting men.

    (5)   Men have a higher incidence of antisocial behavior.

 g.   Planning for the homeless

    (1)   Homelessness and criminalization are concerns for many people with chronic mental illness.

    (2)   It is believed between 25%-33% of the homeless population is chronically mentally ill.

    (3)   The new "revolving door" is not within the state hospital but has been now described as the county jail with the criminal justice system being described as the newest mental hospital.

 h.   Four types of planning

    (1)   Strategic planning is a continuous, systematic process of making risk-taking decisions today with the greatest possible knowledge of their impact on the future usually done for the next 5 year period.

    (2)   Functional planning is a specialty service planning such as planning for a staff development department.

    (3)   Operational planning is everyday work management, develops shorter term goals from both long-range and short-range plans.

 i.   Steps in preparing a planning project proposal, for example starting an adolescent therapy group for an outpatient practice setting.

    (a)   Describe the current business or the current outpatient practice.

    (b)   Analyze the strengths and weakness within the outpatient setting of starting the proposed adolescent group.

    (c)   Analyze the opportunities and threats outside of the setting of starting the proposed adolescent group. For example are other outpatient settings also conducting the same group?

    (d)   Describe the product or group therapy including all staff, facility, and financial resources.

    (e)   Describe how the program will be marketed.

    (f)   Describe how the program fits into the organizational chart.

    (g)   Show a projected time line or the steps and dates when the project or group therapy will begin.

    (h)   Describe how much the program will cost and how much revenue the program will produce.

2. Directing

    a.   Defined as coordinating or activating work

    b.   The manager directs work activities such as issuing assignments, orders, and instructions that permit the worker to understand what is expected as well as contribute to the attainment of organizational goals.

    c.   The manager needs to establish work guidelines, manage time efficiently, resolve conflict, facilitate collaboration, and negotiate for needed resources.

    d.   The manager needs to create a motivating climate for staff by using motivation theories.

        (1)   Reinforcement Theory—B. F. Skinner's Behavior Modification. To motivate staff, managers need to:

            (a)   Create a consistent, visible reward system.

            (b)   Reward positive staff behaviors or the behaviors will be extinguished.

(2) Herzberg's Two Factor Motivation Theory (Swansburg, 1996). Assumptions are:

    (a) People want to work and do that work well

    (b) Worker can be motivated by work itself

    (c) It is possible to separate personal motivators from job dissatifiers

    (d) Job motivators (satisfiers) present in work itself and encourage workers to do the work well. Include achievement, recognition, the work itself, responsibility, advancement, possibility for growth, status, company policy

    (e) Maintenance factors (hygiene factors) keep workers from being dissatisfied but do not motivate. Includes salary, supervision, job security, positive working conditions, personal life, interpersonal relations/peers

e. The role of the manager in creating a motivating climate (Marquis & Huston, 1994)

    (1) Communicate clear expectations to staff

    (2) Develop the idea of working as a team

    (3) Request staff input for decisions that affect staff

    (4) Give positive reinforcement

    (5) Be fair and consistent with all employees

    (6) Allow employees to make as many autonomous decisions as possible

    (7) Integrate the uniqueness of each individual into meeting organizational goals

    (8) Explain your own and organizational decisions to staff

f. Resolving conflicts

    (1) Conflicts are inevitable outcomes of social interactions.

    (2) Levels of conflict include intrapersonal, intragroup, intra territorial, interpersonal, intergroup and interterritorial.

    (3) Diagnosing the conflict (Swansburg, 1996)

(a) What is the issue in question?

(b) What are the size of the stakes?

(c) How interdependent are the parties?

(d) Are the parties in a continuing relationship?

(e) What is the power and work structure of the parties?

(f) How involved are third parties?

(g) How do the parties perceive the progress of the conflict?

(4) Conflict resolution strategies

(a) Avoidance or keeping the conflict quiet

Ignoring the conflict—when issue is trivial or symptomatic of a more basic issue

Imposing a solution—when a quick decision is needed or when an unpopular decision is going to be made and the group can not reach a decision

(b) Defusion or cooling the emotions of the parties involved

Smoothing—playing down its importance and magnitude, gives people time to cool down and gain perspective, used when conflict is with issues not related to work

Appealing to superordinate goals—when there are important goals that both parties can not meet without the other's help

(c) Containment allows some conflict to come out into the open, but in tightly controlled manner

Bargaining—when two parties have relatively equal power

Structuring the interaction—when a third party is needed so that the conflict does not escalate

(d) Confrontation is openly discussing all areas of conflict with the end result of finding a solution to conflict

Integrated problem solving—when there is limited trust among parties and unlimited time to problem solve

Redesigning the organization—when sources of conflict come from work processes and the work can be divided into more self-contained work groups

3. Organizing

    a. Organizational theory-Open Systems Theory

        (1) Apply open systems theory to organizations

            (a) An organization is greater than the sum of its parts.

            (b) Permeable boundaries exist between the organization and its environment.

            (c) The input, throughput, and output processes are goal oriented, focused on accomplishing organizational work.

            (d) The components of the throughput (work) process are the workers, the work itself, the formal support processes and the informal support processes.

            (e) The organization is dependent on the environment for resources to do the work and to accept its work.

            (f) The organization is constantly adapting.

            (g) Over time, the organization will become larger and will become increasingly complex and specialized.

    b. Organizing patient care delivery

        (1) Many nursing units organize patient care based on the existing delivery system or by the latest trend.

   (2) Patient care delivery systems include case management, primary nursing, team nursing, functional nursing and any variation of these.

   (3) Factors to be considered in the decision of selecting the optimal patient care delivery system include (Marquis & Huston, 1994):

     (a) Quality or care and cost-effectiveness

     (b) Patient and family satisfaction

     (c) Nursing and other discipline satisfaction

     (d) Consistent with organizational philosophy and goals

     (e) The nature of work that needs to be accomplished

 c. Organizing the budget

   (1) Managers are concerned with following types of budgets:

     (a) Personnel budgets reflecting the amount of money spent on staffing including full time personnel, part-time personnel, and personnel hired as needed.

     (b) Operating budgets reflect expenses that fluctuate up or down when services are provided such as electricity, supplies, rent, and repairs.

     (c) Capital expenditure budgets reflect large purchase items which have use over a year such as hospital beds, or a desk

   (2) Stages of the budget include:

     (a) Planning the budget usually 6 months to a year

     (b) Reviewing and justifying the final budget

     (c) Implementing the budget

     (d) Monitoring and reviewing the budget

 d. Organizing Nurse and Client Empowerment

   (1) Empowerment is a process which changes the distribution of power and enables others to recognize and use

their talents and contributions so that they experience their own personal power.

(2) Nursing empowerment is creating an empowering climate for nurses and staff (Gunden & Crissman, 1994). Empowerment is created by:

(a) Fostering trust—manager needs to demonstrate constancy, congruity, reliability, and integrity

(b) Feedback—manager needs to receive and give realistic feedback including fostering opportunities for staff to make decisions, and providing inspiration

(c) Communication—manager needs to encourage open communication about organizational communication

(d) Goal setting—manager needs to work with staff to set goals for their work and for their professional development

(e) Positivity—manager needs to create a positive climate so that the staff can accomplish their goals

(3) Client empowerment creates an empowering climate for patients

(a) Nurses should assist all vulnerable groups to achieve a greater sense of empowerment.

(b) Clients who are empowered have a greater sense of hope and are more able to make autonomous decisions about health care which may increase their health.

(c) Nursing interventions for assisting clients to feel more empowered include active listening, letting clients know their rights, initially acting as an advocate for them if needed, reassuring them that fears are normal, mutually setting reasonable goals, helping them identify their strengths, being culturally sensitive, and teaching health promotion and disease prevention.

(d) The empowerment model of recovery is a health

promotion model in which individuals define their own needs and are active collaborators with a variety of people in their own healing. (Fisher, 1994)

(e) The empowerment model of recovery is based on experiences of consumers in recovery and on the independent living movement which is a grassroots movement for social justice and civil rights led by people with disabilities.

(f) Nurses can apply the principles of the empowerment model of recovery as follows:(Fisher, 1994)

   (i) Facilitating recovery through education and instilling hope

   (ii) Developing alternatives to hospitalization

   (iii) Providing state funding for involuntary admissions under the public safety budget rather than the health care budget

   (iv) Maximizing consumer involvement in all aspects of treatment; establishing self-help and consumer-run services

   (v) Ensuring that consumers are genuinely and effectively involved in activities to protect human rights and improve the quality of services

   (vi) Favoring the role of personal care attendants rather than case managers (who are too controlling)

   (vii) Viewing the life experience of recovery from a serious psychiatric disability as an asset in hiring, not a liability

   (viii) Promoting consumer control and choice in housing and financial, educational, vocational, and social services

   (ix) Providing staff training based on the needs of consumers

   (x) Basing quality improvement of mental

health services on outcome measures designed by survivors and consumers

4. Evaluating

    a. Evaluation is the systematic attempt to assess worth and value for decision-making purposes.

    b. Program Management and Evaluation

        (1) For program improvement use formative evaluation or receive intermittent feedback throughout the program's performance

        (2) For program judgement at the end of program use summative evaluation

    c. Types of measurement in evaluation:

        (1) Resources for program—structure of people, equipment, setting

        (2) Judgements of process performance

        (3) Concerns and issues of all stakeholders or those having an interest in the program

        (4) Goals and objectives of program and whether the goals and objectives were met

        (5) Intended and unintended program outcomes

    d. Methods of measurement.

        (1) Empirical research designs with statistical analysis

        (2) Questionnaires and surveys of stakeholders for attitudes, satisfaction, and goal attainment

        (3) Comparison to other similar programs

        (4) Review of documents, policies, and procedure manuals

        (5) Cost analysis for effectiveness, benefits, feasibility

        (6) Interviews of individuals or focus groups

        (7) On-site observation of process and structure

    e. Continuous Quality Improvement (CQI)

        (1) CQI is a philosophy for evaluating and managing the quality of health care services.

(2) To successfully integrate CQI into a mental health setting, staff must understand the philosophy and processes of CQI in a collaborative, multidisciplinary setting.

(3) Total Quality Management is a management philosophy that incorporates the concept of continuous quality improvement by allowing all levels of personnel within an organization to actively participate in decision making.

(4) The definition of ''quality'' has broadened from a property of the product to being defined by the customer which helps focus mental health care to customer focus.

(5) Deming (1986) wrote that to increase quality, management should:

    (a) Create an organizational culture that wants to continually improve its services

    (b) Eliminate quotas, slogans and awarding contracts based on price alone

    (c) Promote self-improvement of workers and management

(6) To be effective over time, CQI involves:

    (a) Staff working together to improve the work process. Employees can only be as productive as their work process is organized.

    (b) All staff using a continuous, rational approach for problem-solving over time. It involves every employee on every level working together.

    (c) Feedback mechanisms are built into work processes so that work can be monitored and improved. When quality is improved, mistakes occur less, resulting in less cost.

    (d) A plan systematically attacking problems identified by staff, and patients

f. Peer Evaluation

(1) Peer evaluation has been shown to be a valuable part of a total performance evaluation plan and can include multiple ratings of different peers.

    (2)   Peer evaluation identifies strengths and weaknesses of an employee, identifies competency, increases self-awareness, improves and evaluates the enactment of professional roles.

    (3)   The three phases of peer review are:

        (a)   Employees become familiar with peer review

        (b)   Objectives are defined; employees try different peer review techniques; objectives are further refined.

        (c)   Peer evaluation becomes fully operational

  g. Self Evaluation

    (1)   Nurses should be continually involved in self evaluation or identifying their own strengths and weaknesses in a professional role. Nurses are accountable to the public and profession.

    (2)   Self evaluation has been found to be threatening if an employee must discuss findings in a group of other employees

    (3)   Advanced practice nurse self-evaluates practice based on client outcomes (ANA, 1996)

  h. Evaluation of Care and Legal Issues (Stuart & Sundeen, 1996) (Fontaine & Fletcher, 1995)

    (1)   Nurses' ability to provide safe care is enhanced by knowledge of the law, ANA Code for Nurses, the state's "nurse practice act", and Standards of Psychiatric Practice.

    (2)   An important concept in psychiatric nursing is understanding the legal framework for the delivery of mental health care in the state in which the nurse practices.

    (3)   State law may also vary regarding admissions, discharges, patient rights, and informed consent.

    (4)   Types of admissions to psychiatric units:

        (a)   Voluntary admission—signed standard admission form indicating patient voluntarily seeks help

(b) Involuntary admission or commitment—patient did not request hospitalization and admission was initiated by hospital or court

Emergency Involuntary Admission

State laws differ as to procedures for petitioning for admission, psychiatric evaluation of the client, treatment available and length of detainment (usually 2–3 days)

Clients are restricted from leaving and may be forced to take psychotropic medication.

Clients' right to consult with attorney to prepare for hearing must be enforced

Indefinite Involuntary Admission

Civil hearing is convened to determine need for continuing involuntary treatment

"Clear and convincing evidence" of "mentally ill and dangerous to self and others" must be demonstrated

(5) Clients do not lose their legal rights because they are admitted to a psychiatric facility.

(6) Malpractice is the failure of professionals to provide the proper and competent care resulting in harm to the patients, judged by national standards of care by other members of their profession.

(a) Nurses should be familiar with the following resources which help define standards of care:

Code for Nurses with Interpretive Statements

Standards of Addictive Nursing Practice

Documents published by the Joint Commission on Accreditation of Health Care Organizations (JCAHO) and Federal Agency Guidelines (USPHS) (AHCPR)

Statements from the American Hospital Association

> Policies and Procedures of the employing agency
>
> Nurse practice statutes of the state
>
> For Advanced Practice Registered Nurses—Scope and Standards of Advanced Practice Registered Nursing of the American Nurses Association

   (b)   If standards are not clear in a particular instance, a lawyer should be consulted.

   (c)   Malpractice suits usually come from angry patients who have had poor results from treatment.

   (d)   Malpractice lawsuits involving nurses usually include administration of medications or treatment, communications, and supervision of patients.

   (e)   Most malpractice suits are filed under the law of tort which is a private civil wrong committed by one individual against another for which money damages are collected by the injured party from the wrongdoer.

(7)   Battery is a harmful or offensive touching of another's person.

(8)   Assault is a threat to use force without actual bodily contact although the person must have the opportunity and ability to carry out the threat immediately (words alone are not enough).

(9)   Negligence is an act or an omission to act that breaches the duty of due care and results in or is responsible for a person's injuries.

(10)   For psychiatric-mental health nurses, the most common causes of negligence are implementation of suicide precautions and assisting in electroconvulsive therapy.

(12)   Informed consent is the client's right to receive enough information to make a decision about treatment and to communicate the decision to others.

(a) In an absence of the consent, a health care provider can be held liable in a civil lawsuit for battery, assault, and professional negligence.

(b) In the case of an emergency situation, consent may not be obtained because a delay would endanger the client's health and/or safety, and client may be treated without legal liability.

(c) To give informed consent, the patient should be told the diagnosis, differential diagnosis, nature of diagnostic and therapeutic procedures to be performed, the prospect of success from the treatment, prognosis or expectations, and alternative courses of treatment if available.

(13) Clients must be informed of the potential risks of medications and have the right to refuse medications. If the physician or nurse believes the patient needs the refused medication, the physician can take the decision to the courts to rule whether client is incompetent.

(14) Competency is a legal determination that a client can make reasonable decisions about treatment and other areas of his/her personal life.

(15) Communication, both written and oral, is a legal responsibility. Specific charting, e.g. on suicide precautions, document the nurse's actions.

(16) There are federal rules regarding chemical dependence confidentiality so that staff members can not disclose any admission or discharge information.

(17) All 50 states have enacted child abuse reporting statutes which generally include a definition of child abuse, a list of persons required or encouraged to report, and the governmental agency designated to receive and investigate the reports.

(18) Some states have enacted adult abuse laws.

(19) Duty to warn or disclose (Tarasoff v. The Regents of University of California, 1976) ruled that a psychotherapist had the duty to warn his or her client's potential victim of potential harm. In 1983, the court stated that the

duty to warn was composed of two elements 1) duty to diagnose and predict the client's danger of violence 2) the duty to take appropriate action to protect the identified victim. The duty to warn supercedes the client's right to confidentiality.

(20) Some general areas of health care litigation in multi-disciplinary psychiatric-mental health private practice—informed consent, faulty diagnosing resulting in wrong treatment, physical restraint and bodily harm, confidentiality and defamation, failure to warn those threatened by clients, limitation of ability to perform a needed service and failure to refer to another professional, misuse of therapy, and inappropriate termination and abandonment of client

- The Consultative Liaison Role As a Leadership Role in Health Care Delivery

  1. This Master's degree nursing role which evolved from consultative roles, requires the ability to integrate expert psychiatric-mental health knowledge into all health care settings (American Nurse Association, 1996).

  2. In community mental health model, Caplan (1970) defines consultation as a specific professional process between two systems. The consultee system has a problem and requests assistance. The consultant system gives the assistance.

  3. Role characteristics include collaborative professional relationships, not supervisory relationships, where the user/consultees choose whether or not to accept professional advice.

  4. The psychiatric liaison nursing role provides and coordinates psychiatric care and maintains a therapeutic environment for clients admitted with a physical symptom or dysfunction.

  5. Psychiatric liaison nurses, as members of the health care team, provide direct care, including psychotherapy, health teaching, anticipatory guidance, and somatic therapy to individuals, groups, and families.

  6. Psychiatric consultation liaison nurses may provide indirect care

such as consultation, education, maintenance of a therapeutic environment, systems evaluation, and program development for work unit and/or organizational issues.

7. The consultation liaison nurse provides support and guidance in assisting the user/consultee to solve the problem and gain more understanding of the issues.

8. Consultation liaison nurses may fill roles in a variety of settings—independent private practitioners who are self-employed, nurses who are contracting out services to an organization based on a fee for service arrangement, and/or staff members of an organization.

9. In general, the nurse consultant will deal with three problem areas.

    a. A problem with a specific patient

    b. A specific service program problem

    c. An organizational problem

10. Phases of the interactive consultative liaison process are (Lehmann, 1996):

    a. Orientation phase

        (1) Identifying the overt and covert expectations of the consultee

        (2) Clearly defining the problem so that the staff have realistic expectations for the consultation

        (3) Communicating confidentiality

        (4) Writing a written contract

            (a) Represents an exchange between the consultee and consultant

            (b) Clearly writes services expected and method of payment signed by each party. It is not so much a legal document but an agreement between two professional systems

            (c) Contains a brief description of problem, expected outcomes or goals, estimated time to be devoted to project, amount of compensation for consultant's time, key department and personnel related to consultant, and name of contact person from consultee agency

b. Working phase.

    (1) After contract is formalized, further assessing the problem

    (2) Selecting interventions for the problem. At this point, the nurse consultant may have completed the consultation depending upon the terms of the contract

c. Termination phase.

    (1) Writing a formal summary written report

    (2) Including in the written report—purpose, dates, time, and activities of consultation; statement of identified problem, assessment and diagnoses of problem, proposed interventions for problem resolution, alternative problem-solving approach, and evaluation criteria and findings if available

Questions
Select the best answer

1. Today, the goal of most inpatient hospitalizations is:

   a. Assessment
   b. Rehabilitation
   c. Psychotherapy
   d. Crisis stabilization

2. The main difference between inpatient and outpatient treatment is:

   a. Therapeutic milieu
   b. Care giving activities
   c. Integrating and coordinating care
   d. Evaluating outcomes

3. In the last thirty years, public mental hospital settings':

   a. Inpatient census and admissions have increased over 75%
   b. Inpatient census has declined over 75%, admissions have doubled
   c. Admissions of younger, violent patients have declined
   d. Inpatient census has increased by 50%, admissions have decreased

4. In 1963, a fundamental change in the mental health delivery system occurred because of the following mental health legislation:

   a. Omnibus Reconciliation Act
   b. Community Mental Health Center Act
   c. Social Security Act
   d. Americans with Disabilities Act

5. In general, discharged public mental health patients had the following problem MOST frequently in working with community mental health centers:

   a. Had difficulty working in family therapy
   b. Wanted to immediately live independently in the community
   c. Had difficulty keeping appointments
   d. Became involved in a revolving door with long jail times

6. In working with discharged public mental health patients, the community mental health program that was most essential was:

   a. An inpatient unit

b. Geriatric services

c. Drug abuse treatment

d. 24 hour crisis intervention

7. Mobile crisis services, including services in private homes, hospital emergency rooms and residential programs, help provide:

a. Group therapy

b. Improved access to care

c. Family psychotherapy

d. Long-term rehabilitation of chronic patients

8. One important function of a partial hospitalization program is to:

a. Stabilize the patient in an inpatient setting

b. Transition patients from the inpatient to outpatient setting

c. Provide 24 hour 7 day a week crisis intervention

d. Provide mobile crisis services at the patient's home

9. For maximum treatment effectiveness, partial hospitalization nurses should consider the following group therapy issue:

a. Acutely ill patients need an intensive group-orientated psychotherapy

b. Low level and high level patients have the same group needs

c. High level patients may dilute intensive group-orientated psychotherapy for low level patients

d. Low level patients may dilute intensive group-orientated psychotherapy for high level patients

10. Managed care has created the following health care change:

a. Separating treatment plans for inpatient and outpatient providers

b. Shifting from capitated to fee-for-service reimbursement

c. Evaluating quality and patient outcomes

d. Longer and more intense psychiatric inpatient stays

11. Which of the following is NOT a strategy that health care organizations must use to be successful in managed care?

a. Understand the change in reimbursement

b. Aggressively promote self-care

c. Case manage high cost members

d. Promote its fee for service structure

12. The most prevalent ethical dilemma in managed care is that managed care providers:

    a. Prolong inpatient stays
    b. Limit patient treatments and options
    c. Prescribe too many patient treatments given by too many providers
    d. Prolong life-saving measures in intensive care units

13. For an Advanced Practice Nurse to work competitively in a managed care setting, the nurse should :

    a. Provide cost effective care
    b. Focus exclusively on self-care
    c. Expect referrals from providers providing similar services
    d. Focus on decreasing cost per DRG case

14. In therapy, the nurse should be aware of gender role stereotypes. Which of the following is LEAST influenced by gender role stereotypes:

    a. A person's self esteem and prescribed role in society
    b. The nurse-client therapy relationship
    c. Nursing roles with other disciplines
    d. Lateral peer nursing roles

15. When staff nurse assumes a nurse manager's position, the nurse assumes the following type of power:

    a. Referent
    b. Expert
    c. Legitimate
    d. Coercive

16. A nurse can use the following strategy for acquiring power in an organization:

    a. Increase visibility
    b. Inform patients about their rights
    c. Write letters to the media about the organization
    d. Complain about management to other staff members

17. The most effective strategy for psychiatric-mental health nurses to use as change agents in mental health policy is:

    a. Serve on a legislative committee
    b. Write the media about mental health issues

c. Advocate for patients in the hospital

d. Notify the patient of his/her rights

18. A major mental health legislative debate includes:

a. Giving parity of insurance coverage to mental health clients

b. Creating Medicaid coverage to include managed care

c. Restricting hospital consolidation

d. Caring for the elderly

19. The most influential legislation to give patients access to health care was the:

a. Omnibus Reconciliation Act

b. Community Mental Health Center Act

c. Social Security Act

d. Americans with Disabilities Act

20. Healthy People 2000 focuses the U.S. on the following mental health promotion:

a. Decreasing polypharmacy in mental health care

b. Reducing children and adolescent suicide

c. Promoting deinstitutionalization

d. Increasing social supports for the indigent

21. The MOST significant barrier for Advance Practice Psychiatric-Mental Health Nurses in practicing within health care organizations is:

a. Perferred Provider Organizations (PPOs) restrictive hiring policies

b. Lack of clients

c. Limited autonomy in organized practice settings

d. Limited liaison roles

22. Advanced Practice Nurses can use the following strategy for obtaining third party reimbursement:

a. Volunteer and serve on committees related to health care issues

b. Increase visibility and assume authority in interactions in health care organizations

c. Network with elected officials who can submit and pass reimbursement legislation

d. Empower staff and clients by sharing knowledge and involving them in decisions

23. Paying a set amount of money for mental health services for a defined group of people is referred to as:

    a. Fee-for-service reimbursement
    b. Capitation
    c. Prospective payment reimbursement
    d. Sliding scale reimbursement

24. Which role should be performed by an Advanced Practice Nurse with a graduate degree?

    a. Case management
    b. Consultation
    c. Budgeting
    d. Coordinator of patient care

25. Which nursing activity demonstrates an indirect nursing care function?

    a. Teaching patients
    b. Supervising staff
    c. Crisis intervention
    d. Group therapy

26. To consider beginning a solo private practice, what factor would be most important?

    a. Experience as an Advanced Practice Nurse
    b. Survival with the economic uncertainties of private practice
    c. An intensive personal support system
    d. Total responsibility for professional accountability

27. Which are key factors in establishing a viable private practice?

    a. Adapt a financial management system, obtain insurance, market successfully
    b. Create support groups, establish criteria for using consultants, successful marketing
    c. Establish criteria for using consultants and employees, adapt a financial management system
    d. Create professional support groups, pay courteous attention to referrals

28. The strongest predictor of private practice charges for Psychiatric-Mental Health Clinical Specialist is:

    a. A private practice psychologist's charges who have comparable experience

    b. The price above what your clientele is willing to pay

    c. A private practice social workers charges who have equal education requirements

    d. The charges that third-party payers are saying are "reasonable and customary"

29. In private practice, an advantage to capitation as compared to fee for service reimbursement is:

    a. The clinician receives money for each service provided

    b. The clinician will receive money for referrals

    c. Reimbursement is not based upon diagnosis

    d. The client can see any provider

30. Which of the following are NOT leaders' tasks?

    a. Renewing

    b. Distracting members from goals

    c. Envisioning goals

    d. Serving as a symbol

31. According to Hersey and Blanchard's Leadership Theory, leadership strategies are based upon:

    a. The ability of the leader

    b. The level of readiness of the follower

    c. The leader's charisma

    d. The organization's goals and objectives

32. The four classical functions of managers are:

    a. Planning, organizing, leading, and evaluating

    b. Visioning, planning, leading and supervising

    c. Planning, directing, organizing and evaluating

    d. Changing, visioning, bargaining and supervising

33. Epidemiology is useful in mental health care because it:

    a. Shows that the relationship between physical and psychiatric disorders do not vary in different populations

    b. Allows attention to be focused on identifying causes of mental illnesses

    c. Allows attention to be focused on giving different populations different levels of social support

    d. Shows that the relationship between patterns of diseases vary in human beings and animals

34. An example of a host risk is:

    a. Ethnicity
    b. Toxic chemicals
    c. Population density
    d. Social support

35. An example of an agent risk is:

    a. Life-style behaviors
    b. Age
    c. Levels of stress
    d. Pesticides

36. An example of an environmental risk is:

    a. Religion
    b. Bacteria
    c. Housing
    d. Race

37. Which combination gives the most complete community assessment?

    a. Community's educational level, safety, social support
    b. Community's politics, recreation, and safety
    c. Community's physical environment, social support, and economics
    d. Community's transportation, safety, and communication channels

38. Nurses who screen workers for depression are using which type of intervention?

    a. Primary intervention
    b. Secondary intervention
    c. Tertiary intervention
    d. Quality intervention

39. Nurses are creating and implementing a plan to assist nursing home residents deal with homesickness. They are using which type of intervention?

a. Primary intervention
b. Secondary intervention
c. Tertiary intervention
d. Quality intervention

40. Which of the following populations are often in need of mental health services, but neglected because of lack of programs?

a. Geriatric population
b. Adolescent and children
c. Substance abusers
d. Mentally ill in jail

41. Two criteria for home visits by psychiatric nurses are:

a. Need for treatment and geographical location of patient
b. Type of diagnosis and family services resources available
c. Need for treatment and homebound status of patient
d. Patients' ability to pay and need for treatment

42. Which population is at high risk because members ignore warning signals and engage in risk-taking behaviors?

a. Children
b. Women
c. Men
d. Aged

43. The following is important to consider in planning women's issues and mental health:

a. Women are more likely to make a serious attempt to kill themselves than cry for help
b. Women have a depression rate twice men
c. Major health problems include accidents and acute illness
d. Women's suicide rate is four times higher than men

44. The "new" revolving door with mental health patients is:

a. Community mental health centers
b. The public mental hospital
c. The acute care inpatient unit
d. The jail

45. The following type of planning is 3-5 year long range planning:

    a. Strategic
    b. Operational
    c. Functional
    d. Capital

46. The following type of planning addresses everyday work management:

    a. Strategic
    b. Operational
    c. Functional
    d. Capital

47. In preparing a proposed plan for a new program, the important factor the nurse should consider is:

    a. The evaluation plan containing both quality and patient outcomes measures
    b. The need for the program
    c. Marketing strategies for the program
    d. The fit of the program into the organizational chart

48. The nurse manager knows that positive reinforcements for productive staff behaviors are important in the workplace. Which theory most supports this statement?

    a. Maslow's Need Theory
    b. Skinner's Behavior Modification Theory
    c. Herzberg's Two Factor Theory
    d. Hersey and Blanchard's Life-Cycle Theory

49. Based on Herzberg's Motivation Theory, which is most important for the nurse manager in creating a motivating work environment for the staff?

    a. Physiology needs are lower level needs and are being met
    b. Consistent, clear rules guide the staff in producing the work
    c. The work itself should be interesting to the worker
    d. Staff must understand the mission of the work

50. A nurse manager wants to create a motivating climate for staff. Which strategy best accomplishes this goal?

    a. Allow staff to create the budget for the department

    b. Allow staff input into decisions which affect their work

    c. Give all staff a 10% raise

    d. Allow staff more sick time

51. Two staff members approach you and state that they are arguing over the up-coming political election. The best strategy for the nurse manager is:

    a. Bargaining, so that the argument will not escalate

    b. Confrontation, so the issue can be resolved expeditiously

    c. Redesigning the organization, because the work group needs to be more self contained

    d. Smoothing, because the issue is trivial and not related to work

52. The evening charge nurse complains repeatedly to you, the nurse manager, that day shift personnel do not complete admitting new patients who enter the unit late on day shift. What is the best conflict management approach?

    a. Redesigning the organization, because the conflict is within the work process

    b. Avoidance, because the issue is trivial

    c. Smoothing, because it gives people time to calm down

    d. Structuring, because an objective third party is needed

53. When choosing an optimal patient care delivery system, desired outcomes include:

    a. Short length of stay, physician satisfaction, and least expensive nursing care

    b. Cost effective nursing care and administration satisfaction

    c. Patient, administration, and managed care satisfaction

    d. Patient satisfaction, quality nursing care, and cost effective nursing care

54. The Clinic needs a new computer. This expense will come out of what type of budget?

    a. Technology

    b. Capital

    c. Personnel

    d. Operating

55. For the nurse manager, the second stage of a budget is:

    a. Monitoring and reviewing the budget

    b. Implementing the budget

c. Planning the budget

d. Reviewing and justifying the budget

56. The purpose of evaluating programs is to:

    a. Assess cost effectiveness
    b. Assess community needs and desires
    c. Assess stakeholders' involvement for decision making purposes
    d. Assess worth and value for decision making purposes

57. In evaluating a program, an essential component to measure is whether:

    a. Goals and objectives of program are met
    b. Cost containment strategies are finished
    c. Formative evaluation is used
    d. Employees are motivated

58. Continuous Quality Improvement (CQI) can be defined as a philosophy for:

    a. Checking quality at set intervals
    b. Evaluating and managing quality
    c. Providing quality at the lowest possible cost
    d. Determining quality over time

59. Which of these nursing interventions most exemplifies the CQI process:

    a. Interdisciplinary teams working together to solve patient discharge problems
    b. The nurse manager creates a plan to decrease costs over time
    c. Nursing administrators decide to give all staff raises
    d. The nurse management team collaborates to monitor sick time usage

60. In the Scope and Standards of Advanced Practice Registered Nursing, self-evaluation is based upon:

    a. Peer evaluation
    b. Consultation
    c. Patient outcomes
    d. Interdisclinary process

61. Psychiatric mental health nursing practice may vary from state to state because of laws governing:

    a. Child abuse reporting

    b. Informed consent

    c. Nurse practice acts

    d. The ANA Code for Nurses

62. When a patient is an involuntary admission to the psychiatric unit, the nurse knows the patient:

    a. Requested hospitalization

    b. Can sign out Against Medical Advice

    c. Has his/her legal rights taken away

    d. Has restricted freedom

63. Malpractice can be shown if the nurse:

    a. Gives a reasonable standard of care

    b. Does not harm the patient

    c. Fails to give competent care

    d. Gives quality care but the patient has a poor outcome

64. Which patient right can be suspended with justified documentation?

    a. Right to treatment in least restrictive environment

    b. Right to freedom from restraints and seclusion

    c. Right to warn others of danger

    d. Right to access courts and attorneys

65. In most states, the amount of time that a person can be under an emergency commitment is:

    a. 12 to 24 hours

    b. 24 to 36 hours

    c. 48 to 72 hours

    d. 3-5 days

66. A health care worker telephones a substance abuse unit and asks the nurse if Mr. A. Smith is a patient there and can he talk with him. The nurse replies:

    a. Here is Mr. Smith's telephone number, please call him

    b. Mr. Smith is in a group and cannot talk with you now

    c. No information can be given

    d. Please talk to Mr. Smith's caseworker

67. On an inpatient unit, the patient commits suicide because an intensive suicide

watch was not continued throughout the shift. The nurse breached which legal concept?

a. Informed consent
b. Negligence
c. Battery
d. False imprisonment

68. A therapist has a duty to warn. This involves informing:

a. A patient about possible side effects of medications
b. A patient about tardive dyskinesia
c. A patient about their right to refuse treatment
d. A potential victim of potential harm

69. A nurse manager gives the staff the ability to create their own work schedules. This is an example of:

a. Risk management
b. Goal setting
c. Self realization
d. Empowerment

70. Nursing interventions which enable client empowerment include:

a. Suggesting hospitalization if client does not comply with medication regime
b. Assisting patients in not disclosing their psychiatric hospitalizations
c. Promoting consumer choice in treatment
d. Promoting family therapy

71. A consultation liaison nurse's role includes:

a. Supervision of staff
b. Support and guidance
c. Organization of patient care delivery
d. Monitoring the CQI process

72. A characteristic of a liaison contract is:

a. A legally binding contract between two professional systems
b. Set up for a five year period
c. A permanent document that can only be modified by the Court
d. An agreement between two professional systems

73. The nurse manager wants to empower the staff and uses the following strategy:

    a. Creates staff committees with authority to resolve departmental problems
    b. Creates staff committees to develop goals for other departments
    c. Provides education and training to provide opportunity for advancement
    d. Implements employee suggestion program with monetary incentives

74. Which of the following is an indirect care intervention of a psychiatric consultation nurse?

    a. Health teaching
    b. Psychotherapy
    c. Anticipatory guidance
    d. Systems evaluation

75. The nurse manager discovers that nurses on the substance abuse unit are recapping their used needles. He/she immediately stops this practice because of violation of:

    a. Continuous Quality Improvement (CQI) programs
    b. Risk management
    c. Cost containment programs
    d. Ethics

Answers

1. d	26. b	51. d
2. a	27. a	52. a
3. b	28. d	53. d
4. b	29. c	54. b
5. c	30. b	55. d
6. d	31. b	56. d
7. b	32. c	57. a
8. b	33. b	58. b
9. d	34. a	59. a
10. c	35. d	60. c
11. d	36. c	61. c
12. b	37. c	62. d
13. a	38. b	63. c
14. d	39. a	64. b
15. c	40. d	65. c
16. a	41. c	66. c
17. a	42. c	67. b
18. a	43. b	68. d
19. c	44. d	69. d
20. b	45. a	70. c
21. c	46. b	71. b
22. c	47. b	72. d
23. b	48. b	73. a
24. b	49. c	74. d
25. b	50. b	75. b

BIBLIOGRAPHY

American Nurses Association (1996). *Scope and Standards of Advanced Practice Registered Nursing.* Washington DC: Author

American Nurses Association (1994). *Statement on psychiatric-mental health clinical nursing practice and standards of psychiatric nursing practice.* Washington DC: Author

Anderson, E.T., & McFarlane, J. (1995). *Community-as-partner: Theory and practice in nursing.* Philadelphia: J. B. Lippincott Company.

Berdahl, A. (Ed.). (1996). 1996 state health policy survey. *Health System Review* 11/12, 36–52.

Billings, C. V. (1993). Nuts and bolts of reimbursement: How to bill for your services. In P. Mittelstadt, (Ed.), *The reimbursement manual: How to get paid for your advanced practice nursing services (pp181-186).* Washington DC: American Nurses Publishing.

Buerhaus, P. I. (1994). Economics of managed competition and consequences to nurses: Part II. *Nursing Economics, 2*(12), 75–80, 106.

Caplan, G. (1970). *The theory and practice of mental health consultation.* New York: Basic Books.

Chowanec, G. D. (1994). Continuous quality improvement: Conceptual foundations and application to mental health care. *Hospital & Community Psychiatry, 45*(8), 789–792.

Cleverley, W. O. (1997). *Essentials of health care finance* (4th ed.). Gaithersburg, MD: Aspen Publishers.

Deming, W. E. (1986). *Out of Crisis.* Cambridge, MA: Massachusetts Institute of Technology.

Easterling, A., Avie, J., Wesley, M. L., & Chimner, N. (1995). *The case manager's guide: Acquiring the skills for success.* American Hospital Publishing, Inc.

Fisher, D. B. (1994). Health care reform based on an empowerment model of recovery by people with psychiatric disabilities. *Hospital & Community Psychiatry, 45*(9), 913–915.

Fontaine, K. L., & Fletcher, J. S. (1995). *Essentials of mental health nursing* (3rd ed.). Redwood, CA: Addison-Wesley Nursing.

Geller, J. L., Fisher, W. H., & McDermeit, M. (1995). A national survey of mobile crisis services and their evaluation. *Psychiatric Services, 46*(9), 893–897.

Godschalx, S. (1996). Advantages of working in a capitated mental health system. *Psychiatric Services, 45*(5), 477–478.

Gunden, E., & Crissman, S. (1994). Leadership skills for empowerment. In E. C. Heine & M. J. Nicholson (Eds.). *Contemporary leadership behavior: Selected readings (4th ed., pp. 231–236).* Philadelphia: J. B. Lippincott.

Hillard, J. R. (1994). The past and future of psychiatric emergency services in the U.S. *Hospital & Community Psychiatry 45*(6), 541–543.

Hollingsworth, E. J., & Sweeney, J. K. (1997). Mental illness expenditures for services for people with severe mental illness. *Psychiatric Services. 48*(4):485–490.

Jones, L. C., & Trabeaux, S. (1996). Women's health. In M. Stanhope, & J. Lancaster (Eds.), *Community health nursing: Promoting health of aggregates, families, and individuals (4th ed., pp. 545–564).* St. Louis: Mosby.

Lehmann, F. G. (1996). Consultative liaison psychiatric nursing care. In G. W. Stuart. & S. J. Sundeen, (Eds.), *Principles and practice of psychiatric nursing (5th ed., pp 851–862).* St. Louis: Mosby.

Marquis, B. L., & Huston, C. L. (1994). *Management decision making for nurses (2nd ed.).* Philadelphia: J. B. Lippincott.

Marshall, S. (1994). The larger mental health environment. In C. Houseman, (Ed.), *Psychiatric certification review guide for the generalist and clinical specialist in adult, child, and adolescent psychiatric and mental health nursing (pp. 491–542).* Potomac, MD: Health Leadership.

Merwin, E., Fox, J., & Bell, P. (1996). Certified psychiatric clinical nurse specialists. *Psychiatric Services, 47*(3), 235.

McFarlane, B. H., & Blair, G. (1995). Delivering comprehensive services to homeless mentally ill offenders. *Psychiatric Services, 46*(2), 179–183.

McCloskey, J., & Grace, H. K. (1994). *Current Issues in Nursing* (4th ed.). St. Louis, MO: Mosby.

Peplau, H. E. (1990). Evolution of nursing in psychiatric settings. In E. M. Varcarolis (Ed.), *Foundations of psychiatric mental health nursing (pp. 87–111).* Philadelphia, PA: W. B. Saunders.

Ozarin, L. D. (1995). Community mental health centers: Success or failures? *Psychiatric Services, 46*(5), 431.

Rosie, J. S., Azim, F. A., Piper, W. E., & Joyce, A. S. (1995). Effective psychiatric day treatment: Historical lessons. *Psychiatric Services,* 46(10), 1019–1026.

Sebastian, J. G. (1996). In M. Stanhope, & J. Lancaster (Eds.), *Community health nursing: Promoting health of aggregates, families, and individuals* (4th ed., pp. 623–646). St. Louis: Mosby.

Swansburg, R. C. (1996). *Management and leadership for nurse managers* (2nd ed.). Sudbury, MA: Jones and Barlett Publishers.

Stanhope, M., & Lancaster, J. (Eds.). (1996). *Community health nursing: Promoting health of aggregates, families, and individuals* (4th ed., pp. 437–449). St. Louis: Mosby.

Streff, M. B. (1994). Third-party reimbursement issues for advanced practice nurses in the /90s. In J. McCloskey, & H. K. Grace (Eds.). *Current issues in nursing* (4th ed.). St. Louis: Mosby.

Stuart. G. W., & Sundeen, S. J. (1996). *Principles and practice of psychiatric nursing* (5th ed.). St. Louis: Mosby.

Talley, S., & Caverly, S. (1994). Advanced-practice psychiatric nursing and health care reform. *Hospital & Community Psychiatry, 45*(6), 545-547.

U.S. Department of Health and Human Services. (1990). Healthy people 2000, Washington, DC: Public Health Service.

Worley, N. K. (1996). Community psychiatric nursing care. In G. W. Stuart & S. J. Sundeen (Eds.), *Principles and Practice of Psychiatric Nursing,* (5th ed., pp. 831–849). St. Louis: Mosby.

INDEX

For information on Certification Review Courses, Home Study Programs and Review Books contact:

Health Leadership Associates, Inc.
Post Office Box 59153
Potomac, Maryland 20859

1-800-435-4775

REVIEW BOOK/AUDIO CASSETTE ORDER FORM
HEALTH LEADERSHIP ASSOCIATES, INC.

PLEASE PRINT OR TYPE

NAME: _____

ADDRESS: Street _____ Apt. # _____ City _____ State _____ Zip Code _____

TELEPHONE: _____ (HOME) _____ (WORK)

Section 1: AUDIO CASSETTES

Professional "live" audio recordings of Review Courses are approximately 15 hours in length unless otherwise noted and include detailed course handouts. Continuing Education contact hours are available for these audio cassette Home Study Programs.

QTY	REVIEW COURSE TITLE	PRICE	
____	Acute Care Nurse Practitioner	$150.00	_____
____	Adult Nurse Practitioner	$150.00	_____
____ **	Childbearing Management	$ 45.00	_____
____	Clinical Specialist in Adult Psychiatric and Mental Health Nursing	$150.00	_____
____	Family Nurse Practitioner (Consists of ANP, PNP & Childbearing Management Courses)	$330.00	_____
____ *	Gerontological Nurse	$ 75.00	_____
____	Gerontological Nurse Practitioner	$150.00	_____
____	Home Health Nurse	$150.00	_____
____	Inpatient Obstetric/Maternal Newborn/ Low Risk Neonatal/Perinatal Nurse	$150.00	_____
____	Medical-Surgical Nurse	$150.00	_____
____ **	Menopause Lecture	$ 30.00	_____
____	Midwifery Review	$150.00	_____
____ *	Pediatric Nurse	$ 75.00	_____
____	Pediatric Nurse Practitioner	$150.00	_____
____ *	Psychiatric and Mental Health Nurse	$ 75.00	_____
____ **	Test Taking Strategies and Techniques	$ 20.00	_____
____	Women's Health Care Nurse Practitioner	$150.00	_____

* 8 Hour Course, ** 2-4 Hour Course

SUB TOTAL: _____

Maryland Residents add 5% sales tax: _____

CEU FEE ($25/course, except FNP course $35): *OPTIONAL*

Shipping: 2-4 Hour Course $ 5.00 _____

All other Courses $10.00 _____

TOTAL: _____

PAYMENT DUE   METHOD OF PAYMENT

☐ Check or money order (US funds, payable to Health Leadership Associates, Inc.) A $25 fee will be charged on returned checks.

☐ Purchase Order is attached. P.O. # _____

☐ Please charge my: ☐ MasterCard ☐ Visa ☐ AMEX ☐ Discover

Credit Card# _____ Exp. date _____

Signature _____

Print Name _____

REVIEW GUIDES & AUDIO CASSETTES

1) Section 1 Total $ _____
2) Section 2 Total $ _____
3) Section 3 Total $ _____

TOTAL PAYMENT DUE $ _____

Section 2: REVIEW BOOKS

QTY	BOOK TITLE	PRICE	
____	Adult Nurse Practitioner Certification Review Guide (3rd edition)	$ 47.75	_____
____	Family Nurse Practitioner Certification Review Guide Set (Includes ANP,PNP, and Women's Health Care NP Guides)	$123.25	_____
____	Gerontological Nursing Certification Review Guide for the Generalist, Clinical Specialist, and Nurse Practitioner (revised edition)	$ 47.75	_____
____	Pediatric Nurse Practitioner Certification Review Guide (3rd edition)	$ 47.75	_____
____	Psychiatric Certification Review Guide for the Generalist and Clinical Specialist in Adult, Child, and Adolescent Psychiatric and Mental Health Nursing (2nd edition)	$ 47.75	_____
____	Women's Health Care Nurse Practitioner Certification Review Guide	$ 47.75	_____

SPECIAL OFFERING

____	TODAY and TOMORROW'S WOMAN – MENOPAUSE: BEFORE AND AFTER (Girls of 16 to Women of 99) (Author: Virginia Layng Millonig)	$ 19.95	_____

SUB TOTAL: _____

Maryland Residents add 5% sales tax: _____

CEU FEE ($20 per book, except FNP Set $35): *OPTIONAL*

Shipping: $9.00 FNP Set: _____

$5.00 for one book: _____

$2.00 for each additional book: _____
(Except $1.00 for each add'l. *Today and Tomorrow's Woman*)

TOTAL: _____

For orders of 10 or greater call 1-800-435-4775.
(All prices subject to change without notice)

Section 3: REVIEW BOOK/AUDIO CASSETTE DISCOUNT PACKAGES

A discounted rate is available when purchasing Review Book(s) and Audio Cassettes together. When purchasing packages, indicate Book/Audio Cassette selections in sections 1 and 2. Calculate amount due in this section.

QTY	PACKAGE SELECTION	PRICE	
_____	8 Hour Course / 1 Review Guide	$120.00	_____
_____	15 Hour Course / 1 Review Guide	$190.00	_____
_____	FNP Package	$415.00	_____

FNP Package consists of Adult NP, Pediatric NP, Women's Health Care NP Guides & Audio Cassettes of the ANP, PNP, and Childbearing Management Courses.

SUB TOTAL: _____

Maryland Residents add 5% sales tax: _____

CEU Fee ($35 per package, except FNP Package $45) *OPTIONAL*

TOTAL: _____
(Shipping charge included in package rate)

RETURN POLICY

Due to the nature of the material contained in the review books and audio cassettes, returns on books ONLY will be accepted one week post delivery. No returns on audio cassettes except for defective audio cassettes which will be replaced.

MAIL TO:	Health Leadership Associates, Inc. P.O. Box 59153 Potomac, MD 20859
OR PHONE:	(800) 435-4775; (301) 983-2405
OR FAX:	(301) 983-2693